Covid-19 Pandemic

Christian Aspalter
Editor

Covid-19 Pandemic

Problems Arising in Health and Social Policy

Springer

Editor
Christian Aspalter
BNU-HKBU United International College
Zhuhai, Guangdong, China

ISBN 978-981-99-2496-7 ISBN 978-981-99-2497-4 (eBook)
https://doi.org/10.1007/978-981-99-2497-4

This Springer imprint is published by the registered company Springer Nature Singapore Pte Ltd.
The registered company address is: 152 Beach Road, #21-01/04 Gateway East, Singapore 189721, Singapore

Only great pain, the long, slow pain that takes its time ... compels us to descend to our ultimate depths ... I doubt that such pain makes us 'better;' but I know it makes us more profound ... From such abysses, from such severe sickness, one returns newborn, having shed one's skin ... with merrier senses, with a second dangerous innocence in joy, more childlike and yet a hundred times subtler than one has ever been before.

(from: The Gay Science)

Friedrich W. Nietzsche (1844–1900)

Foreword by Alan Walker

The Damaging Consequences of Zombie Politics

This multi-layered, multidisciplinary, multinational, and data-rich collection succeeds superbly in exposing the reasons why so many and varied countries failed in their responses to the Covid-19 Pandemic and why some, such as Taiwan and Thailand, managed to negotiate it with relative success. The book focuses on the Covid-19 Pandemic but provides so much more: indeed, this focus may be seen as a lens through which to expose the manifold deficiencies of institutionalized welfare, which desperately needs to be defended against neoliberal attacks, but also needs radical reform. The book's authors raise fundamental questions about the purposes of welfare systems globally, not only the most fully developed Western welfare states. Invariably, in their present anachronistic forms they fail to ensure fundamental human rights for all, let alone equal citizenship and even basic levels of social quality. Furthermore, it is clear that the deeply gendered nature of health and welfare systems continues to be particularly damaging for women's health and wellbeing, and their equal opportunities for personal and professional development.

The unifying red thread running through the book comprises, first, the many inadequacies of national and international responses to the Covid-19 Pandemic and, second, in the face of their dehumanizing effects, there is a consistent plea for a greater policy emphasis on the quality of human life. The book's varied analyses are framed by the idea, borrowed from economists, of "*zombie politics*." These are anachronistic approaches that echo a bygone era and which are quite unsuited to the current global challenges. It is the combination of this outdated zombie approach with those global challenges—rapid societal ageing, digitalization, and global heating—each of which merits new political and policy paradigms, which results in the inadequacy of policy responses. The same zombie critique applies to many more policy areas where the same out of time and place formulation is evident: gender, race, family, children, young people, mental health, employment, education, social security, and so on. In other words, outdated approaches to social policy across the world were ripe for critical analysis, and that is what this book succeeds in providing.

It is anachronistic politics, guided by neoliberal ideology that has encouraged inequality to increase exponentially across the world, for societal ageing to be defined as an economic and social problem, for deadly global heating to continue apace, and which is also responsible for the inadequate responses to the Covid-19 Pandemic.

The US serves as a stark warning of the hugely negative effects of the lethal combination of neoliberalism and *zombie politics*. The richest country in the world has been transformed into one of the most unequal, with income inequality higher than any other OECD country. The US also leads the world in wealth inequality. Neoliberalism there has supercharged capitalism's inexorable drive toward inequality—hidden by deceitful rhetoric about "individual responsibility," "land of opportunity," and "dead hand of the state." This was possible only because of the long-term undermining of public sector values and hollowing out of public services, coupled with economic and social policies that eulogized wealth accumulation while stigmatizing and excluding those who could not, or would not, conform to the individualist's mantra of self-reliance.

This was indeed fertile ground upon which Covid-19 might prosper, and so it did: since late 2021 the US experienced the highest cumulative rate of deaths from Covid-19-related causes of any developed country in the world (90 percent of which were older people). It was not simply that the US was unprepared for the pandemic, it represented an open invitation for Covid-19 to do its worst. This included not only excessive deaths from Covid-related causes but also, among other awful things, exacerbation of "deaths of despair." If the richest country in the world was so ill-equipped to respond to the pandemic, what chance was there for the less developed world? Yet, perhaps surprisingly, some, such as Taiwan and Thailand, did manage to limit the worst effects of Covid-19. The lesson appears to be that those countries that put a high value on human life and, therefore, public health were able to manage the pandemic more successfully than those that failed to guarantee fundamental human rights to health and welfare.

If the US stands as a warning against the neglect of the social and the duty of any state to protect the health of its citizens, the service that was most often in the eye of the Covid storm, long-term care (LTC) also provides an indictment against neglect. Almost everywhere LTC, or social care, services have for decades been the "Cinderellas" of welfare systems. For a variety of reasons but, especially, the deeply gendered and ageist nature of welfare systems, services that mirror family provision (or women's domestic labor) and focus on older people are invariably neglected and, therefore, under-funded and under-staffed. Long before the pandemic it could have been predicted that LTC would be ill-prepared, and so it proved, with devastating consequences especially for older people and their families.

While the bulk of this book examines, in granular detail, these negative consequences of the Covid-19 Pandemic and policy responses to it, providing much to both appall in terms of the effects and regret in terms of the policy failures; there are also many positive indications of how much better the outcomes might have been if governments had focused on human health and wellbeing, and on providing an environment of social quality in which everyone has an equal chance to flourish.

Alan Walker
Professor of Social Policy
University of Sheffield
Sheffield, UK

Foreword by Joe C. B. Leung

Professor Christian Aspalter is an internationally renowned and prolific scholar on comparative social policy. This forthcoming edited book is another masterpiece examining how different countries cope with the Covid-19 pandemic crisis and its effectiveness, as well as the impacts on different vulnerable population involved. The application of "zombie politics" to conceptualize the common and dehumanized failures of the government policy-making mechanism as "out-of-place and especially out-of-time policies" is vivid and ingenious.

Indeed, the Pandemic has exposed the inadequacies of most government capacity in the world to cope with emergency crises in general, and the shortcomings of our healthcare system in specific. The immediate and long-term socio-economic impacts and their repercussions in both developed and developing countries are profound. More importantly, it has further aggravated impending social issues. As described in this book, these social issues include socio-economic inequalities, poverty, mental health, informality of employment, women status, migrant workers, and elderly care. Country and regional examples include the United States, Indonesia, China, Taiwan, Thailand, Hong Kong, and Italy.

Finally, this inspiring book, using distinctive conceptualization, in-depth, and comparative case studies, allows readers and policymakers to learn from our policy failures, prevent zombie paradigms, and hopefully get out of the shadow of the pandemic effectively.

Joe C. B. Leung
Honorary Professor
Department of Social Work and Social Administration
The University of Hong Kong
Hong Kong, Hong Kong

Contents

Contributors

Christian Aspalter Department of Social Sciences, Beijing Normal University-Hong Kong Baptist University United International College, Zhuhai, Mainland China, China

Marco Betti Dipartimento di Scienze della Comunicazione, Università degli Studi di Teramo, Teramo, Italy

Maria Letizia Bosoni Catholic University of Milan, Milan, Italy

Shiau-Fang Chao Department of Social Work, National Taiwan University, Taipei, Taiwan

Isabella Crespi University of Macerata, Macerata, Italy

Wannaphong Durongkaveroj Faculty of Economics, Ramkhamhaeng University, Bangkok, Thailand

Ghee W. Ho Department of Life Sciences, Beijing Normal University-Hong Kong Baptist University United International College, Zhuhai, China

Selma Kadi European Centre for Social Welfare Policy and Research, Vienna, Austria

Varvara Lalioti Department of Political Science and Public Administration, National and Kapodistrian University of Athens, Athens, Greece

Kai Leichsenring European Centre for Social Welfare Policy and Research, Vienna, Austria

Wan-I Lin Department of Social Work, National Taiwan University, Taipei, Taiwan

Tao Liu School of Public Affairs, Zhejiang University, Hangzhou, China

Franca Maino Dipartimento di Scienze Sociali e Politiche, Università degli Studi di Milano, Milano, Italy

Sara Mazzucchelli Catholic University of Milan, Milan, Italy

Thomas F. Remington Department of Government, Harvard University, Cambridge, USA;
Political Science Department, Emory University, Atlanta, USA

Andrea E. Schmidt National Public Health Institute, Vienna, Austria

Heidemarie Staflinger Chamber of Labour for Upper Austria, Linz, Austria

Johnston H. C. Wong Department of Social Sciences, Beijing Normal University-Hong Kong Baptist University United International College, Zhuhai, China

Tauchid Komara Yuda Department of Social Development and Welfare, Universitas Gadjah Mada, Yogyakarta, Indonesia

Part I
Introductory and Overarching Theory Part

Chapter 1
Introduction: The New Age of Zombie Politics

Christian Aspalter

Abstract This introductory chapter is shortly venturing into the overarching issue of zombie politics. Vigilent and keen observers around the world have had the chance to witness a great many applications of the theory and concept of zombie politics over the last couple of years. This chapter is introducing this concept to the study of the global Covid-19 Pandemic, as out of place and especially out-of-time policies, including strategies on grand scale and every single measure and its integral aspects on a micro scale, have become a commonplace in most countries dealing with and being affected by the Pandemic. The second part of this introductory part will introduce each following chapter of this book, drawing attention to unique and interesting aspects of, and profound conclusions provided in these chapters that cover most important and consequential topics for all people around the world, using theoretical, comparative and case study approaches to investigate, explain and remedy different aspects of the Covid-19 Pandemic.

Keywords Zombie politics · Covid-19 Pandemic · Out-dated ideas in policy-making · Health policy · Social policy

It just strikes one, time and again, when one wakes up in the morning, or when one tries to simply go to work, or to the supermarket and buy some vegetables, the feeling of general anxiety and insecurity, the thoughts of what are the rules, what am I allowed to do today, where am I allowed to go, am I allowed to go to work and try pay my bills, pay back my housing loan, how to prevent forceful removal of oneself and one's beloved family from one's home, for one reason or the other.

Life and living have changed. We arguably, or how is it possible *not* to argue that we, live in a new more fierce, more volatile, and inhumane world, meaning our *live-worlds* (cf Habermas 1981) have changed. On the job, in the supermarket, in the very

---

C. Aspalter (✉)
Department of Social Sciences, Beijing Normal University-Hong Kong Baptist University United International College, Zhuhai, China
e-mail: christian@uic.edu.cn

C. Aspalter (ed.), *Covid-19 Pandemic*,
https://doi.org/10.1007/978-981-99-2497-4_1

sanctuary of our home, nothing is sacred anymore. Rules set by robotic *administrators*, aloof committees that are more than ecstatic to sit down and rule every aspect of people's lives, knowingly (in any active or passive manner) or not. *Politicians* and self-proclaimed, or chosen by this or that politician (it does not matter), *experts* become the new gods who sit over and rule over our every aspects—our ever-so private aspects and facets—of our lives, families, interpersonal relationships, and (who would have imagined that before) our every bit of physical movement, and the way we breath in our air (and how much of it).

This experience, these new *lifeworld realities*, has been in the last couple of years shared by billions around the globe.

First, ignorance-filled politics, then fear-driven politics, all helped to boost and augment—in successive overlapping, and progressively reinforcing, waves—not a new phenomenon, but an entirely grown out of proportion phenomenon, that of zombie politics. The term zombie politics sprang from old, out-of-date practices that linger on in politics and policymaking, long after their rationale and need for existence has vanished, long after they ceased to fulfill their goal and effectiveness. This phenomenon was first acknowledged in economics, and then in the field of public policy (cf Giroux 2010, 2021; Quiggin 2012; Krugman 2020; Peters and Nagel 2022).

Each distinct phase of the Covid-19 Pandemic, in each distinct political arena, saw coming of out-of-date/out-of-time policies, policy stands, and policy strategies—i.e. out-of-date/out-of-time practices and believes that formed and fleshed out, cemented and perpetuated *lost-in-time policy paradigms.* While sometimes, some things (paradigms, strategies, policies, rules/regulations, and practices) were in place in the right place and at the right time, some of them always, and sometimes all of them together, were *out of time and out of place*, i.e. we always had to and have to deal with *out-of-time-and-place* paradigms, policy strategies and their produced policy practices.

This, if it would not have been so consequential, also consequential in the sense of a great many (when put them altogether) people—i.e. babies, birth-giving mothers, dialysis-needing people, people who ran out of their life-sustaining medicines, people who needed emergency and other health care, people who starved and starved to death due to food shortages and shortages of human contact—being totally affected by it, has become not an entirely new, not a new, but on a different-level new *New Normal.*

At the same time, other developments, path-altering developments, are thrown into the mix of meta factors that keep changing and speeding up the change of policy needs, and with it the making, fast and fluid transition and perpetuated presence of zombie politics. These include super-forceful developments other than the Covid-19 Pandemic, like e.g.: (a) super-fast and super high levels of societal aging combined with free-falling total fertility rates of societies around the globe, (b) super-digitalization and AI-ification of society and politics, and especially the economy, the supposed-to-be-*human* workplaces, and (c) the ongoing earth-altering changing weather patterns and the accompanying frequency, severity and geographical spread of extreme weather phenomena (i.e. the first *taste* of climate change).

The arrival of these new meta factors give rise to a new age, *the Age of Zombie Politics*, *if* we do not learn to prevent zombie paradigms, its affiliated zombie strategies and practices, i.e. to sense, understand and then to eliminate and prevent them altogether in a continuous, all-encompassing, all-and-ever-present effort, with textbook mechanisms and new organizational/political institutions (like e.g. real and constantly applied critical thinking, standing and other ad-hoc zombie-politics-and-practice-preventing expert and political committees and new respective political institutions). Without the general honest admission of policymakers and policymaking, and administrative/juridical, institutions that—due to numerous factors and meta-factors—*zombie policy paradigms and practices* that are out-of-place, out-of-time, no matter how much out of time *do exist, and do exist most frequently in all sorts of expected and unexpected places (even in most important policy areas and cases)*, there is no real chance of preventing this new Age of Zombie Politics.

Self-criticism is not everyone's strong suit, or attained or easily-attained familiar cultural/political/personal characteristic. This is clear. Nevertheless, it is of most importance that we work in this direction of realizing, analyzing, and reacting to and proacting towards the reduction and minimization of acts and incidences of zombie rules and regulations, zombie laws, zombie institutions, their zombie practices and ways to operate and legitimate (make up rationales, i.e. excuses, for) the very same.

While at the beginning of the Pandemic in general policy-makers did not respond or not respond in the right or in the right amount, at the right time, in the right place, in the right way, and hence were out of touch with the time and place they were in, they operated in, later on, especially in the later phases of the Pandemic, this turned into a fallacy of responding to new waves of distinctively altered viruses with *remedies* (no matter if they were right or wrong in the previous place and time, to different degrees, or not) *or better perceived remedies of the past* (or out-of-place remedies). This included the whole shebang of policy-making, together with the rationales used and abused, as well as the strategies and committees that started to work into the direction of quickly becoming self-supporting and self-prolonging living entities. In other words, *ideas live*, and *all administrative/legislative policies and their respective institutions live*—i.e. they quickly or instantly behave as if they are a distinct living entity.

Zombie paradigms and practices can be found in the whole spectrum of policy areas covering gender policies, family policies, child custody and divorce laws and practices, employment policies, education policies, social security policies and institutions that are being implemented and maintained (beyond their natural/effective/efficient live expectancies), and the same is true for anti-poverty policies; especially when one dares to step back and look at them from a distance, a comparative and historically comparative perspective, zooming in and focusing on their economic and social side-effects and follow-on effects (e.g., national fertility, the decline of the family system, perpetuated/cemented-in/artificially-spread poverty, and so forth).

This book has been designed to shed light on the inner and overall workings and outcomes of the Covid-19 Pandemic. A strong theoretical and meta-analytical stream of papers at the beginning of the book will work on (in multiple ways) comparative and/or topical issues and developments, while the second part of the book has descended to the country-level operational theatres of Covid-19 developments, covering policies and outcomes, from humanitarian, integrative and contextual perspectives.

After this critical (reflective, meta-analytical) thinking-based introduction, Chap. 2 drags open the curtain of confinement that has hindered, smothered and made barely possible or likely critical, fully-informed—'real rational,' i.e. science-based ("complete-evidence-based")—thinking, evaluation and policy action. From the very first day of the Covid-19 Pandemic, the truth about every aspect of the Pandemic has been hijacked. Narratives have been designed and redesigned, employed and reemployed, at the (power-guided) free will of policy-makers, and hand-selected, non-voted-for, 'experts' (whoever wanted to be called an expert, for whatever, and whoever wanted them to take over decision-making on behalf of elected or chosen governments and politicians, for whatever reason, e.g. blame-avoidance and/or power-concentration and control-sharpening). This chapter is offering a new light, and new perspectives and findings that are poised to *bring humanity back in.*

In the following chapter, Chap. 3, Thomas F. Remington of Harvard University takes on and investigates the Bermuda Triangle of spatial inequality, socio-economic inequality and—what concerns us most here—health inequality. Geography is the key, the utmost important, variable that determines the lengths of our lives, the quality of our lives, the resources available, the choices made, all of it. Small, relatively very small differences in geographic realities are most consequential for people's life-courses and life outcomes. And, this is a universal truth, i.e. this holds for every country on earth, in every corner, for every population group that there is. The super-rich empirical evidence provided by Thomas F. Remington in this chapter truly speaks for itself.

Chapter 4, also by Thomas F. Remington, opens up a thorough and most-exiting crime scene investigation into the causes of the rather unique phenomenon of rising deaths of despair—and here again especially, but not exclusively due to drug overdose—in the United States. The investigation concludes that the Covid-19 Pandemic has reinforced already-strong economic and spatial inequalities, which led to a greatly widened gap between the rich and the poor in general and between rich regions and localities on the one side and poor regions and localities on the other. As the consequence, the narrowing of opportunities and with it the associated loss of hope led to most devastating social-psychological impacts on people's lives, ending in surge of gun purchases, gun homicides, and fatal drug overdoses.

In the next chapter, Chap. 5, Jason L. Powell investigated the historical and cultural crime of modern-day societies to classify older people as weak, as a burden, as vulnerable and in need of "protection." These fixed explanations and rationales have, over centuries and decades, permeated into every fabric of modern-day policymaking, be it in social policy in general or in health policy in particular. Being written by the world's foremost expert on this very topic, the chapter leads to the conclusion that social policy and health policy makers and administrators are urged to, in a wholesome and preventative manner, in most humane and ethical ways, shape acceptable forms of aging whilst older adults need to be given realistic and workable opportunities to self-monitor and design their paths towards and through old-age, and effectively deal with biomedical, socio-cultural and linguistic suppression, i.e. dominance, control and sub-ordination.

In Chap. 6, which is entirely related to the previous chapter, Franca Maino and Marco Betti apply an international comparative perspective in analyzing the effects of the Pandemic on long-term care systems and policies in aging societies. All in all, the increased need for long-term care today and in the decades to come is necessitated by the combined forces of particularly new changing social patterns, such as smaller household size (smaller families), different forms of residential choices and patterns, and continued increases in female labor force participation. There are many important takeaways from the experience of long-term care systems and their older adults during the course of the Covid-19 Pandemic. Long-term care systems were, in general, non-prepared or ill-prepared for any major health emergency. The preference of most elderly to stay at home and get home-based care services has not been supported by the long-term care systems in place, and policymakers in charge.

Chapter 7 by Johnston H.C. Wong and Ghee W. Ho executes a comparative analysis on older people's experience in four cities around the world, namely Wuhan, Hong Kong, Milan and London. This chapter by Wong and Ho provides extremely valuable data and, in addition, improves the comparability of policymaking and human experiences across the globe during the Pandemic. The chapter among other things sheds light on the problem of out-of-date policies, and dehumanizing policies, especially with regard to one of the in most countries fastest-growing and/or largest population group, i.e. older people. Policy neglect and policy failures as uncovered by the Pandemic are most severe, most consequential in terms of losses of human lives and losses of life quality, human decency and humanity itself. At last, the authors point to the existence and differences of so-called *health welfare regimes*.

In the following, Tauchid Komara Yuda (in Chap. 8) is chasing innovatively and effectively the root causes of policy changes, longer-term and larger-scale social policy and health policy changes in Indonesia. Two separate crises are being compared, as case studies, across time, so to speak. Whereas the Asian Financial Crises in Indonesia led to a tug-of-war between politicians' clientelistic interests and extremely competitive democratic elections, which led to the establishment and extension of the social security for more and then eventually all of the population, the Covid-19 Pandemic caused regress instead of progress in terms of the political driving forces behind policy formation, in health and social policy alike. As a result of the Pandemic, the entrenched system of oligarchic power was used by the oligarchs to reorganize, and thus extend, their power and power relations.

Next comes a very exiting analysis of relative poverty, and especially a special form of relative poverty, i.e. secondary poverty. Secondary poverty is not caused by low (relative) incomes, but conversely by high expenditures, e.g. due to natural disasters, medical emergencies, long-term care emergencies, and so forth. In Chap. 9, Tao Liu masterfully examines relative poverty and secondary poverty in the case of Mainland China, putting it fully into the broad-based wider social policy and economic policy context. China's welfare regime, so Tao Liu, has employed a comprehensive repertoire of economic, fiscal, and social policies in responding to the Covid-19 Pandemic. This included increased overall monetary liquidity, and lowering taxation and social insurance premiums, as well as a range of irregular special responsive social policies, including the extension of unemployment insurance and social assistance coverage in terms of recipients and time of benefit payments (e.g. by means of de-bureaucratization and digitalization).

Chapter 10, written by Shiau-Fang Chao and Wan-I Lin, meticulously depicts the development of prompt and highly effective responses of the government to the Covid-19 Pandemic in Taiwan. Even though, Taiwan in general was very successful in managing the Covid-19 Pandemic (as a whole), the Pandemic still disproportionally affected older people in Taiwan. Thus, the chapter, in addition, also examines the experience of older people with special needs, such as people with special health care needs and/or disabilities, and residents in long-term care facilities, and the policy responses implemented by the Taiwanese government. On top, Shiau-Fang Chao and Wan-I Lin also provide a very strong and comprehensive catalogue of specific normative policy recommendations to mitigate the effects of disasters associated with the Covid-19 virus and to sustain the physical, mental and social well-being of older people in Taiwan and around the world.

Wannaphong Durongkaveroj, in Chap. 11, takes on the problems of the informal workforce that in most developing countries make up the majority of the workforce. Wannaphong Durongkaveroj's strong and rich data, and sharp analysis, examines the most severe problems that the majority of the population in developing countries, like Thailand, is facing. Due to the lack of social protection and job contracts, and thus the lack of social protection coverage, informal workers *en mass* have been losing their jobs and their living standards abruptly declined, pushing millions of people and their families into dire poverty. As a consequence, the Thai government needs to rise the benefit levels of temporary cash handouts to informal workers, plus extending the very same, i.e. bringing in the informal workforce, which carries the brunt of labor input to the production- and tourism-driven economy, into the realm of institutional, broader and more secure/generous, welfare state system coverage and benefits.

The case of Italy is being investigated at close range by Isabella Crespi, Sara Mazzucchelli and Maria Letizia Bosoni (Chap. 12). After depicting the development of the Covid-19 Pandemic itself, and the government's responses to it, Crespi, Mazzucchelli and Bosoni draw attention to the needs and sufferings of women and families not only as a consequence of the Pandemic, but also, and above all, the consequences of the government's manifold—not or not fully reflected and in most cases unrelenting—responses to the Pandemic. For sure the Pandemic hurt and killed people on a large scale, but also sure is the maltreatment and discrimination of families, children and mothers in particular, due to government policies that are supposed to help and rescue people, and not hurt and damage them. The authors of this brilliant chapter conclude in the future policies that are in full or in part aimed at supporting women and families are to be embedded into and adjusted to the context of all kinds of women's and families' needs and special situations, in order to address the existing severe inequalities and imbalances.

Connecting to the previous chapter, Chap. 13, written by Varvara Lalioti, investigates the issue of women's employment during the Covid-19 Pandemic, taking the example of Greece. In this study, Lalioti describes in full the unfolding of the Covid-19 Pandemic in Greece, and the government response to the pandemic, including their evaluation by both, researchers and the public. Then, the chapter investigates in detail the effects of particular policy measures regarding job retention schemes, measures to address work-life balance, repayable advance payments to enterprises, as well as mandatory rent reductions for business properties in the economic sectors that were more hit by the Pandemic. While pointing out ongoing and persisting problems for women employment in Greece, Lalioti points out also the positive side-effects of the Pandemic, e.g. the new, possible reevaluation of women's role as the core workforce in the essential occupations, in education, social and health care.

The next chapter (Chap. 14) focuses on yet another cornerstone in the overall analysis of the Covid-19 Pandemic and its concomitant social policy and health policy implications. Here, Kai Leichsenring, Selma Kadi, Andrea E. Schmidt and Heidemarie Staflinger have joined forces to provide an utmost meticulous and important examination of the government's policy responses to the Pandemic, with a strong, special emphasis on the situation of the long-term care service industry, and expressly the dire conditions, under which care workers had to work even before the onset of the Pandemic, which of course largely worsened with the very same. Migrant workers in Austria, as in many other European countries, and here particularly the Western half of Europe, carry the brunt of care-work services, and all of whom hence find themselves in double-dreadful positions and exposed to double-precarious conditions. As a result of the Pandemic, the government too lately and too lightly tried to manage the dire conditions of care workers, and chiefly migrant care workers. General responses included e.g. an additional week of annual leave for those who are over 43 years of age, and an increased authority given to care assistants in caring out care services. Other specialized responses included e.g. tailored language courses for migrant care workers, and easier access to work permits. The chapter closes with an appeal to a European solution on a European level that effectively and timely addresses the shortage of and the conditions faced by professional care workers, migrant (live-in) carers and informal carers.

The final chapter of this book (Chapter 15) goes on to give a larger picture, and provide a larger conclusion, applying a more lay-back (not-so-close-up) perspective. A *meta conclusion* is offered, to arrive at the overall takeaway, hovering on top of so many chapter-based takeaways. In public policy—and social policy including health policy—science there need to be a greater understanding and theoretization of problem-cum-policy cycles, in a comparative (global and historical) fashion, with a prime focus on social problems that underlie and interact with these policy cycles. Also, a very short appraisal about the outcomes of policy strategies applied during the Pandemic (for more data and results, cf Chap. 2), which led to different patterns of pandemic and its intertwined social/health problems cycles, is given, that is based on most recent, and more comprehensive, data available so far (cf also OECD, 2022, 2021).

This book will not answer *every* question one can ask about the Covid-19 Pandemic and its dehumanizing effects on people all over the world. It is not designed to do that. And, it would be preposterous to think than any one book can that at all.

The book has chosen to focus on social policy and health policy issues, people's problems at large, which are of medical, psychological, financial, social, etc. nature. The experts in this book have been chosen meticulously, these are the very best that there are in the world on this particular topic they wrote on. The assortment of the contributors, too, is global in terms of geography, but also global in terms of topics covered, as much as that is possible in any one single book. The book is very up-to-date, empirically and theoretically most informative.

Finally, I would like to express my greatest gratitude for the hard, hard and most excellent work of the contributors of this book. It was a great pleasure working with all these experts, some I know very well for a very long time, and it is the greatest honor of having been able to set up this wonderful book with all these renowned and excellent contributors, which will stand its ground, scientifically speaking, for a very long time.

References

Giroux, Henry A. 2010. Zombie politics and other late modern monstrosities in the age of disposability, *Policy Futures in Education*, 8(1), https://journals.sagepub.com.

Giroux, Henry A. 2021. *Zombie politics and culture in the age of casino capitalism.* New York: Peter Lang.

Habermas, Jürgen 1981. *Theorie des kommunikativen Handelns: Zur Kritik der funktionalistischen Vernunft*, Volume 2, Frankfurt a.M.: Suhrkamp.

Krugman, Paul. 2020. *Arguing with zombies: Economics, politics, and the fight for a better future.* New York: W.W. Norton.

OECD. 2021. *Health at a glance 2021.* Paris: OECD.

OECD. 2022. *Health at a glance: Europe 2022.* Paris: OECD.

Peters, B. Guy and Nagel, Maximilian 2022. *Zombie ideas: Why failed policy ideas persist*, https://www.ippapublicpolicy.org.

Quiggin, John. 2012. *Zombie economics: How dead ideas still walk among us.* Princeton: Princeton University Press.

Chapter 2
The Human Face of the Pandemic

Christian Aspalter

Abstract This paper is aiming to fill a relative gap in science, and social policy science in particular. That is, a greater focus on the 'quality' of humanity is needed, i.e. dignity and quality of life, compassion and care. Scientists, and science as such, in fact can oppose turning society, governance, and the health care systems into mechanic, solely-rules-driven, unreflective, detached-from-life, detached-from-humanity kind of systems. Not only need national constitutional laws be respected, humanity needs to be respected too, all the way during the Pandemic and in every aspect of the Pandemic. Covid-19 fears and protection of life arguments have been used as tools to *also unnecessarily* take away freedoms that humanity fought centuries and millennia for. This paper hence tries to look behind the curtain of public and social media, beyond the excuses for all sorts of rules and doctrines established over the past couple of years. Apart from looking at and analyzing international/global empirical data from the Pandemic and its human aftermath, this paper at its core provides a deeper look at the root cause of a number of Pandemic-related social problems and health problems—i.e. systemic inequalities—from a theoretical and empirical point of view, and that also worldwide. In essence, it is a review of humanity and how it fared during the Covid-19 Pandemic, a glimpse of a review of humanity, but nevertheless.

Keywords Covid-19 pandemic · Performance of governments · Comparison of outcomes · Inequality · Dignity · Freedom · Humanity

Rules and regulations have taken center stage since the first wave of the Covid-19 Pandemic, or simply the Corona Pandemic (as it is called by common people), in the world as we know it. This article is a mere attempt to shift the focus away from rules and regulations that are geared and/or sold to protect one's own health, lower (or possibly prevent) the risk of getting the virus (or passing it on) and hence to protect

C. Aspalter (✉)
Department of Social Sciences, Beijing Normal University-Hong Kong Baptist University United International College, Zhuhai, Mainland China, China
e-mail: christian@uic.edu.hk

C. Aspalter (ed.), *Covid-19 Pandemic*,
https://doi.org/10.1007/978-981-99-2497-4_2

society. Among all these rules and regulations, laws, prohibitions and permissions (and proofs/tests) needed, the human and especially human freedom has suffocated and been robbed of space, time in space, movement in space, and the quality thereof and the quality that comes along with or is attached to the very same (cf Shimwell 2020; Peisah et al. 2020; Santos 2021; Raposo 2021; ENNHRI 2022; Delvac 2022).

The 'quality' of humanity ("*Menschlichkeit*" or condition of humanity) has undoubtedly suffered, and been pushed back to yet much lower limits and standards, enforced in the name of protection and greater public good. The virus, a new enemy (that is for sure) of public life, private life and human freedom, has been taking center stage, and the human, human existence, the essence of human life and existence has been pushed under water, locked into the backrooms and basements of what used to be the fringes of public and private human lives and livelihoods.

Of course, there are always lots of good reasons (and that in any direction) when one just looks for them and repeats and pushes them to the utmost—through public media and hence social media, through rules and regulations, dominant thoughts, believes, attitudes and opinions that are not to be doubted and questioned in any way, in any form, howsoever lightly and indirectly.

This article is not about those rules and regulations, but rather about what is left from the human, from humanity, the human spirit and face. It applies the method of non-statistical *thematic meta-analysis* (Aspalter 2021a). And as such, it is philosophical and inspirational (and informing at best). Non-statistical meta-analyses in policy sciences (social policy and/or public policy) can be e.g. of thematic, historical, or philosophical nature (cf Aspalter 2021a). They are set to guide current and future research works and the scientific enterprise of social policy (as in our case here). Meta-analyses are greatly needed, as they are still super-rare in absolute and relative terms.

There need to be more spaces for thought and philosophical pondering, in public policy and social policy alike. As a social policy scientist and professional, the author does take more than just a keen interest—a core interest, one could say—in the overall, total well-being and welfare of the people, families and communities that (a) have been become victims of the virus, and (b) victims of sub-optimal, and more often than one could have expected counterproductive—or just meaningless—rules, regulations, and governance decision-making. These often aimed at suppression and creating fear for the purpose of increasing political hegemony of dominant/ruling elites and stiffing different opinions, thoughts and reasoning.

The devil often, but not always, lays in the detail(s). Sometimes it is obvious that taking a mountain hike only with one's own children is not extra dangerous, even at the height of the pandemic, especially e.g. if the mountain is situated next to one's home, or very nearby. It is obvious that in general parents should be allowed to visit their own children, even if they reside with the other parent after divorce, also at the height of the pandemic. It is obvious that *the virus* does not know if the owner has already walked the dog more than 150 m away from home, or not. Also, the virus does not get more dangerous after e.g. ten o'clock in the evening or after midnight, as it cannot tell time (cf e.g. also Simões 2022; Čović and Nikolić 2021).

There are a lot of good—even when very tough, depending on time, and extent of the problems a country and society is facing, and the context in general—rules and regulations, including appropriate lockdowns.

But, on the other hand, there are also quite a shockingly high number of useless and dehumanizing rules and regulations, or at least bits and elements thereof, which also add up, over longer periods of time, and in sum, in terms of overall dehumanizing effects (cf e.g. Choi 2022; Burrowes 2020a, b; Sandel and Reckford 2020; Fenner 2020). Rebecca Hilsenrath, the Equality and Human Rights Commission Chief Executive, put it to the point:

> We are walking a tightrope. We need to find the balance between saving lives from coronavirus, and allowing people the hard won freedoms that are the framework for those lives—such as a right to a private and family life, to freedom of assembly, and to an education. This must go hand in hand with an economic recovery that provides everyone with an adequate standard of living. (EHCR 2020).

The usefulness of rules and regulations, laws and policies, are highly dependent upon *contexts* of specific spaces and specific times, including e.g.:

1. different waves of the pandemic;
2. phases within each wave of the pandemic;
3. different variants of the virus;
4. different health care system capabilities;
5. the availability of vaccines;
6. amount and effect of vaccines available;
7. the presence, extent and vulnerability of people with pre-existing conditions (hypertension, diabetes, cardiovascular disease, overweight and obesity, cf. e.g. Li et al. 2021a);
8. degree of aging and especially degrees of unhealthy aging in respective societies;
9. prevalence and degrees of multiple co-morbidities, and so forth.

These dehumanizing aspects of unwarranted rules and regulations—or fractions thereof—are part of, and act as catalysts of, universal dehumanizing aspects regarding economic and social inequality, economic and cultural oppression, intellectual and spiritual oppression alike (cf Aspalter 2021b). These are:

> the universal chains that enslave us in a myriads of dehumanizing conditions (Mohan 2012: 2).

On the Causal Relationship Between Inequality and Systemic Poverty

It is hard to measure '*humanity*' ('*Menschlichkeit*,' or *the essence and art of being human*) and *human 'quality'* (i.e. human dignity *and* quality of life), in quantitative terms at least. The opposite, dehumanization, however is much easier to grasp and put into numbers (for the international audience, and for any keen government and scientific observer alike).

If we conceptualize welfare as the absence of diswelfare and/or absence of inequality, oppression, poverty, disease, disability, discrimination, injustice, neglect, agony and despair, we are having a much better chance of encapsulating the realities of human suffering across the globe, in the majority of places (countries, regions, countries, remote/backward/forgotten areas) with the majority of human-kind living in those places—what people (and scientists) have come to call the '*developing world.*'

Most of today's world is called the *developing* world, or *developing* countries, which is an expression created by the super-powerful and super-super-rich to make the for-centuries-and-in-multiple-ways-enslaved-and-oppressed feel better about, hopefully forget about, and/or do not pay attention to the multiple historical and systemic inequalities that cause and maintain their disadvantaged, desolate and dire conditions (cf Frank 1966, 1991; Wallerstein 1979; Cardoso and Faletto 1979; Hopkins and Wallerstein 1980; as well as Myrdal 1965, and Rothschild 1971).

However, when subsequently reversing this definition of the concept of welfare back again, we can understand welfare as any government action, policy and program that improves *existential human conditions* (cf Dixon 2010; Mohan 1987; cf also Mohan 1985, 1986, 1992, 1993, 2007; Mohan and Sharma 1985). The Covid-19 Pandemic, but also a great deal of policies, rules and regulations, that were brought up and reasoned to combat the very same, have reversed and worsened these *existential human conditions.* These existential human conditions are threatened, eroded, annihilated and made impossible by the twin evils of humanity: inequality and poverty.

> Across our planet, poverty and inequality have explosively grown, in recent decades (Piketty 2014, 2006, 2000), and much more so also in the time of the Covid-19 Pandemic (CSRI 2022; Collins 2022; FIA 2021).
>
> Most of the scientific world, and with it social policy, has not yet come to acknowledge the fact that *inequality is* in all its numerous forms of manifestations *a chief cause of poverty* (cf Remington 2023a, b; Aspalter, 2023; USAID, 2021; Casas Herrera 2017; Gould 2014).
>
> As if this were not enough, it has also been empirically proven that inequality in all its manifesting and interlocking aspects also has colossal self-propelling and self-perpetuating properties (cf Remington 2023a, b).

Providing a general theory of mass poverty and systemic poverty, *the theory of super inequality* (Aspalter 2022a, 2023) also stresses that different dimensions of *systemic inequalities*—together with institutional, political, cultural, environmental and geographic inequalities of opportunities and unequal distribution of abilities and limitations—*cause multi-faceted systemic povertization processes* (cf Brady 2009; Aspalter 2021b, 2023; Remington 2023a, b).

> These povertization processes are set up and maintained by the economic, political and cultural elites of society.

Povertization processes are twofold in their effects, as the super-super-rich and super-powerful elites: (1) enrich themselves and shield themselves from losses; (2) enslave, impoverish, incarcerate and drain the life energy and financial sources out of the masses (the working and middles classes at the same time), and (3) practically exclude and prohibit them (a) from taking part in financial and asset gains and accumulation, as well as (b) from the vast majority of advantageous education and good health prospects.

The perpetuating outcome of these aggregating povertization processes is systemic poverty in all its forms and aspects. Thus, mass poverty and all kinds of systemic poverty is now being explained by this new *Theory of Super Inequality* (Aspalter 2022a), which is mainly built on the theoretical foundations (but also other philosophical and importantly empirical foundations) of a number of key meta theories themselves, especially:

(1) *Luhmann's theory of social communication* (i.e. his version of social system theory) (Luhmann 1984, 1998),
(2) Foucault's *theory of the constant and all-encompassing 'civil war' matrix* of asymmetric and in multiple ways systemically skewed power relations and knowledge (i.e. 'power of knowledge' that is used for and against people, i.e. for the rich and powerful, and against the poor and moderately well off) (Foucault 1975, 2009, 2010, 2014; Lukes, 2005; Rabinow, 2010),
(3) Tilly's *durable inequality theory* (Tilly 1998),
(4) Weber's *open versus closed relations theory* (Weber 2019), and so forth.

By itself, it is rather obvious that the Covid-19 Pandemic did not invent *new* forms and *new* reasons of inequality and poverty—i.e. super inequality, mass poverty and systemic poverty in all its forms for all kinds of people wherever they are. That is to say,

> the Pandemic acts as a multiplier and catalyst of super inequality, and hence mass poverty and systemic poverty.

In other words, the Covid-19 Pandemic triggered *new amplitudes* and opened up *new pathways* of oppression within the old *skewed power relations matrix* (what Foucault called *the 'civil war' matrix*), and its many sub-matrices (cf e.g. also Ciuffetelli Parker and Conversano 2021; UN 2020a, b).

Policymaking for Survival *and* Dignity

In a nutshell, this paper is about the *human face* of the Pandemic—or a short appraisal or meta-analysis of how humans fare in the Pandemic. It is however merely depicting the gist of the existential human conditions facing the outcomes of the Pandemic and the overall picture of what has been and is still going on around the world. In doing so, it calls for establishing, safeguarding, and fostering *human dignity* across all major aspects of *existential human conditions* (human well-being), because, simply and unmistakenly put: "[s]urvival without dignity is dehumanization" (Mohan 2012: 94).

Social policy, and public policy in general, consequently must always have its eyes set on both survival *and* dignity; such as health policy must always set its eyes on life-expectancy, the quality of life *and* human dignity at the same time, of individuals themselves and society at large.

In general, *inequality*—in all its despicable forms—*is the nemesis of human dignity*, as inequality is the means that makes possible, generates and sustains dehumanizing poverty, and its associated processes of povertization, which are multifaceted (cf Aspalter 2022a):

1. *education polarization*, regarding both access and contents of education (cf e.g. Bourdieu 1973, 2002; Collins 1979),
2. *wealth polarization* (cf Piketty 2014) and *income polarization* (cf Kim and Aspalter 2021a, b),
3. *monopolization and privileged rewards associated with access to finance and power relations* (cf Tilly 1998; Murphy 1988; Collins 1975; Weber 2019),
4. *exclusion and punishments delivered through taxation, fees, and social security financing, inflation and devaluation of savings and pensions, cold progression in taxation, plus exclusion from finance and economic opportunities* (cf Brady 2009, 2019; Brady et al. 2016; Huang et al. 2021; Remington 2023a; Aspalter 2022b, 2023),
5. *exclusion from social and cultural harmony* and positive social and cultural participation (cf Nietzsche 1887; Mohan 1987, 2011),
6. *technologically facilitated and/or caused oppression of the poor and vulnerable* (Eubanks 2018),
7. expulsion from economic, social and cultural life through *mass incarceration* as a systemic means of oppression and weakening of the masses, i.e. working and middle classes alike (cf Foucault 1975, 2009, 2010, 2014; Lukes 2005; Rabinow 2010, as well as DeFina and Hannon 2009; Brady 2009: 5), and so forth.

The public responses to the Covid-19 Pandemic across the world have been varied, and at times highly contrasting to one another—also within comparable situations, i.e. comparable conditions and contexts (see above). The *societal follow-on effects of policy responses* to the Covid-19 Pandemic are still less (or least) understood and less (or least) studied. These have been highly varied—while they also needed to be varied according to different phases of different waves in different societal contexts, health contexts, health care resources contexts, and vaccination contexts.

Who are the population groups most suffering from the Pandemic in terms of follow-on effects? Unquestionably, the ones directly affected by the virus, and those who are family members, friends and helping hands of those who have been directly affected by the virus, are the ones bearing the brunt of the Pandemic's fallout. But, there are more groups, especially the elderly, the vulnerable in general, minorities and the poor in general, and women and children in general (cf e.g. Crespi et al. 2023; Chao and Lin 2023; UNICEF 2022; Morales and Ali 2021; Kretchmer 2020; Peisah et al. 2020; Robinson 2020). The elder generation, the poor and the vulnerable, for instance, were and are subject to social exclusion and institutional (mandated) isolation and hence loneliness. Women and mothers were and are the ones affected most by needing to care, or simply choosing to care, for loved ones, family members, the elder parents and grandparents, the sick, and the children who are out of school and out of kindergarten or are sick themselves as well.

> Lockdowns and school closures around the world have particularly put women in jeopardy "due to increased home and childcare duties as schools and restaurants closed, and family incomes fell. Single mothers suddenly faced with round-the-clock childcare duties and possible job loss provide one illustration of the kind of challenges faced. Such stresses may show up in wealth effects as well as health and social impacts." (Shorrocks et al., 2021: 14)

In addition, across the entire population across all age groups—and here again particularly children and youths(!)—people have been subject to rocketing prevalence of mental health problems, including all kinds of major mental health problems that are common in post-industrial/digital societies. Figures 2.1 and 2.2 cut across countries with different economic development levels and different levels of risk factors regarding mortality and severe cases of Covid-19 infections, depicting their prevalence of anxiety and depression respectively, when compared from just before the Pandemic, with the first year of the Pandemic.

The fact that Mexico stands out twice in this comparison of mental health problems and its increases during first phase of the Covid-19 Pandemic shows that its record-high levels of prediabetes/diabetes, overweight/obesity and high blood pressure (in other words, all problems that are part of the metabolic syndrome) are the key problem behind not just mental health problems, but also *other* main problems related to the Covid-19 Pandemic. Figure 2.4 sums up that conundrum.

Modern mass diseases, non-communicable diseases (NCDs), are the main problem behind the Covid-19 Pandemic and all the problems it poses directly for people's health—but also predominantly people's poverty and misery. With initial higher levels of modern mass diseases, i.e. Covid-19 risk factors, the resulting levels of health problems after the onset of the Pandemic are particularly large, often

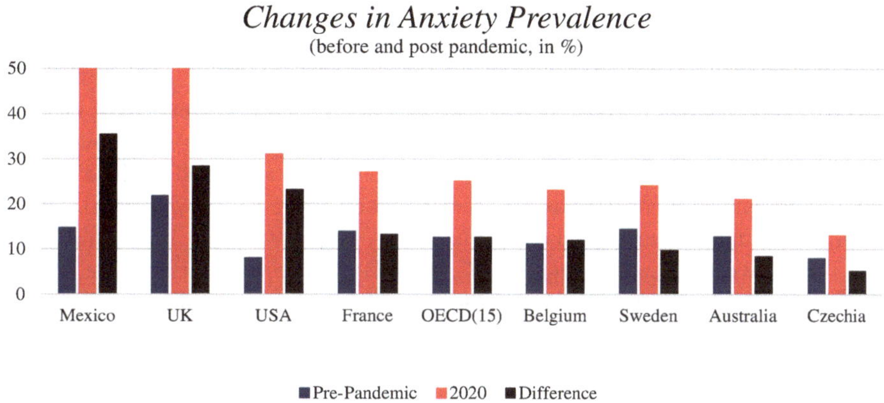

Fig. 2.1 Rising anxiety levels since the onset of the pandemic. *Source* Compiled and calculated from OECD (2021)

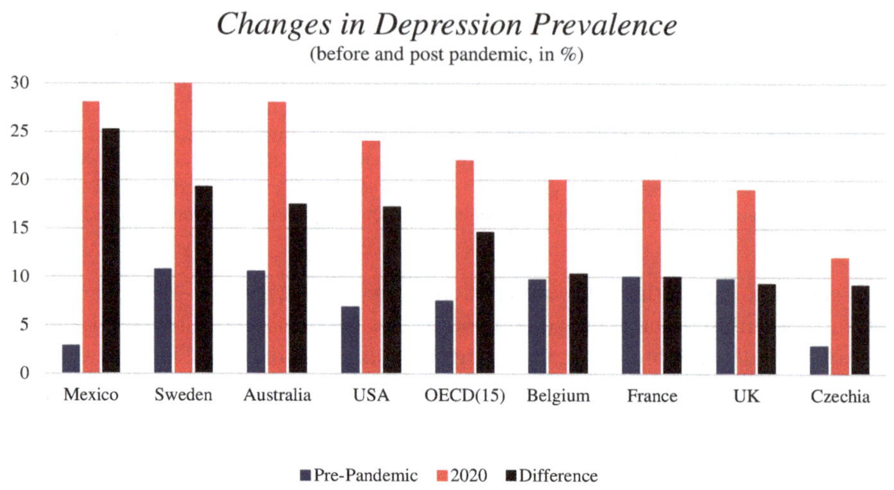

Fig. 2.2 Rising depression levels since the onset of the pandemic. *Source* Compiled and calculated from OECD (2021)

resulting in a failure of health care systems' capacity to keep emergency and essential health care services (including cancer screening, routine operations, etc.) running. The resulting piling up of risk factors, eventually leads to rising mortality, rising poverty—which indeed can be referred to *spiraling effects* of the Pandemic that started way before the onset of the Pandemic itself.

Furthermore, unemployment, employment losses and income losses—and hence largely increased levels of poverty and economic insecurities—are also the direct result of the effects of the Pandemic—and so are increased levels of inequality and poverty, both of which have been staggering throughout all parts of the world (cf ENNHRI 2022).

These need to be incorporated into any ad hoc and in advance evaluation of responses to the Pandemic, as well as the evaluation of overall outcomes of Pandemic itself and the policy responses, in total and one by one.

The direct effects of loss of employment, loss of self-employment, loss of income and loss of one's home during the Pandemic, and especially during lock-downs and other periods of intense policy measures, in turn are being amplified by the different overall (aggregate) response measures' direct impact on people's physical and mental health, social support, and social interaction of any kind (family life, community life, etc.). These we can call *self-amplifying effects of the Pandemic responses*—i.e. *effects that amplify other effects* of rules, regulations and policies put in place.

To be sure, poverty, income losses, homelessness, income insecurity, and existential insecurities of all kinds directly exacerbate health and social problems, such as e.g. anxiety, despair, loneliness, depression, anger, violence, overweight, additional alcohol consumption, lack of exercise, lack of social support, and this list goes on and on (cf e.g. Figs. 2.1 and 2.2). This is especially the case for the lower income groups of any society, and here again especially in poor and poorer countries across the globe.

As more data is yet to come in for the early phase of the Pandemic, and any major data sets for the mid- and later phases of the Pandemic are yet to be compiled and analyzed, the search for conclusions and findings here is merely at its very beginning.

Attacking Global Human Dignity: The Appalling Rise of Inequality Across the Globe

Nonetheless, when continuing with our above analysis of institutional inequality and systemic forms and venues of poverty, *there is a group of people—the super-super-rich and the super-powerful (the elites)—that actually thrived and used the Pandemic as a huge opportunity portal and platform.*

> Wealthy people in general were "relatively unaffected by reductions in the overall level of economic activity and, more importantly, they have also benefited from the impact of lower interest rates on share prices and house prices." (Shorrocks et al. 2021: 23).
>
> [T]he elite [is] manipulating our fear as we witness the defense of mankind against an elitist coup for the purpose of taking away fundamental rights and freedoms, conquered after several centuries of fighting (Burrowes, cited in Čović and Nikolić 2021).

It is no secret that the super-super-rich and the super-rich got so much wealthier during the Pandemic (cf e.g. Scholz 2022), due to rising real estate prices, rising stock market values, new arising business opportunities (e.g. hygiene and medical equipment, online businesses, delivery services) and so forth.

> With a single exception—the share of the top 1% in 2014—the inequality rise in 2020 was significantly greater than that recorded in any year this century. (Shorrocks et al. 2021: 25).
>
> The bottom 50% of adults in the global wealth distribution together accounted for less than 1% of total global wealth at the end of 2020. In contrast, … the top percentile alone has nearly half (45%) of all household assets. (Shorrocks et al. 2021: 25).

The story that has however for the very most part evaded public and academic scrutiny is *the resulting global wealth inequality shift*. The super-super-rich and the super-rich in the poor and poorer countries (what people and scientists reflexively call 'developing countries') gained extraordinarily more from the Pandemic, as a whole, than their counterparts in the rich (so-called 'more developed') countries (Table 2.1).

It is for this reason that the poor and the average masses in the poor and poorer countries, as a logical and inevitable consequence thereof, have suffered disproportionally more than the poor and average people have suffered in the rich countries. It is a great pity that yet again, the rich countries have been more at the center of attention of the global media and academia at the same time. Hence, more attention to the poor and their problems (and their causes) in poor countries need to be given by the global community; governments, media and academia alike.

Table 2.1 Change of wealth inequality during the first year of the pandemic—a shift in global wealth inequality

	Wealth Gini coefficient		Wealth share of Top 1%		
	2019	2020	2019	2020	Relative increase (%)
Brazil	88.2	89.0	46.9	49.6	5.75
China	69.7	70.4	29.0	30.6	5.51
UK	71.4	71.7	22.4	23.1	3.12
India	82.0	82.3	39.5	40.5	2.53
Japan	64.2	64.4	17.8	18.2	2.24
Russia	87.3	87.8	57.1	58.2	1.92
Italy	66.4	66.5	21.8	22.2	1.83
USA	85.1	85.0	35.0	35.3	0.85
Germany	77.9	77.9	29.4	29.1	−1.02
France	69.9	70.0	22.4	22.1	−1.33

Source Credit Suisse Research Institute (2021), *Global Wealth Databook*

Policymaking and Its Comparative Performance During the Pandemic

Far from having been debated nearly enough, and being pushed aside and under the rug again and again, by mainstream media and the governments (and academia) worldwide, are (i) the highly diverse levels of outcomes of the Pandemic and (ii) the highly diverse performances of government policies and strategies to address and fight the Pandemic.

More than just interesting, i.e. high intriguing indeed, is the similarity in the outcomes of neighboring countries in certain regions in e.g. Europe. Scandinavian countries on the one hand have very different outcomes, and so do e.g. Eastern Central European countries. The loss of (normally increasing) life expectancy at birth in e.g. OECD countries in Fig. 2.3 is highly telling.

Of course, this comparison also reflects different levels of and exposure to preconditions for extreme dire infection courses and infection outcomes, i.e. high levels of diabetes and prediabetes, high rates of obesity and overweight, high shares of *unhealthily-aged* elder populations (i.e. people that have pursued and are pursuing unhealthy lifestyles, in particular food and exercise choices, in the past and/or present), and so forth (cf e.g. NHLBI 2020; Li et al. 2021b; Ritchie et al. 2022).

In general, the reported numbers—and the reporting rules, guidelines and incentives—vary greatly across countries due to different practices, standards, definitions, and very different cut-off points in terms of calling an infection an infection.

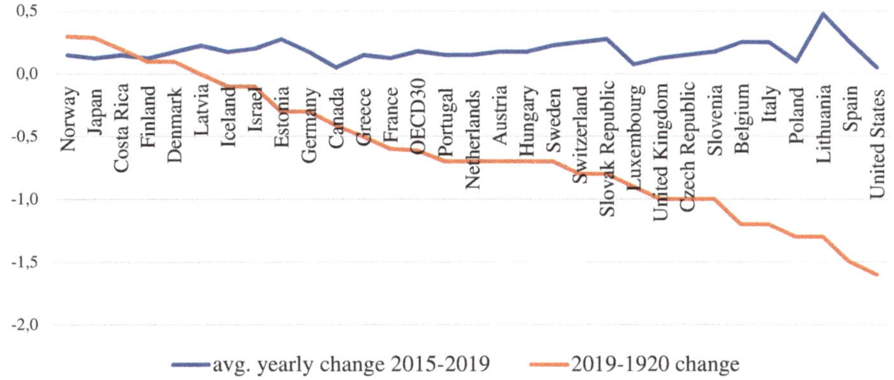

Fig. 2.3 Average life expectancy (at birth) growth and its change during the first year of the pandemic *Source* OECD Global Health at a Glance (2021)

These two factors need to be kept in mind when looking at Fig. 2.4. Nevertheless, the overall comparison given in this figure still holds a commanding perspective for comparative, analytical and learning purposes.

The rankings that can be derived (from Fig. 2.4) are, hence, not all-telling and not all-inclusive, but rather (strongly) indicative and direction-giving in terms of understanding what happened, how the world—i.e. humanity—fared in general and across different countries and regions of the world.

Figure 2.4 has been using a new statistical approach in measuring exactly the distances of relative performances of different countries with regard to different indicators (measures of performances). The indicators used for Fig. 2.4 include the number of excess deaths, 'official' Covid-19 deaths, 'official' Covid-19 cases, as well as vaccination rates (OECD 2021), each with equal weighting. The Standardized Relative Performance (SRP) Index as developed earlier by Aspalter (2006) can be used to show the exact spread of compound performances of countries across a wider spectrum of indicators.

In Fig. 2.4, the most commonly used indicators have been incorporated into the comparison of performances across different countries during the first phase of the Pandemic (the year 2020 and larger parts of 2021). These can however be extended and triangulated with different performance indicators, as well as different forms of performance indicator evaluations altogether. In addition, data of the last one and a half years (and beyond) can be added and the current findings yet again triangulated further.

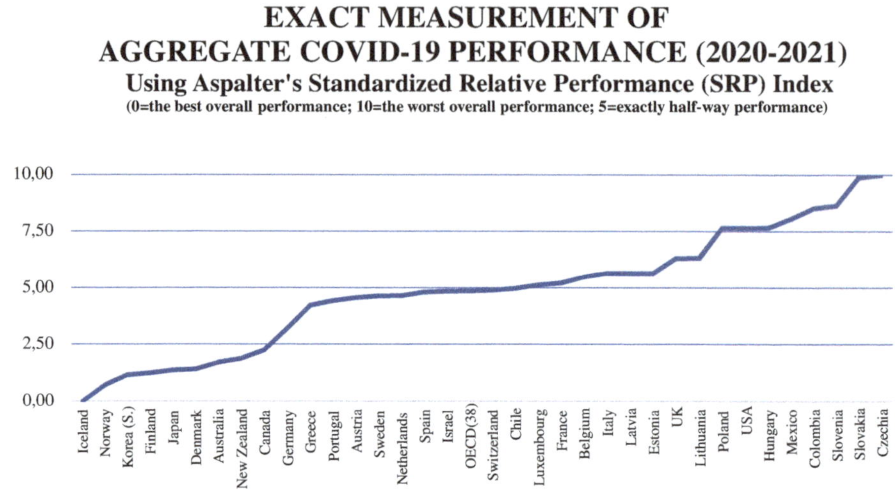

Fig. 2.4 Aggregate Performance in Terms of No. of Excess Deaths, 'Official' Covid-19 Deaths, 'Official' Covid-19 Cases, as well as Vaccination Rates. *Notes* The method of comparison used has been developed by Aspalter (2006), it is designed and able to compare directly different indicators, even when they use different measurement units and dimensions. We can compare number of deaths, with number of infections, etc. by looking directly at their relative performance distance to the best performer and the worst performer within each particular group of countries. The formula for *Aspalter's Standardized Relative Performance (SRP) Index* is: ((CV-LV)/(HV-LV))*10; where CV stands for the current value that is being standardized, LV for the lowest value in each particular column, HV for the highest value in each particular column. Here, the lowest value must always become 0, and the highest value must always become 10. To begin with, negative values have to be turned into positive values, and negative and positive indicators need to be pointing in the same direction (that is, in our case the SRP value for vaccinations, which is a good thing per se, has been turned upside down, by calculating 10 minus the calculated SRP value). Indicators *can* be combined, as in our case here, by e.g. averaging the SRP values for all the indicators of each country and then using the above formula *again* (so that there will be another 0 for lowest value, and 10 for highest value). It is good to re-standardize the final values again (using the above formula once more) *in order to* be better able to judge the mid-point cases, which then exactly lay at 5; on top, 7.5 then exactly stands for 75% of exact distance in terms of relative performance to the highest value performer, and 2.5 then stands exactly for 25% of relative performance distance from lowest to highest value performer. Depending on the researcher, 10 can stand for the worst value, or aggregate worst value; or the opposite thereof, depending on each researcher's preference, and the context of the data/indicators that one works with. Based on data from OECD (2021), for intermediate results that were used to calculate these final results above see the Appendix at the end of this chapter

General Conclusions and Takeaways

The biggest lesson that one can derive from the experience and the literature on the Pandemic is perhaps that truth is very political (because it is used in that way). Elements of truths, i.e. versions of truths, have been used constantly in a barrage of words of wars and ideologies on more than one political and ideological side—as well as on more than one societal/social side.

The masses, the common people, as well as the common researcher alike, have been exposed to constant kidnapping of truths to serve either side of ideas and convictions; politically convenient truths and elite-serving truths. The worst of it all is perhaps the forceful categorization of (accidental or not) opponents and (eager or not) supporters of this or that side of the truth, or interpretation (or yet better: world views or political views) of the respective truths. People, media and governments have called those who do not support this or that view, deniers, refusers, crazy and many more such words. The truth, and with it to a great extent science, has been hence hijacked, used and abused constantly almost, and in many ways (cf e.g. the theory and past works of Chomsky 1987, 2002; Herman and Chomsky 2002).

> The most important thing that one could take away from the Pandemic is that: *opinions are opinions, and that 'not' all people have to have the same opinion.* If this is not allowed, freedom is not allowed. If this is questioned, or put on hold, then freedom is not anymore.
>
> Human freedom then certainly, and definitely, would be a thing of the past.

The facts, on which science is to be based always, and to be held accountable to always, are not so easy, and not so quickly, to be told (read, analyzed, interpreted and doublechecked). After two and a half years of the Covid-19 Pandemic, the comparison of responses in general reveals that Scandinavian countries on the whole fared much better, and so did countries in e.g. East Asia. One could argue that equality (in the case of Scandinavia) played a vital role, first people protecting themselves, and more importantly in governments providing better and more humane responses to the Pandemic. Scandinavia has been marked by a high level of self-responsibility of people themselves and remarkably low government restrictions and interventions into people's lives and human rights. In East Asia, some countries have played out a different strategy with fast and/or strong government responses, also achieving remarkably low Covid deaths (in international/global comparison), with strongly varying approaches of government policies and strategies in dealing with the Pandemic.

Poorer countries and countries with strong prevalence of high-risk factors of Covid-19 related mortality due to diabetes/prediabetes, obesity/overweight and high blood pressure prevalence fared the worst. Then there were many rich countries who applied strong and far-reaching measures, but also encountered horrendous side-effects of their measures in place in terms of: (i) physical and mental health deterioration (including emotional health and behavioral problems), (ii) economic/social deterioration, i.e. intense rises in poverty and inequality, and (iii) in large parts unnecessary trampling of fundamental human rights of movement, exercise, family support, self-determination, etc.

There is more than one conclusion, more than one takeaway from the Pandemic. There are hideous winners and abysmal losers in several different ways. It is safe to say, that longevity without *quality* is not the only goal in policymaking, we *must* also take care of mental health, poverty, inequality, unemployment, social rights, economic rights, human rights, and all essential human conditions all along. That is to say:

humanity without *quality*—without its qualities (dignity, freedom, compassion, and so forth)—ceases to be humanity.

Appendix: Aggregate Country Performances During the Early Phase of Covid-19 Pandemic: Using Aspalter's SRP Index

	Excess deaths, 2020–21	Registered Covid-19 deaths, 2020–21	Registered Covid-19 cases, 2020–21	Vaccination rates, 2020–21	Vaccination rates, 2020–21	Together	Together as SRP indexes
	Standardized	Standardized	Standardized	Standardized	Values reversed	Average	Standardized again
Iceland	0.98	0.25	2.03	9.09	0.91	1.043	0.00
Norway	0.00	0.47	2.20	6.47	3.53	1.547	0.70
Korea (S.)	0.70	0.11	0.34	3.70	6.30	1.862	1.14
Finland	1.31	0.56	1.58	5.78	4.22	1.917	1.22
Japan	2.25	0.37	0.80	5.35	4.65	2.016	1.36
Denmark	1.00	1.41	3.87	8.08	1.92	2.049	1.40
Australia	1.03	0.10	0.22	2.33	7.67	2.257	1.69
N. Zealand	1.04	0.00	0.00	1.53	8.47	2.377	1.86
Canada	2.96	2.26	2.70	7.29	2.71	2.660	2.25
Germany	2.54	3.56	3.19	5.93	4.07	3.339	3.20
Greece	3.55	3.86	3.86	5.00	5.00	4.067	4.22
Portugal	4.86	5.41	6.55	10.00	0.00	4.205	4.41
Austria	3.27	3.93	5.25	5.14	4.86	4.305	4.55
Sweden	1.74	4.62	7.04	5.93	4.07	4.365	4.63
Netherlands	3.51	3.31	7.27	6.59	3.41	4.374	4.64
Spain	4.47	5.56	6.60	8.72	1.28	4.480	4.79
Israel	2.20	2.41	9.42	5.97	4.03	4.515	4.84
OECD(38)	3.75	4.18	5.27	5.12	4.88	4.521	4.85
Switzerland	2.84	3.89	6.17	4.77	5.23	4.534	4.87
Chile	5.10	5.66	5.45	7.77	2.23	4.609	4.97
Luxembourg	2.44	4.24	7.88	5.68	4.32	4.723	5.13
France	3.49	5.37	6.57	6.30	3.70	4.783	5.21
Belgium	3.49	7.12	6.84	7.56	2.44	4.972	5.48
Latvia	3.14	4.31	5.32	2.48	7.52	5.072	5.62
Italy	5.13	6.97	4.93	6.72	3.28	5.074	5.62
Estonia	3.53	3.10	7.53	3.86	6.14	5.078	5.63
UK	3.96	7.27	7.31	6.28	3.72	5.566	6.30
Lithuania	4.66	5.12	7.67	5.17	4.83	5.568	6.31
USA	5.99	5.93	8.32	4.19	5.81	6.515	7.63
Poland	8.32	6.44	4.81	3.51	6.49	6.516	7.63

(continued)

(continued)

	Excess deaths, 2020–21	Registered Covid-19 deaths, 2020–21	Registered Covid-19 cases, 2020–21	Vaccination rates, 2020–21	Vaccination rates, 2020–21	Together	Together as SRP indexes
	Standardized	Standardized	Standardized	Standardized	Values reversed	Average	Standardized again
Hungary	5.71	10.00	5.30	4.86	5.14	6.536	7.66
Mexico	10.00	5.90	1.76	0.35	9.65	6.826	8.06
Colombia	5.49	7.00	6.13	0.00	10.00	7.157	8.52
Slovenia	5.49	7.38	8.94	2.85	7.15	7.241	8.64
Slovakia	7.20	7.46	9.36	1.51	8.49	8.129	9.88
Czechia	7.91	9.24	10.00	4.28	5.72	**8.217**	10.00

Note All excess deaths data had been transformed first, to turn them all into positive values, as Norway had a negative excess death rate in that period.
Source Author compilation from OECD (2021).

References

Aspalter, Christian. 2006. Freedom, dehumanization and welfare: An Asian perspective. *Journal of Comparative Social Welfare* 22 (2): 95–114.

Aspalter, Christian. 2021a. *Classifying different types of meta analyses and meta syntheses—Developing methodology in social policy and public policy research.* https://papers.ssrn.com.

Aspalter, Christian. 2021b. *Understanding systemic social problems: Moving beyond the limits of Leibenstein's x-efficiency theory—An essay in theoretical behavioral social policy.* https://papers.ssrn.com.

Aspalter, Christian. 2022a. Super inequality: A general theory of mass poverty. *Social Development Issues* 44 (2): 1–19.

Aspalter, Christian. 2022b. *The declaration of independence from financial and economic oppression and welfare dependency.* https://papers.ssrn.com.

Aspalter, Christian. 2023. *Ten worlds of welfare capitalism: A global data analysis.* Singapore: Springer.

Bourdieu, Pierre. 1973. Cultural reproduction and social reproduction. In: *Knowledge, education, and social change*, ed. R. Brown. London: Tavistock.

Bourdieu, Pierre. 2002. Cultural power. In: *Cultural sociology*, ed. L. Spillman. Oxford: Blackwell.

Brady, David. 2009. *Rich democracies, poor people: How politics explains poverty.* Oxford: Oxford University Press.

Brady, David. 2019. Theories of the causes of poverty. *Annual Review of Sociology* 45: 155–175.

Brady, David, Agnes Blome, and Hanna Kleider. 2016. How politics and institutions shape poverty and inequality. In: *The Oxford handbook of the social science of poverty,* eds. D. Brady and L.M. Burton. Oxford: Oxford University Press.

Burrowes, Robert J. 2020a. *The elite's Covid 19 coup against a terrified humanity: Resisting powerfully.* Global Research, April 13. https://www.globalresearch.ca.

Burrowes, Robert J. 2020b. *Observing elites manipulate our fear: Covid-19, propaganda and knowledge*, March 30. https://www.nationofchange.org.

Cardoso, Fernando H. and Enzo Faletto. 1979. *Dependency and development in Latin America.* Berkeley: University of California Press.

Casas Herrera, Julián Augusto. 2017. Inequality as determinant of the persistence of poverty. In: *Poverty, inequality and policy,* ed. G. Staicu. London: IntechOpen.

Chao, Shiau-Fang and Wan-I Lin. 2023. *Chapter 10*, this volume.

Choi, Jae-Wook. 2022. The rules vs. humanity. *Korea Joong Ang Daily*, January 10, https://koreajoongangdaily.joins.com/2022/01/10/opinion/columns/Covid19-death.

Chomsky, Noam. 1987. *On power and ideology: The Managua lectures.* Boston: South End Press.

Chomsky, Noam. 2002. *Media control: The spectacular achievements of propaganda.* New York: Seven Stories Press.

Ciuffetelli Parker, Darlene and Palmina Conversano. 2021. Narratives of systemic barriers and accessibility: poverty, equity, diversity, inclusion, and the call for a post-pandemic new normal. *Frontiers in Education*, July 15, https://www.frontiersin.org

Collins, Chuck. 2022. *Report: Taxing the world's richest would raise US$2.52 trillion a year.* https://www.fightinequality.org/news/billionaire-pandemic-tax.

Collins, Randall. 1975. *Conflict sociology: Toward an explanatory science.* New York: Academic Press.

Collins, Randall. 1979. *The credential society: An historical sociology of education and stratification.* New York: Academic Press.

Ćović, Ana and Oliver Nikolić. 2021. *The right to freedom of movement during the Covid-19 pandemic.* Institute of Comparative Law. https://eskup.kpu.edu.rs/dar/article/view/280/202.

Crespi, Isabella, Sara Mazzucchelli, and Maria Letizia Bosoni. 2023. *Chapter 12*, this volume.

CSRI, Credit Suisse Research Institute. 2022. *Global wealth databook 2021.* Zürich: Credit Suisse.

DeFina, Robert F., and Lance Hannon. 2009. The impact of mass incarceration on poverty. *Crime & Delinquency* 59 (4): 562–586.

Delvac, Kelly Shea. 2022. Human rights abuses in the enforcement of coronavirus security measures. *The National Law Review* 12(171). https://www.natlawreview.com.

Dias Simões, Fernando. 2022. Covid-19 and International freedom of movement: A stranded human right? *Yale Journal of Health Policy, Law, and Ethics* 20 (2): 362–432.

Dixon, John. 2010. Comparative social welfare: The existential humanist perspective and challenge. *Journal of Comparative Social Welfare* 26 (2–3): 177–187.

EHRC, Equality and Human Rights Commission. 2020. *Covid-19 restrictions and the effect on human rights*, September 22, https://www.equalityhumanrights.com.

ENNHRI, European Network for National Human Rights Institutions. 2022. *A human rights-based approach to Covid-19 economic response and recovery.* ENNHRI: Saint-Gilles/Sint-Gillis.

Eubanks, Virginia. 2018. *Automating inequality: How high-tech tools profile, police, and punish the poor.* New York: St. Martins Press.

Fenner, James. 2020. *Covid rules are destroying our humanity*, October 1, https://www.spiked-online.com/2020/10/01.

FIA, Fight Inequality Alliance. 2021. *Billionaire pandemic tax.* https://www.fightinequality.org/news/billionaire-pandemic-tax.

Foucault, Michel. 1975. *Surveiller et punir: Naissance de la prison.* Paris: Gallimard.

Foucault, Michel. 2009. *Security, territory, population,* ed. M. Senellart. London: Palgrave Macmillan.

Foucault, Michel. 2010. *The government of self and others.* London: Palgrave Macmillan.

Foucault, Michel. 2014. *Wrong-doing and truth-telling: The function of avowal in justice*, eds. F. Brion and B. E. Harcourt. Chicago: University of Chicago Press.

Frank, André G. 1966. The development of underdevelopment. *Monthly Review* 18 (4): 17–31.

Frank, André G. 1991. The underdevelopment of development. *Scandinavian Journal of Development. Alternatives* 10 (3): 5–72.

Gould, Elise. 2014. *Inequality is the main cause of persistent poverty.* Economic Policy Institute. https://www.epi.org/blog/inequality-main-persistent-poverty.

Herman, Edward S. and Noam Chomsky. 2002. *Manufacturing consent: The political economy of the mass media.* New York: Pantheon.

Hopkins, Terence K. and Immanuel Wallerstein. 1980. *Processes of the world system*. Beverly Hills: Sage.
Huang, Jin, Margaret S. Sherraden, and Michael Sherraden. 2021. Toward finance as a public good. In *CSD working paper*, No. 21–03. Center for Social Development, Washington University, https://doi.org/10.7936/p8dd-p256.
Kim, Jinsoo and Christian Aspalter. 2021. Income polarity and the end of social insurance. In: *Financing welfare state systems in Asia*, ed. C. Aspalter. Oxon: Routledge.
Kretchmer, Harry. 2020. *6 ways to protect human rights during lockdown—According to the UN*, May 1. https://www.weforum.org.
Li, Chaoyang, Nazrul Islam, Juan Pablo Gutierrez, Ben Lacey, Ronald L. Moolenaar, and Patricia Richter. 2021a. Diabetes, obesity, hypertension and risk of severe Covid-19: A protocol for systematic review and meta-analysis, *BMJ Open*, 11(11), November 26. https://pubmed.ncbi.nlm.nih.gov/34836901.
Li, Pengfei, Yining Wang, Maikel P. Peppelenbosch, Zhongren Ma, and Qiuwei Pan. 2021b. Systematically comparing Covid-19 with the 2009 influenza pandemic for hospitalized patients. *International Journal of Infectious Diseases* 102: 375–380.
Luhmann, Niklas. 1984. *Soziale Systeme*. Frankfurt a.M.: Suhrkamp.
Luhmann, Niklas. 1998. *Die Gesellschaft der Gesellschaft*. Frankfurt a.M.: Suhrkamp.
Lukes, Steven. 2005. *Power: A radical view*. London: Palgrave Macmillan.
Mohan, Brij. 1985. Paradigms of social welfare policy. In: *New horizons of social policy*, ed. B. Mohan. Cambridge: Schenkman.
Mohan, Brij. 1986. Unraveling comparative social welfare. In: *Toward comparative social welfare*, ed. B. Mohan. Cambridge: Schenkman.
Mohan, Brij. 1987. *Denial of existence: Essays on the human condition*, Springfield: C.C. Thomas.
Mohan, Brij. 1992. *Global development: Post-material values and social praxis*. New York: Praeger.
Mohan, Brij. 1993. *Eclipse of freedom: The world of oppression*. New York: Praeger.
Mohan, Brij. 2007. *Fallacies of development: Crises of human and social development*. New Delhi: Atlantic.
Mohan, Brij. 2011. *Development, poverty of culture, and social policy*. New York: Palgrave Macmillan.
Mohan, Brij. 2012. *Agony and ecstasy: My omnibus*. Bloomington: iUniverse.
Mohan, Brij and Prem Sharma. 1985. On human oppression and social development. *Social Development Issues* 9 (1): 12–24.
Morales, Daniel R. and Sarah N. Ali. 2021. Covid-19 and disparities affecting ethnic minorities. *The Lancet* 397 (10286): 1684–1685.
Murphy, Raymond. 1988. *Social closure: The theory of monopolization and exclusion*. Oxford: Clarendon Press.
Myrdal, Gunnar. 1965. *The political element in the development of economic theory*. Cambridge: Harvard University Press.
NHLBI, National Heart Lund and Blood Institute. 2020. *High blood pressure, obesity, and diabetes common in patients hospitalized with Covid-19*, April 22. https://www.nhlbi.nih.gov/news.
Nietzsche, Friedrich. 1887. *Zur Genealogie der Moral: Eine Streitschrift*, Leipzig: C.G. Naumann.
OECD. 2021. *Health at a glance 2021*. Paris: OECD.
Peisah, Carmelle, Andrew Byrnes, Israel Doron, Michael Dark, and Gerard Quinn. 2020. Advocacy for the human rights of older people in the Covid pandemic and beyond: A call to mental health professionals. *International Psychogeriatrics* 32 (10). https://www.cambridge.org/core/journals/international-psychogeriatrics.
Piketty, Thomas. 2000. Theories of persistent inequality and intergenerational mobility. In: *Handbook of income distribution*, eds. A. B. Atkinson and F. Bourguignon, vol. 1, New York: North Holland.
Piketty, Thomas. 2006. The Kuznets curve yesterday and tomorrow. In: *Understanding poverty*, eds. A. V. Banerjee, R. Benabou and D. Mookherjee. Oxford: Oxford University Press.

Piketty, Thomas. 2014. [2013] *Capital in the twenty-first century*. Cambridge: The Belknap Press of Harvard University Press.
Rabinow, Paul. 2010. *Michel Foucault: The Foucault reader*. New York: Vintage.
Raposo, Vera Lúcia. 2021. Quarantines: Between precaution and necessity: A look at Covid-19. *Public Health Ethics*. doi: 10.1093/phe/phaa037.
Remington, Thomas F. 2023a. *Chapter 3*, this volume.
Remington, Thomas F. 2023b. *Chapter 4*, this volume.
Ritchie, Hannah, Edouard Mathieu, Lucas Rodés-Guirao, Cameron Appel, Charlie Giattino, Esteban Ortiz-Ospina, Joe Hasell, Bobbie Macdonald, Saloni Dattani, and Max Roser. 2022. *Mortality risk of Covid-19*. https://ourworldindata.org/mortality-risk-Covid.
Robinson, Andrew. 2020. *Husband says 'inhumane' Covid hospital rules stopped him seeing wife before she died*. Mirror. https://www.mirror.co.uk/news/uk-news.
Rothschild, Kurt W. 1971. *Power in economics*. Harmondsworth: Penguin.
Sandel, Megan and Jonathan T.M. Reckford. 2020. *Housing is the prescription we need*. UN Habitat, August 11. https://www.habitat.org/stories.
Santos, Broja. 2021. *(Re)Defining freedom: Covid-19*, April 29. https://www.ie.edu/insights.
Scholz, Benjamin. 2022. *Das hässlichste Gesicht der Pandemie*. https://www.freitag.de.
Shimwell, Morgan. 2020. *Coronavirus and compulsory isolation 'pits human rights against public safety*, March 6. https://www.weforum.org.
Shorrocks, Anthony, James Davies, and Rodrigo Lluberas. 2021. *Global wealth report 2021*. Zürich: Credit Suisse.
Tilly, Charles. 1998. *Durable inequality*. Berkeley: University of California Press.
UN, United Nations. 2020a. *Covid-19 pandemic exposes global 'frailties and inequalities:' UN deputy chief*. UN News. https://news.un.org/en/story/2020a/05/1063022.
UN, United Nations. 2020b. *Covid pushes millions more children deeper into poverty, new study finds*. UN News. https://news.un.org/en/story/2020b/09/1072602.
UNICEF. 2022. *The impact of Covid-19 on children's mental health*. https://www.unicef.org/india.
USAID. 2021. *A briefer: Gender inequality causes poverty*. https://banyanglobal.com/wp-content/uploads/2021/03/Gender-Inequality-Causes-Poverty-Briefer.pdf.
Wallerstein, Immanuel. 1979. *The capitalist world economy*. Cambridge: Cambridge University Press.
Weber, Max. 2019. Open and closed relationships. In: *Social stratification*, ed. D. B. Grusky. New York: Routledge.

Part II
Theme Chapters on Social Problems Raised by the Pandemic

Chapter 3
Socio-economic and Geographic Inequality of the Effects of the Pandemic

Thomas F. Remington

Abstract Since late 2021, the US has experienced the highest cumulative rate of deaths from Covid-19-related causes of any developed country in the world. Why this is the case invites serious analysis. The thesis of this chapter is that the high rate of economic inequality in the US—together with the social and geographic inequalities that are closely associated with economic inequality—explains a large part of the difference. A large body of research has demonstrated the very high, and rising, levels of inequality in wealth and income in the US. Not only labor market income inequality, but also post tax-and-transfer income inequality, are higher in the US than in any comparable OECD country. In turn, as a result of the recursive relationship between top-end income growth and wealth accumulation, wealth concentration has risen as well. Wealth inequality in the US is also highest among the countries in the advanced industrial world. The chapter outlines a model of a three-way relationship among socio-economic, health, and spatial inequalities. Each of the links in this triangle is related through a web of recursive relationships in which each element is both a cause and outcome of the other two. Together, moreover, they exert a longer-term effect on public values and attitudes, and the resulting realignment of political forces. The shifting of American policies and institutions away from provision of public goods and services, toward economic policies that favor the accumulation of incomes and wealth at the top and stagnation of economic conditions for the middle and bottom parts of the distribution, and toward ideological polarization and negative partisanship, in turn feed back into the deepening of all three types of inequality. The severe impact of Covid-19 on the US, both in death rates and economic well-being, reflects the confluence of these trends.

Keywords Covid-19 pandemic · Socio-economic inequalities · Health inequalities · Spatial inequalities · American politics

---

T. F. Remington (✉)
Department of Government, Harvard University, Cambridge, USA
e-mail: tremington@fas.harvard.edu

Political Science Department, Emory University, Atlanta, USA

C. Aspalter (ed.), *Covid-19 Pandemic*,
https://doi.org/10.1007/978-981-99-2497-4_3

Introduction

Since late 2021, the United States has experienced the highest cumulative rate of deaths from Covid-19-related causes of any developed country in the world. Why this is the case invites serious analysis. The thesis of this chapter is that the high rate of economic inequality in the United States—and the social and geographic inequalities that are closely associated with economic inequality explains a large part of the difference. A large body of research has demonstrated the very high, and rising, levels of inequality in wealth and income in the United States (see *inter alia* Hacker and Pierson 2020; Saez and Zucman 2014, 2019, 2020; Saez 2019; Boushey 2019; Piketty et al. 2018; Sitaraman 2017; Stiglitz 2013, 2015; Noah 2012; Frank 2009). Not only labor market income inequality, but also post tax-and-transfer income inequality, are higher in the United States than in any comparable OECD country. In turn, as a result of the recursive relationship between top-end income growth and wealth accumulation, wealth concentration has risen as well. Wealth inequality in the United States is also highest among the countries in the advanced industrial world.

The chapter outlines a model of a three-way relationship among socio-economic, health, and spatial inequalities. Each side is related to the other two through a web of reciprocal causal relationships. Their interaction, moreover, has a longer-term effect on public values, attitudes, policies and institutions. The shift away from provision of public goods and services, toward retrenchment and privatization reinforces the accumulation of incomes and wealth at the top and stagnation of economic conditions for the middle and bottom parts of the distribution, and toward ideological polarization and negative partisanship, in turn feed back into the deepening of all three types of inequality.

These trends help explain the particularly severe impact of Covid-19 on the United States. The extremely high death rate from Covid underscores the point that the very high level of deep poverty and its associated disadvantages in the United States left the US, and particularly its poorest and most vulnerable citizens, highly vulnerable to the infection. Research shows that there is a direct relation between socio-economic status and health, whether measured as the number of healthy days people experience in a month or in terms of their overall health status (Case and Deaton 2020; Payne 2017; Marmot 2007). Health levels vary systematically for all ethnic and ethnic categories by income and education. This is true of geographic inequality as well. For example, even controlling for other individual-level factors, people in lower-income counties have worse health (Shaw et al. 2016).

Figure 3.1 offers a simple graphic representation of the three-way relationship among socio-economic inequality, health inequality, and geographic inequality.

It is important to emphasize that economic inequality itself—apart from poverty and its concomitant effects—not only reinforces health inequality, but worsens overall public health and contributes to the maintenance of rising economic inequality. Ample evidence confirms that inequality plays a part in worsening public health, above and beyond the effects that can be directly attributed to low income, poor education, poor housing, and other attributes of poverty (Graham and Pinto

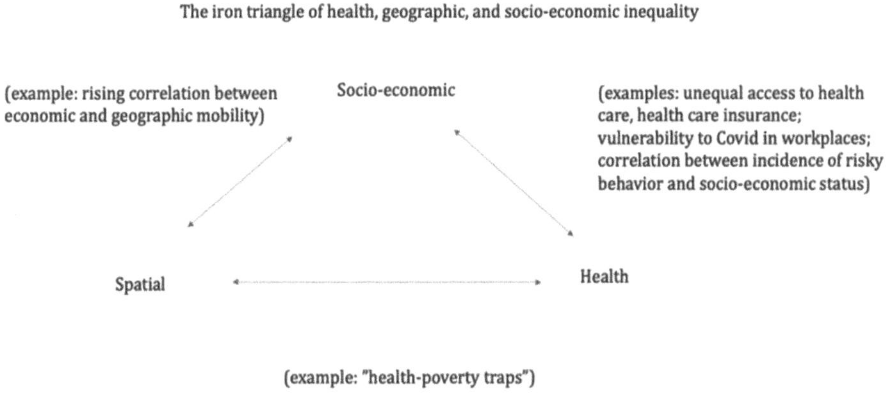

Fig. 3.1 The triangle of health, geographic, and socio-economic inequality

2021; Case and Deaton 2020; Pinker 2018; Payne 2017; Bor et al. 2017; Mankiw 2013; Marmot 2007; Wilkinson and Pickett 2011; Wilkinson 1992).

I will return to this point below. The fact that socio-economic status, spatial location and health are closely interrelated has deepened the impact of the Covid-19 Pandemic, because inequality undermined public health more generally well before the pandemic struck. These factors jointly contributed to the crisis of Covid-related mortality in the United States once the pandemic began in 2020.

The introductory section of the chapter examines each side of the triangle, then addressing their indirect effects on policies, institutions, and public attitudes. First, I will describe the growing overlap between socio-economic inequality and geographic inequality, documenting its effects on health as well as political attitudes and behavior. I will present figures representing the growth of inequality of income and wealth, which has taken a marked upward turn since the late 1970s. Next, I will summarize existing research on the unequal incidence of poor health, and particular Covid mortality, across socio-economic groups, and, third the way inequalities of health and socio-economic condition are increasingly correlated with territorial location (state, county, census zone, even neighborhood). I begin by comparing the United States to other high-income democracies with respect to Covid-related mortality rates and economic inequality. Then I demonstrate the trends in the United States toward rising inequality in incomes and wealth.

In the next section, I will document the reverse relationship between spatial inequalities in economic, social, and political conditions and their effects on American public policy and institutional change. Because of the strongly anti-majoritarian features of the American institutional system, a powerful and motivated coalition of minority interests has allied itself with an extreme wing of the Republican Party to reshape those institutions in such a way as to reinforce the anti-majoritarian features. These shifts include active efforts to redraw legislative district boundaries for state legislatures and the US House of Representatives; to restrict voting access for the groups most likely to vote for Democrats; to appoint to the federal judiciary and

Supreme Court as many Republican-leaning and conservative judges as possible; and to reshape campaign finance law to favor the doctrine that "money equals speech." Meantime, over a similarly long period of time, conservative ascendancy has also resulted in the gutting of administrative bodies and rules that were set up to protect public interests, among them the federal public health system, antitrust law, regulation of the mass media, public education, enforcement of rules regarding public safety and health, social services, the criminal justice system, even the US Census on which so many other policies and institutions rest. The consequence was that the United States deliberately left itself vulnerable to a devastating world-wide pandemic.

This iron triangle has also fed back into the political system by eroding public confidence in government—indeed in science generally—as well as feeding partisan-ideological polarization (cf Abramowitz and McCoy 2019). As polarization has risen, extremism has grown as well, particularly among a right-wing segment that feeds on resentments and grievances around race, immigration, blocked opportunity, and other themes that are readily exploited by right-wing political elites. Reinforced by the segmentation of media eco-systems, this cultural polarization has left a deep gap in behavior during the Covid pandemic, reflected in the wide gap in vaccination rates between Republicans and Democrats, and between rural and urban areas. These gaps then are mirrored in the substantial difference in mortality rates across the same cleavages.

The increasing influence of the alliance of wealthy interests with policymakers has had multiple effects on the economy and society, among them the long and gradual hollowing out of the systems for provision of public health care in the United States as a result of the trends toward the retrenchment of public goods and services, the growing privatization of health care and health care insurance. Rising inequality has also contributed to the increased political polarization and mistrust of authority that have severely hampered the public's willingness to comply with voluntary and mandatory public health protective measures, such as vaccinations, social distancing, and mask-wearing. In the United States, as in many countries, lower levels of trust in government has resulted in lower levels of compliance with policy measures designed to mitigate the effects of the virus's spread (Saville and Thomas 2022; Karlinsky and Kobak 2021; Adamecz-Völgyi and Szabó-Morvai 2021; Bollyky et al. 2022; Szreter and Woolcok 2004).

The United States as Outlier in Both Covid-Related Mortality and Economic Inequality

The Impact of the Pandemic

Why does the US have so high a rate of mortality from Covid, higher than any country comparable in level of income and development? Figure 3.2 illustrates the population-adjusted rate of deaths per million population, according to data from the Johns Hopkins Coronavirus Resource Center, as of May 1, 2022.

The US death rate from Covid-19-related causes, as of the beginning of May 2022, exceeded 3% of the population, the highest in the developed world. Although the overall case rate per million population in the United States was lower than in many comparable countries, its death rate was higher. The reasons for this are actively debated. Moreover, the rate of deaths attributed to Covid almost certainly understates actual Covid-related mortality. An authoritative recent estimate based on analysis of mortality rates at the county level suggests that the actual rate of excess deaths during the pandemic is 22% higher than the rate officially recorded as Covid-related (Paglino et al. 2022). The highest levels of under-reporting occurred in the Southeast, Southwest, and rural areas generally.

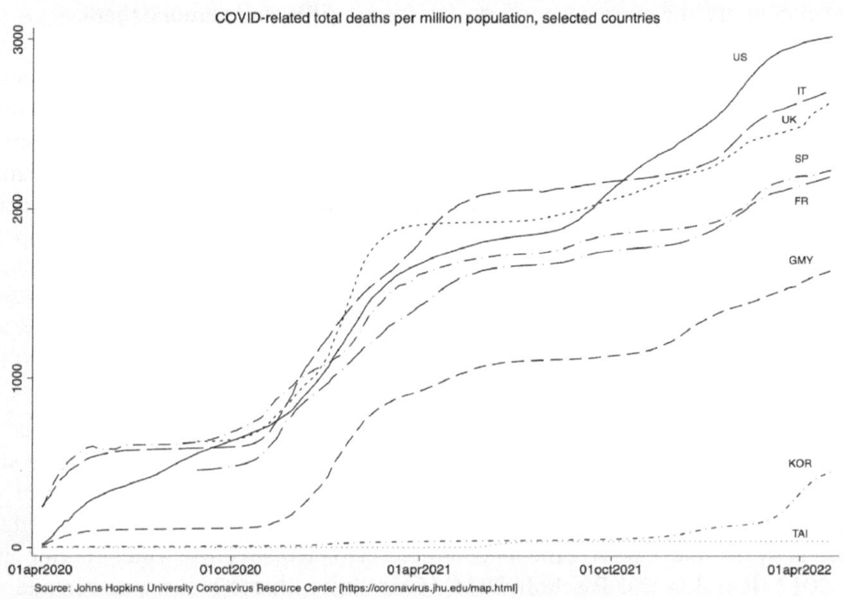

Fig. 3.2 Covid-related deaths per million population, US and comparison countries, April 1, 2020–May 1, 2022

Moreover, recent calculations by a team of researchers at the University of Washington's Institute for Health Metrics and Evaluation indicate that during the global Covid pandemic of 2020 and 2021, the world experienced a 20% higher rate of deaths than would have occurred otherwise and that around two-thirds of these were improperly attributed to other causes than Covid. The United States again ranks among the highest in the developed world in excess mortality during this period, although underreporting was not as widespread as in a few of them, including Spain and Italy. The US rate of pandemic-era excess deaths was about 179 per 100,000 population, although only 130.6 per 100,000 were attributed to Covid. Again, American states varied widely in their rates of excess mortality, from a high of almost 330 per 100,000 in Mississippi to as few as 11 in Hawaii.[2]

Geographic Sorting

The iron triangle model rests on the observation that economic and social inequality, geographic inequality and health inequality are closely interrelated. As I shall show, the US population has become increasingly sorted into territorial units that are increasingly homogeneous within and heterogenous between with respect to income and social characteristics (including partisan ideological tendencies). Crucially, the more micro the spatial unit in question, the greater its homogeneity, and, correspondingly, the more pronounced are spatial differences among them.

Much public attention has been attracted by the differentiation of the country into "Red" (Republican-leaning) and "Blue" (or Democrate-leaning) states. However, states are much more heterogeneous socially and politically than are counties, and counties more heterogeneous than census tracts. A useful index of socio-economic conditions is life expectancy at birth, which reflects a number of social determinants of health. Inequality in rates of life expectancy at birth therefore indicate inequality in multiple social and economic conditions, including economic well-being and opportunity and access to health care. Life expectancy at birth as of 2014 varied by 3.6 years across states, from a high of 80.9 in California and Hawaii, to a low of 77.3 in West Virginia. However, across counties, life expectancy varies from a maximum of 86.83 to a minimum of 66.81, and at the level of census tract, average life expectancy at birth varies by 40 years. In the impoverished coal region of Logan County, WV, it is 56.3, whereas in the Research Triangle region of North Carolina it is 97.5.[3] As differences in the levels of income, education and opportunity widen across neighborhoods, their effects become mutually reinforcing, systematically locking in differences in advantage and disadvantage. More generally, as neighborhoods become more homogeneous by income and race, the inequalities between them grow wider (Taylor and Fry 2012; Reardon and Bischoff 2011). Counties with the highest percentage of people living in the same county where they were born are also those with the worst levels health and well-being (Graham and Pinto 2021).

The Hamilton Project's Vitality index compiles several measures of social and health well-being at the county level.[4] Figure 3.3 presents a scatter plot showing the

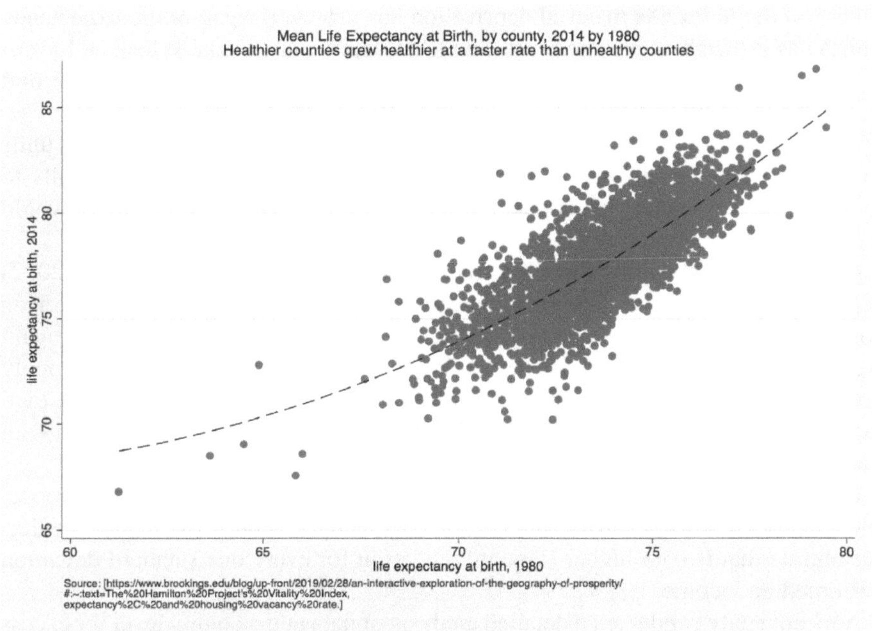

Fig. 3.3 Life expectancy at birth, 2014, by life expectancy, 1980, by county

widening of inequality across counties in life expectancy at birth. The latest year for which data was available was 2014. If we had a full dataset for 2022, it would reflect still greater inequality. The county with the highest mean life expectancy at birth, Mono County, California, recorded a mean of 103.3 years, while the county with the lowest life expectancy, McDowell County, West Virginia, recoded a life expectancy of 67.7—a gap of 35.6 years.[5] Even as the median life expectancy rose, so too did the spread across counties, as reflected in the wider interquartile range.

The curvilinear functional form of the relationship indicates that while most counties experienced improvements in life expectancy rates, counties that had higher rates in 1980 tended to gain ground at a faster rate (cf Fig. 3.3).

The growing confluence of geographic with socio-economic inequality means that advantage is concentrated in some counties, while disadvantage is concentrated in others; fewer and fewer counties are characterized as mixed- or middle-income (Reardon and Bischoff 2011). The same phenomenon can be observed at the higher scale of states and the still more fine-grained scale of census tract. The larger the regional unit we choose, the lower that spatial inequality appears to be, because the more granular the unit, the greater the homogeneity of life circumstances within it. If we look at a broad index of overall deprivation for each county (using criteria of education levels, poverty, income, unemployment, wealth, housing, and others), we find that differences are widening over time rather than narrowing (Singh and Siahpush 2006). The most-deprived decile of counties was about twice as high as the highest on the index. As material deprivation has grown, the gap in life expectancy at birth has grown between the most- and least-deprived counties. When we look at life expectancy at birth and other indicators of well-being by census tract, we find even wider disparities.

The overlapping gaps in life expectancy across social groups and geographic units closely correspond to disparities in death rates from Covid, and more generally to the rate of excess deaths (that is, the number of deaths above the number that would be expected) during the pandemic.

County-by-county, differences in Covid-related death rates (as of January 9, 2022) are strongly associated with the percent of the population that is African American (positive and significant correlation), the percent of the population that is rural (again positive and significant), and with median household incomes (negative and strongly significant). Table 3.1 shows the results of a regression of total deaths from Covid per thousand population on these three variables. Together, they are associated with over 20% of the variation.

Figure 3.4 shows the death rate predicted from this model against median household income. If we standardize the coefficients using Z scores, the model predicts a death rate that is 0.43 higher standard deviation for every one standard deviation lower median income.

A recent study conducted a detailed analysis of data at the county level for excess deaths in 2020 and 2021, comparing them to the average rate of deaths for prior years. The researchers estimate that over those two years, there were about 22% more deaths than were attributed to the Covid-19 virus (Paglino et al. 2022).

Analyzing their data for 2021, about 18% of the variation in rates of excess deaths across counties, adjusting for population, can be accounted for by a small number of social and economic factors, as Table 3.2 indicates.

Table 3.1 County-level variation in Covid mortality

Registered Covid deaths per thousand	Coefficient	Std. error	t	Prob	95% Confidence interval	
Share African American	0.6755764	0.1663172	4.06	0.000	0.35	1.00
Median household income, 2017	−0.0000473	1.99E-06	−23.76	0.000	0.00	0.00
Rural share	0.0022848	0.0008933	2.56	0.011	0.00	0.00
Constant	5.289601	0.1404691	37.66	0.000	5.01	5.57

No of obs: 3102
F (3, 3098): 337
Prob > F: 0.0000
r-sq: 0.2265
Root MSE: 1.2508

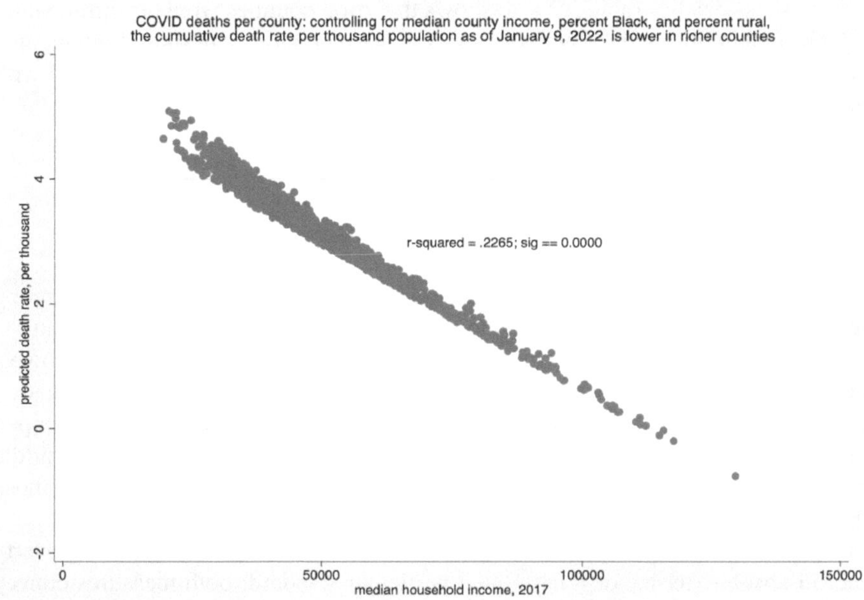

Fig. 3.4 Regression of predicted death rate by median household income, county level

Table 3.2 Excess mortality per thousand population, 2021, county level

Method: OLS					
Variable	Coef	Std. error	t	P > t	Confid. interval
Top decile income share	0.05	0.02	2.58	0.01	0.01–0.08
Income tercile	0.33	0.32	1.04	0.3	−0.30–0.97
Interaction (top decile share * income tercile)	−0.02	0.01	−2.59	0.01	−0.030–0.00
Rural % of population	0.00	0.00	3.31	0.001	0.00–0.01
Poverty rate, 2017	0.07	0.01	7.01	0.000	0.05–0.09
Constant	−0.43				

F(5, 3112) = 141.13
Prob > F = 0.0000
R-squared = 0.1789
Root MSE = 1.8567
No. of observations = 3118

The negative value on the interaction term indicates that the higher the median income of the county, the less that top-end income concentration in it contributes to explaining its rate of excess mortality. However, among counties in the lowest third by income, higher levels of top-decile income concentration are associated with *higher* rates of excess deaths. Table 3.2 also shows that rural counties were hit significantly harder by deaths during the pandemic, as were poorer counties. In short, high income inequality, poverty, and the rural character of the location all were associated with greater excess death.

Economic Inequality

As with the impact of the pandemic, so too the United States is an outlier among developed countries in its level of economic inequality. Economic inequality consists of the combined effects of trends in the distribution of income and wealth at the lowest end of the distribution, as well as in the middle and at the top. As an accounting matter, the reason economic inequality in the US is so high compared to other developed countries is that incomes at the low end are low and stagnating, incomes in the middle are stagnating and there are fewer people in the middle of the distribution, and those at the top are receiving higher and higher incomes.

Consider the relationship between poverty and health. We can define poverty either in absolute terms, or relative to a particular standard; both measures convey useful information. Relative poverty reflects not just whether a household can afford basic necessities, but also whether it can live in dignity and fully participate in society. Moreover, because people evaluate their own status by comparing their current and anticipated future conditions to their own past conditions as well as to the conditions of others in society, relative poverty influences people's attitudes and behavior (Payne 2017; Runciman 1966). Cross-national comparisons of levels of poverty depend on how we define poverty. For example, relative poverty in Germany is high whereas absolute poverty is low. But Germany takes as its benchmark of relative deprivation a family income below 60% of the median, a comparatively high standard. By that measure, 16.5% of households faced poverty in 2016. If the line is lowered to half the median, the share was 9.7%. By the more stringent absolute standard of "severe material deprivation," 3.7% of households were in poverty. In contrast, the number of households in the United States with incomes below the poverty line was 10.5% in 2019, down from 14.8% in 2014. However, the poverty line is low, less than a third of median household income for a 3-person family.[6] Low incomes in the US are therefore very low, just as high incomes are extremely high. Only by analyzing inequality according to multiple standards can we gain a proper appreciation of the actual extent of inequality in the US.[7]

More useful in measuring in equality for our purposes therefore is the data on income shares claimed by different segments—deciles, percentiles and so on—of the population.

Figures 3.5, 3.6 and 3.7 illustrate this point graphically by comparing the US with other members of OECD. Only four Latin American countries have higher top 1% income shares than the US (2021 WID data for pretax income shares) and only the same four and Turkey have higher wealth concentration. Almost 20% of income, and a third of wealth, is controlled by the top 1% of individuals in the US.

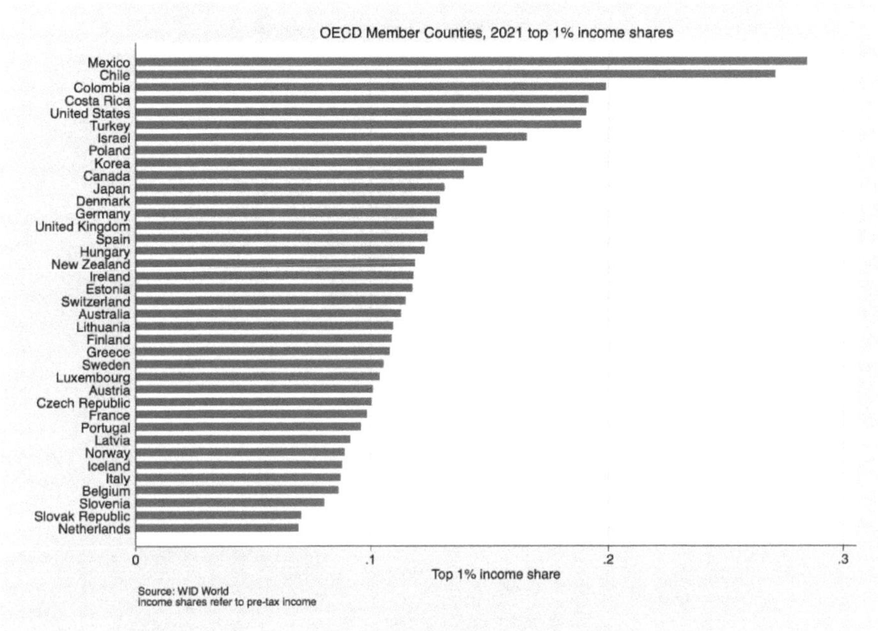

Fig. 3.5 Top 1% income shares, OECD member countries, 2021

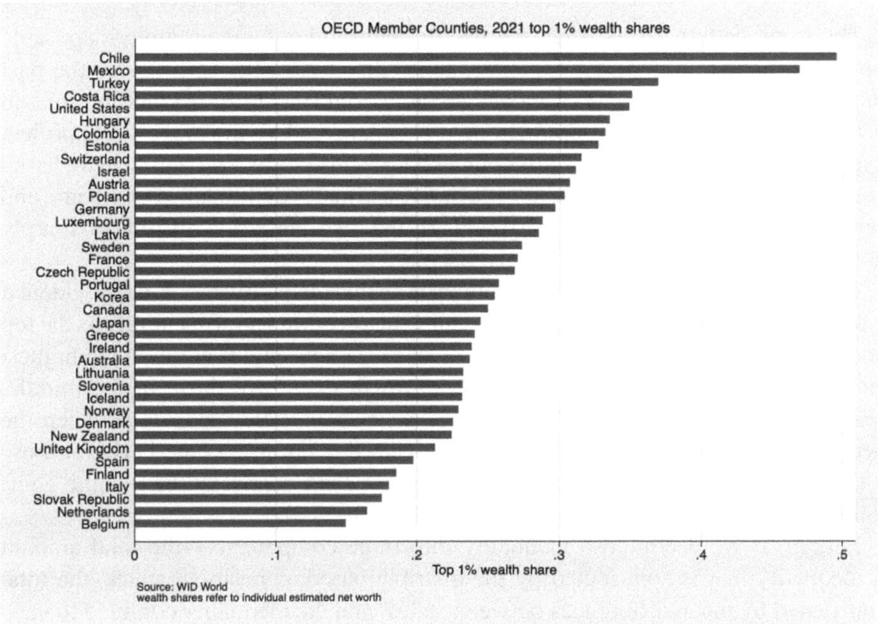

Fig. 3.6 Top 1% wealth shares, OECD member countries, 2021

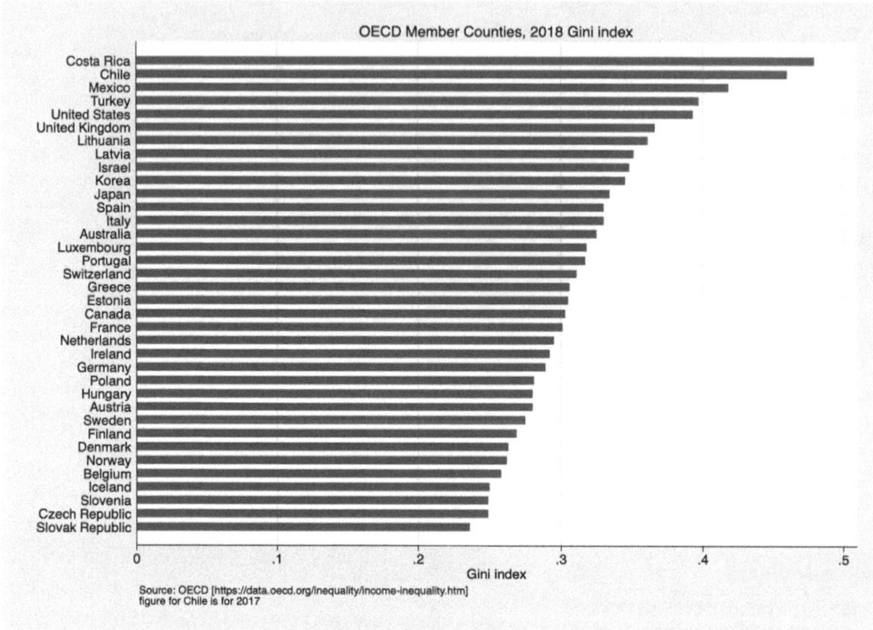

Fig. 3.7 Gini index, 2018, OECD countries

The same pattern holds when we use the Gini index for household disposable (post-tax) income. Moreover, economic inequality has risen sharply over the past four decades, as a great deal of recent research confirms. Both detailed household income survey data and the administrative data analyzed by the WID world project associated with Thomas Piketty, Emmanuel Saez, and Gabriel Zucman (which, based on tax and other administrative data, can derive estimates of the shares of income and wealth accruing to the top-most segments of the distribution) confirm how sharply income and wealth concentration have risen.

Based on US Census data, we can demonstrate that inequality has steadily widened in the post-World War II period. This widening has occurred almost entirely as the top income group (as measured by the income of those households at the in the highest percentiles) has seen much faster income growth than have those in the middle. Census data show that whereas the difference in household incomes between the median and 20th percentiles has hardly budged, the gap in income between those at the 95th percentile and the median has soared, with nearly all the income gains going to those at the 5th and higher percentiles (Fig. 3.8).

Further, if we decompose inequality into three components—the total amount of inequality that is contributed by the distribution common to all states, the total contributed by mean differences between states, and the inequality confined to each state individually—we see a steady rise in the inequality common to all. That is, what had been larger differences across the states in average incomes, is being replaced

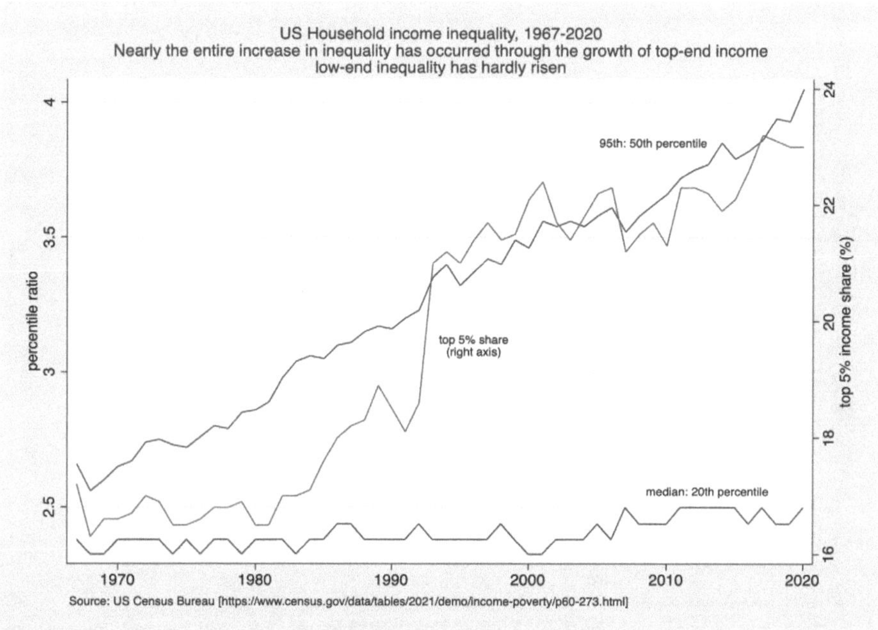

Fig. 3.8 US: trends in growth of income, 1967–2020

by similar gaps between rich and poor in all states. This is a process similar to the conclusions that Branko Milanovic (2016) draws about trends in global inequality—that after a period in which industrialization initially widened, then narrowed income differences across countries, we are now moving to a condition more akin to the pre-industrial era, in which the rich and poor in each country were divided by similar gulfs.

The same trend is demonstrated still more starkly when we examine the rise in income and wealth accumulation at the top and the decline in the income and wealth shares of those at the bottom. These trends hold whether we examine pre- or post-tax income distribution (Fig. 3.9).

Income concentration has risen at a successively faster rate the higher one goes on the distribution, consistent with the Pareto nature of top-end economic inequality.

In fact, post-tax income for the top 1% has risen faster than pre-tax income because the US tax system has grown less and less progressive over time. In fact, considering the total share of income paid in taxes—including federal and state income taxes, payroll taxes, and excise taxes—at the very top of the distribution, the US tax system is regressive (Fig. 3.10).

As income inequality has risen, therefore, the relative share of the taxes paid by those at the top has fallen, whereas the share paid by those in the middle and at the bottom is higher today than it was several decades ago. This indicates that the political influence of the rich relative to the poor has increased. That influence has,

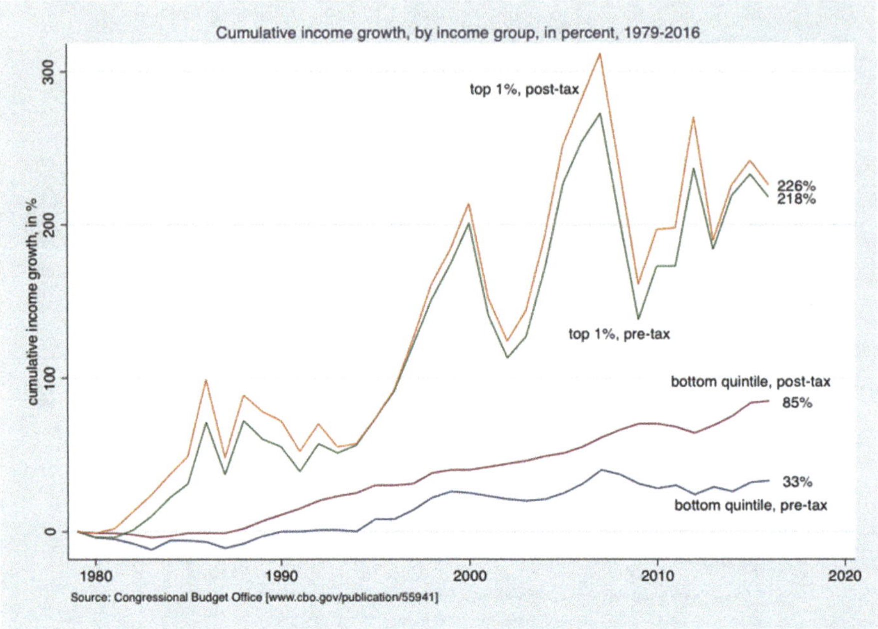

Fig. 3.9 Cumulative income growth, by income group, 1979–2016

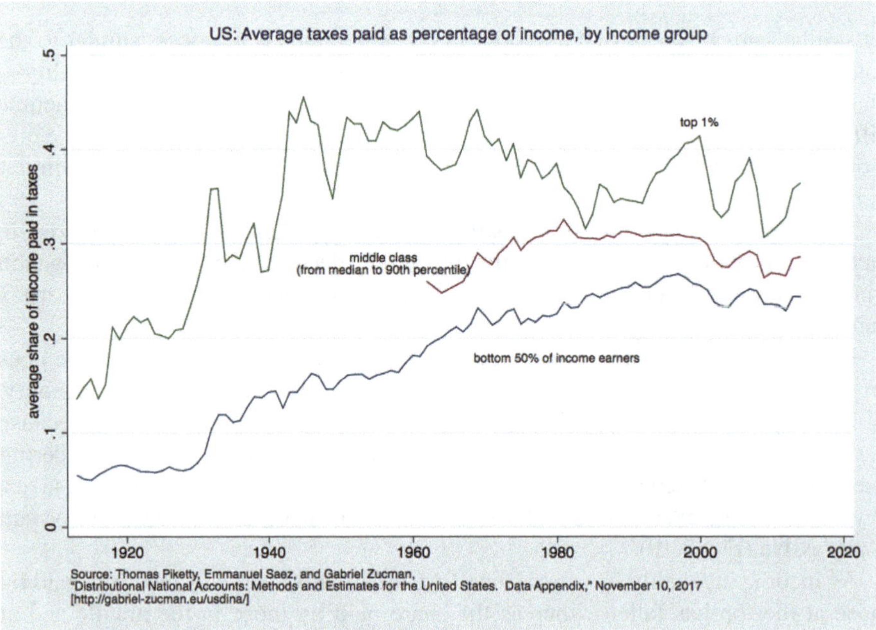

Fig. 3.10 US: taxes paid as share of income, by percentile, 1914–2018

among other things, led to policies tending to reduce public spending on public goods and services such as public education, public health, public safety, and environmental safety. The result is to exacerbate socio-economic, geographic, and health inequalities still further. In the next sections I will explore this recursive relationship in greater detail.

The Pandemic's Differential Effects on Workers

Not only did existing disparities in levels of vulnerability to the pandemic exacerbate inequalities in mortality rates, it also affected different parts of the labor market differentially. The most vulnerable workers experienced faced the deepest setbacks in employment, health and education. The workers most likely to lose jobs as a result of business closings and lay-offs were those in the lowest-wage segments of the job market, particularly in jobs requiring high personal interaction with customers or dependent on the leisure and hospitality sector.

In 2020, as the virus spread in 2020, almost four times as many jobs lost due to Covid were in low-wage positions as in high-paying jobs (CBPP 2021). Many more women lost their jobs than did men. At the outset of the pandemic, more women held jobs than did men, but as of a year later, one million more women than men had lost their jobs (Ruiz 2021). Moreover, women were disproportionately affected by the closing of schools and child-care facilities, forcing many to quit jobs and stay home with children (Alon et al. 2020; Karageorge 2020). Low-wage and high-wage workers, and women and men, also experienced recovery unequally. Most of those working in professional and business services returned to work relatively soon, whereas workers on the front lines of retail trade, and in the healthcare services, leisure and hospitality industries, have seen deep and often permanent employment losses (BLS 2021). By May 2022, unemployment had fallen below its January 2020 level for all groups except African Americans. Figure 3.11 demonstrates the disparity:

A telling indicator of how the pandemic has affected the workforce is the labor force participation rate, defined as the share of the working-age, non-institutionalized, civilian population that is employed or unemployed but seeking work. Labor force participation in the United States is low compared to other high-income economies, and fell significantly from the end of the 1990s until a tightening labor market began pushing wages higher starting in 2016. Using a different methodology, the US Bureau of Labor Statistics reports much lower figures for the United States. According to the BLS, as workers dropped out of the labor force during the pandemic, the rate fell from the already low rate of 63.4 to 61.4%, and still more for African Americans (62.4–60%) (BLS 2021).

According to the March 2022 Bureau of Labor Statistics report, the labor force participation rate in March 2022, at 62.4%, was lower by a full percentage point than the rate two years previously (BLS 2022). Employment recovered differently in different sectors. Whereas the professional and business services industry reached a higher employment level by spring 2022 than spring 2020, total employment in

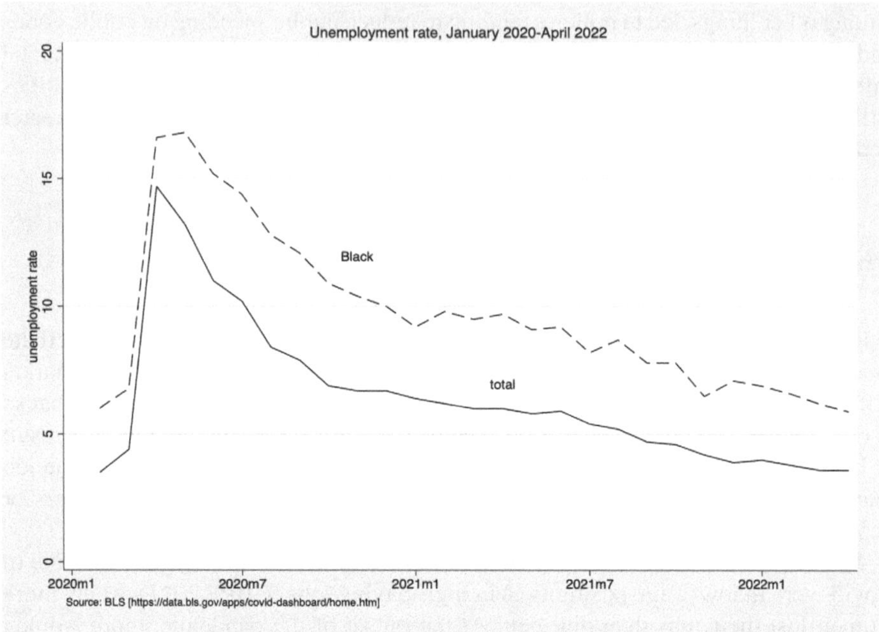

Fig. 3.11 Total unemployment rate, whole civilian labor force and African Americans

leisure and hospitality—with its high concentration of low-wage jobs—remained lower than in 2020 by 1.5 million jobs.

Employment in construction had recovered to its 2020 level, while manufacturing employment was lower. As analysts of the effects of the pandemic on the labor market have made clear, the pandemic tended to accelerate trends toward declining employment in several low-wage job sectors while reinforcing the trend toward higher employment shares in more skill-intensive sectors (Bahar 2020).

The acute shock of the pandemic on employment largely reinforced a longer-term trend toward the hollowing-out of the labor force (that is, the decline in the share of middle-wage-paying jobs) and the increasing share of high-wage jobs and some types of low-wage jobs. This trend has been accompanied by the tendency for the highest-paying jobs to see the highest increases in wages. This trend can be illustrated by Fig. 3.12, using the detailed wage panel data from the Atlanta branch of the Federal Reserve.

Although the largest factor explaining the declining labor force participation rate in recent decades is population aging, the fact that young people—and particularly young men—in their prime working years have been exiting the workforce is a symptom of larger problems in the labor market. Fewer and fewer of the jobs available to low-education workers pay a living wage. As geographic mobility has declined, especially for low-wage workers, more workers are simply dropping out of the labor force altogether (Abraham and Kearney 2018; Krueger 2017).

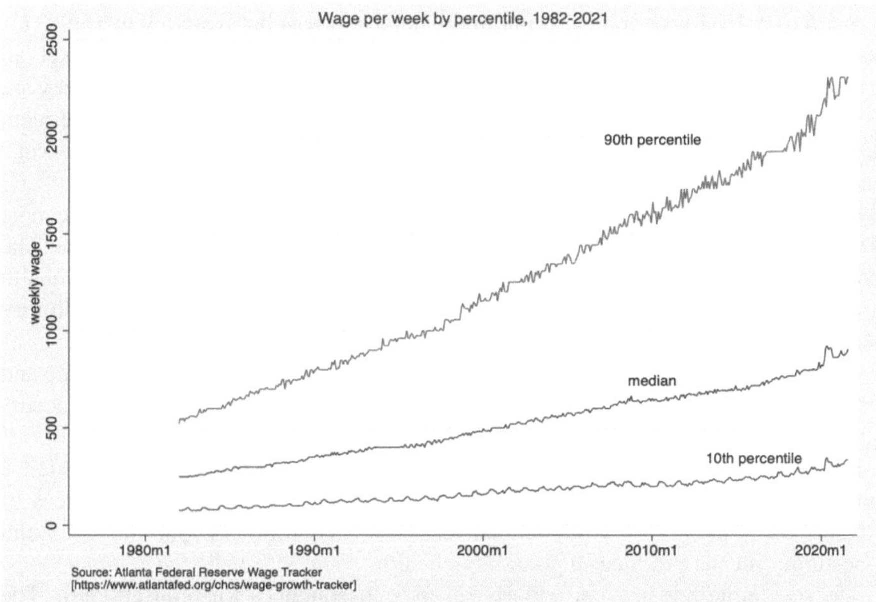

Fig. 3.12 Wage growth by wage level, 1982–2021

This trend suggests also the rise in social anomie and disengagement reflected in rising rates of drug abuse and "deaths of despair," which I will discuss in a separate chapter (Case and Deaton 2021). Here it suffices to point out the association between the loss of employment and employment opportunity and socio-psychic stress, which is evident from the geographic and demographic distribution of deaths from suicide, alcohol abuse, and opioid overdoses, which have been highest among Caucasian American males in the regions hardest hit by the loss of decent-paying jobs.

Low-wage workers compose a very large share of the country's workforce—44% as of January 2020—and have been much more severely affected by the pandemic than higher-earning workers.[8] Lay-offs threaten their security in several ways, including the loss of housing and of health care insurance (Garfield et al. 2020). Even before the pandemic about a quarter of those living in rental housing were paying more than half their gross monthly income on housing rent. By January 2021, about 20% of all renters had fallen behind on their rent payments. 40% of children in renter households faced difficulty with food, housing, or both (Dougherty 2021; CBPP 2021).

Thirty million people work in the retail and hospitality fields, almost 20% of the total US labor force; the great majority of those people work at wage levels below the median wage (77% in retail, 93% in hospitality). These are the most vulnerable jobs: employment is dropping; wages are low; health insurance coverage is sparse; and the Covid-19 pandemic is causing heavy job losses. Whereas the unemployment rate rose from January 2020 to January 2021 from 4 to 6% for all workers, it rose from 2.5 to 3.4% for people working in financial services but from 5.9 to 15.9% for those in leisure and hospitality (BLS 2021). Low wage workers are the least likely to be able to switch to online work; their educational levels tend to be low; and they are disproportionately likely to be female, African American and Hispanic American. The Covid crisis therefore is dealing a severe, multi-faceted blow to the low-wage segment of the workforce.

Low-wage workers are not only the most likely to be laid off, they are also the most likely to lose employment-based health insurance or to lack it in the first place. The pandemic has laid bare the basic fact that the US employment-based system of health care insurance is expensive, inefficient, and highly skewed in quality and accessibility (Metzl et al. 2020). Those who are most exposed to the economic and social stresses of stagnant or falling wages, precarious employment, and overstretched income and health insurance social insurance systems have been the likeliest to lose what access to health care they had.

For industries that were already losing jobs, the pandemic has accelerated a painful transition and intensified the harsh social and economic consequences of high and rising inequality. High inequality in the distribution of economic and social opportunity means produces a gradient in health.

The pandemic has had particularly severe consequences for poor children. The fact that we rely on schools to provide basic food (more than 20 million American children rely on school breakfast or lunch (Sharfstein and Morphew 2020). and nursing services means that closing schools has cost millions of children access to school nurses and nutrition. It has also severely hampered learning. Research on learning losses associated with the switch by schools to remote instruction were more concentrated among the most socially disadvantaged schoolchildren (Goldhaber et al. 2022). Not only were high-poverty-schools more likely to turn to remote instruction, their pupils experienced 50% more learning loss in math than did children in low-poverty schools. Moreover, among high-poverty schools, it was those predominantly attended by African American and Hispanic American pupils that were the most likely to close.

Summing up, the impact of the pandemic has varied systematically by population group, industry, and geography (Bahar 2020).People living in densely populated areas, and particularly in multi-person, multi-generation households or congregant living facilities, are at greater risk for becoming infected and spreading infection more widely. People working in jobs requiring a high, prolonged, and intensive level of face-to-face contact, such as assembly line manufacturing, food processing, retail sales, and personal care services, have likewise been at higher risk. Groups that have been systematically disadvantaged in access to good housing, health care, education, and job opportunities—particularly minority and immigrant groups–are at greater risk from the illness due to higher underlying rates of hypertension, heart disease, diabetes, poor nutrition, and other chronic conditions (Metzl et al. 2020; Owen et al. 2020). Where these risk factors linked to geography, industry, and demography overlap, clusters of illness develop and spread at especially high rates.

Political Polarization

Socio-economic and geographic inequality not only has a direct and deleterious effect on public health, including vulnerability to the pandemic, it also has more subtle, roundabout effects as it erodes public support for public goods provision, trust in government and in science; even acceptance of a common baseline of knowledge about society has eroded due to polarization. Socio-economic inequality has long been deeply interwoven with the American history of ethnic injustice, from slavery, through Jim Crow, residential segregation in major cities, the system of criminal justice and incarceration, and ethnic hostility on the part of Caucasian Americans. Socio-economic inequality is connected as well to many other forms of difference in society in addition to race, including ethnic divisions as they overlap with labor market opportunity, differences between women and men in income and opportunity, differences across states, counties, cities and neighborhoods, differences across educational levels, between immigrant and native-born populations, and in levels of health and well-being. These aspects of inequality have become more mutually reinforcing with time, and, together, feed the trend toward growing political polarization. The deepening tensions over the redistributive implications of democracy contribute to the lock-in of policies that shift the risks and burdens of opportunity from public to private responsibility. As a result, inequality of access to education and health—traditional channels of mobility in American society—has widened.

Because ethnic identity, always a salient dimension in American politics, has again assumed a central role as a signifier of social status, the social identity of Caucasian Americans as Caucasian Americans has gained renewed importance in defining group lines. It has merged with a broadly anti-redistributive economic agenda. Trump skillfully exploited status anxieties among Caucasian American voters on issues loaded with symbolic significance for cultural and ethnic identity—immigration, trade, and ethnicity.[9] The ethnic identity aspects of the rightwing populism movement then join with unwillingness to levy taxes and spend money for the provision of public goods in support of the privatization of public goods—even when, as Heather McGhee has pointed out, lower income Caucasian Americans also suffer. The merger of the ethnic and cultural identity lines with a broad if inconsistent antagonism to taxes then undermines public support for taxing and spending on public goods and wider insurance pools. The harder it is for us to accept those we see as being above and below us as being like us, the less likely we are to support broader spending on public education, public health, even public sanitation, let alone support for expanded social insurance programs, a higher minimum wage, or anti-poverty programs (Sandel 2020; Trounstine 2018; Alesina and Glaeser 2004; Alesina et al. 2001; Easterly 2001). As a result, those channels that equalize opportunity and foster mobility become clogged. The quality of schools, health care, public amenities, and public safety differs more and more sharply across neighborhoods and regions. The smaller the share of middle-class neighborhoods, the more the inequality gap reproduces itself across generations. Mobility across income levels and geographic units is lowest where incomes are lowest, separating enclaves of disadvantage from areas of growth and opportunity (Graham and Pinto 2021).

Therefore, inequality contributes to political polarization through both direct and indirect channels. It concentrates political resources into ideologically-oriented organizations, such as right-wing think tanks, media outlets, law schools and universities; it funnels political money into lobbying and campaign finance. It facilitates the recruitment of loyalists into the executive bureaucracy and judiciary. It manipulates rules of electoral representation in such a way as to over-represent the privileged. The effort to privatize formerly public goods, such as education and the media, is helping to sort the public into sharply opposed partisan-ideological camps living in different social and geographic enclaves.[10] In turn, this social and spatial sorting has reduced the sense of common purpose or a shared political community. It has intensified the long-standing ethnic division in the country. As it further widens the gaps between the life experiences and opportunities of rich from poor, driving people of different socio-economic class into separate worlds, it also undermines notions of fairness as meaning equality of opportunity for people different from oneself. Those who see themselves as doing well tend to see the system as fair, whereas those who are not doing well tend to blame others—the undeserving poor, or immigrants, or elites, or government. Conservative activists are skillful at invoking themes that activate responses of resentment against extending equality of political rights to others, such as the threat of "socialism" and fear of redistribution (MacWilliams 2016; Hetherington and Weiler, 2009). By privatizing public goods and depriving the disadvantaged of opportunities to publicly-provided health care, education, and social protection, conservatives can point to the actual experience people have with dysfunctional public services to back up their claims that government is the problem, not the solution.[11] Attacks on government as intrusive, on the notion of the common good as socialism, feed the mistrust and polarization that are poisoning our public life.

The consolidation of the alliance of those with great wealth and populist impulses built on resentment and relative deprivation—the plutocratic-populist alliance, as Hacker and Pierson (2020) put it—follows a path dependent dynamic. The drive to ensure that policy gains are irreversible leads to a continuous widening of the scope of strategy as its leaders work systematically to deprive potential opponents of political resources, among them voting rights, access to public goods, and even belief in science and reason. At the same time, each generation of leaders must fortify their flanks against threats from the right, driving the movement ever further to the extremes as insufficiently moderate figures are pushed aside by more radical figures who outbid their predecessors by appealing to tribal solidarity.

These conclusions from recent political science research help explain the Trump Administration's response to the Covid pandemic. Trump refused to permit the government's public health organizations to organize a concerted effort to reduce the spread of the virus. Some judges Trump appointed to the federal bench actively impeded federal and state efforts to enact masking mandates. For example, in April 2022, a Trump-appointed judge (who had been rated as unfit for appointment by the American Bar Association) struck down a CDC mandate.[12] The Trump Administration dropped two to three million people from health insurance coverage and politicized bodies such as the CDC and FDA. Trump's policies resulted in some 188,000 deaths in 2020 alone, based on calculations by a team of public health specialists who estimated what the US mortality rate would have been had the US experience death rates equivalent to those of Canada, France, Germany, Italy, Japan, and the UK (Woolhandler et al. 2021).

Summing Up

The overlapping dimensions of inequality—socio-economic, health, and spatial—worsened the impact of Covid on mortality in the United States. This was through both direct channels—the unequal vulnerability to the pandemic's effects across social groups and territorial locations—and indirect pathways. These included the longer-term effect of inequality on political polarization, and, through it, to the progressive abandonment of a governmental commitment to the public good. Decades of eroding provision of public health protection, public education, public safety, and environmental health, left the country poorly equipped to fight the pandemic. Moreover, the pandemic exacerbated political polarization, as politicians took advantage of popular fears and resentments to reinforce their policy agendas. The result of the confluence of these trends has been to leave the United States with the highest death rate from Covid of any developed country in the world.

Notes

1. Examples of those who argue for focusing on poverty *instead* of inequality include Gregory Mankiw and Steven Pinker. However, public health experts such as Richard Wilkinson and Kate Pickett, Michael Marmot, Keith Payne, Anne Case and Angus Deaton demonstrate consequences of socio-economic differences for both aggregate-level and individual-level health outcomes. Moreover, people who face "relative deprivation" are more likely to engage in behavior that in turn contributes to lower economic opportunity and worse health. Therefore, poverty and poor health form "health-poverty traps" that are concentrated in particular places, such as those that have suffered serious consequences from outsourcing and automation of jobs; cf Bor et al. (2017), I discuss this point further below.
2. Interestingly, in several countries, including Iceland, and in Washington DC, the overall death rate was lower than would have been expected. This may be due to patterns of social behavior (masking and social distancing) that reduced total mortality compared to normal years; see Lancet (2022). I calculated the

figures from data compiled by the Institute for Health Metrics and Evaluation, University of Washington; https://ghdx.healthdata.org.

3. State-level figures for 2019; county and census tract level figures are from 2014, the most recent year available. See CDC, Life Expectancy at Birth for US States and Census Tracts, 2010–2015, https://www.cdc.gov/nchs/data-visualization/life-expectancy.
4. Data from https://www.brookings.edu/blog/up-front/2019/02/28.
5. Data from the County Health Rankings and Roadmaps at the University of Wisconsin Population Health Institute, https://www.countyhealthrankings.org.
6. US Census Bureau figures, see Jessica Semega et al. (2020).
7. Note that using the Gini index to measure aggregate income inequality masks a good deal of essential information. Mathematically, it assigns too much weight to gaps in the middle of the distribution and too little to the wide differentials at the bottom and top. In addition, Gini indexes are usually derived from household surveys, which yield underestimates of total inequality. This is, first of all, because since there are relatively few extremely rich households, they are less likely to fall into a survey sample of households. Second, their incomes are subjected to top-coding, which means that the census agency records all households above a particular income threshold as receiving the same maximum income. Therefore, we do not know the distribution of incomes above that threshold. Third, top-end households are the most likely to understate or conceal their actual incomes, both to the surveyors and to the tax authorities, see Atkinson et al. (2011), Osberg (2018), Guyton et al. (2021), Johns and Slemrod (2010).
8. Low-wage workers are defined as those earning less than 2/3 the median hourly wage for full-time, full-year male workers, adjusted for local cost of living. See Escobari et al. (2019).
9. A considerable amount of recent political science research has confirmed the importance of these valence issues for Trump's support, with economic issues of far lower significance. See Reny et al. (2019), Mutz (2018), Abramowitz and McCoy (2019), Green and McElwee (2019).
10. Social identification, with strong emotional and moral content, is driving political polarization more than rational calculation of self-interest. See Mason (2018).
11. A good example is the strong class cleavage dividing Americans over their willingness to be vaccinated against Covid-19. Much more than race or income, educational level is the principal correlate of vaccination resistance. Mistrust of government drives much of the unwillingness to being vaccinated among those with lower educational attainment. A delivery truck driver commented in an interview that "When you're in a high tax bracket, the government protects you. So why wouldn't you trust a government that protects you?" Another women observed of an offer by New York City to pay a US$500 bonus to city workers to get vaccinated, "They are over here shoving money at us. And I'm asking, why are you so eager, when you don't give us money for anything else?," Streedhar and Anand (2021).

12. U.S. District Judge Kathryn Kimball Mizelle struck down the federal mask mandate for airplanes and other modes of public transportation Monday, [April 18, 2022] writing in a 59-page ruling that the CDC had exceeded its authority and failed to follow proper rulemaking procedures, https://s3.documentcloud.org/documents/21636220/047124235804.pdf.

References

Abraham, Katharine G., and Melissa S. Kearney. 2018. Explaining the decline in the U.S. employment-to-population ratio: A review of the evidence. NBER, Working Paper No. 24333, February.

Abramowitz, Alan, and Jennifer McCoy. 2019. United States: Racial resentment, negative partisanship, and polarization in Trump's America. *Annals of the American Academy of Political and Social Sciences* 681: 137–156.

Adamecz-Völgyi, Anna, and Ágnes Szabó-Morvai. 2021. Confidence in public institutions is critical in containing the Covid-19 pandemic. *GLO Discussion Paper Series* No. 861, CERS-IE WP, No. 2021/26, June.

Alesina, Alberto, and Edward L. Glaeser. 2004. *Fighting poverty in the US and Europe: A world of difference*. New York: Oxford University Press.

Alesina, Alberto, Edward L. Glaeser, and B.S. Sacerdote. 2001. Why doesn't the US have a European-style welfare state? *Brookings Papers on Economic Activity* 2: 187–277.

Alon, Titan, et al. 2020. The impact of Covid-19 on gender equality. NBER, *Working Paper* No. 26947, April.

Atkinson, Anthony B., Thomas Piketty, and Emmanuel Saez. 2011. Top incomes in the long run of history. *Journal of Economic Literature* 49 (1): 10.

Bahar, Dany. 2020. A review of metrics to help decision-makers determine the proper pace of reopening. In: *Reopening America: How to save lives and livelihoods*, eds. J. R. Allen, and D. M. West. Washington, DC: Brookings Institution. https://www.brookings.edu/interactives.

BLS, US Bureau of Labor Statistics. 2021. *The employment situation*. US Bureau of Labor Statistics, March.

BLS, US Bureau of Labor Statistics. 2022. *The employment situation*. US Bureau of Labor Statistics, March.

Bollyky, Thomas J., et al. 2022. Pandemic preparedness and Covid-19: An exploratory analysis of infection and fatality rates, and contextual factors associated with preparedness in 177 countries, from Jan 1, 2020, to Sept 30, 2021. *Lancet*, February 1.

Bor, Jacob, Gregory H. Cohen, and Sandro Galea. 2017. Population health in an era of rising income inequality: USA, 1980–2015. *Lancet* 389: 1475–1490.

Boushey, Heather. 2019. *Unbound: How inequality constricts our economy and what we can do about it*. Cambridge: Harvard University.

Case, Anne, and Angus Deaton. 2020. *Deaths of despair and the future of capitalism*. Princeton: Princeton University Press.

CBPP. 2021. *Tracking the Covid-19 recession's effects on food, housing, and employment hardships*. Center on Budget and Policy Priorities Covid Hardship Watch, January 28.

Dougherty, Conor. 2021. Pandemic's toll on housing: Falling behind, doubling up. *New York Times*, February 6.

Easterly, William. 2001. The middle class consensus and economic development. *Journal of Economic Growth* 6 (4): 317–335.

Escobari, Marcela, Ian Seyal, and Michael J. Meaney. 2019. *Realism about reskilling: Upgrading the career prospects of America's low-wage workers*. Washington DC: Brookings Institution.

Frank, Mark W. 2009. Inequality and growth in the United States: Evidence from a new state-level panel of income inequality measures. *Economic Inquiry* 47 (1): 55–68.

Garfield, Rachel, Gary Claxton, Anthony Damico, and Larry Levitt. 2020. *Eligibility for ACA health coverage following job loss*. Kaiser Family Foundation, May 13, https://www.kff.org.

Goldhaber, Dan, et al. 2022. *The consequences of remote and hybrid instruction during the pandemic*. Research Report, Center for Education Policy Research, Harvard University, May 2022, https://cepr.harvard.edu/road-to-Covid-recovery.

Graham, Carol, and Sergio Pinto. 2021. The geography of desperation in America: Labor force participation, mobility, place, and well-being. *Social Science & Medicine* 27: 113612.

Green, Jon, and Sean McElwee. 2019. The differential effects of economic conditions and racial attitudes in the election of Donald Trump. *Perspectives on Politics* 17 (2): 358–379.

Guyton, John, et al. 2021. Tax evasion at the top of the income distribution: Theory and evidence. NBER, Working Paper No. 28542, March.

Hacker, Jacob S., and Paul Pierson. 2020. *Let them eat tweets: How the right rules in an age of extreme inequality*. New York: Liveright.

Hetherington, Marc J., and Jonathan D. Weiler. 2009. *Authoritarianism and polarization in American politics*. New York: Cambridge University Press.

Johns, Andrew, and Joel Slemrod. 2010. The distribution of income tax noncompliance. *National Tax Journal* 63 (3): 405–406.

Karageorge, Eleni X. 2020. Covid-19 recession is tougher on woman, *Monthly Labor Review*, September.

Karlinsky, Ariel, and Dmitry Kobak. 2021. The world mortality dataset: Tracking excess mortality across countries during the Covid-19 pandemic. *medRxiv*, January 27.

Krueger, Alan B. 2017. Where have all the workers gone?: An inquiry into the decline of the U.S. labor force participation rate. *Brookings Papers on Economic Activity*, Fall, 1–87.

Lancet. 2022. Estimating excess mortality due to the Covid-19 pandemic: A systematic analysis of Covid-19-related mortality, 2020–21. *Lancet* 399: 1513–1536.

MacWilliams, Matthew C. 2016. Who decides when the party doesn't? Authoritarian voters and the rise of Donald Trump. *PS: Political Science and Politics*, October, 716–721.

Mankiw, N. Gregory. 2013. Defending the one percent. *Journal of Economic Perspectives* 27 (3): 21–22.

Marmot, Michael. 2007. *The status syndrome: How social standing affects our health and longevity*. New York: Macmillan.

Mason, Liliana. 2018. *Uncivil agreement: How politics became our identity*. Chicago: University of Chicago Press.

Metzl, Jonathan M., Aletha Maybank, and De Maio Fernando. 2020. Responding to the Covid-19 pandemic: The need for a structurally competent health care system. *JAMA* 2020: E1–E2.

Milanovic, Branko. 2016. *Global inequality: A new approach for the age of globalization*. Cambridge: Harvard University Press.

Mutz, Diana C. 2018. Status threat, not economic hardship, explains the 2016 presidential vote. *Proceedings of the National Academy of Sciences* 115 (19): E4330–E4339.

Noah, Timothy. 2012. *The great divergence: America's growing inequality crisis and what we can do about it*. New York: Bloomsbury Press.

Osberg, Lars. 2018. *The age of increasing inequality: The astonishing rise of Canada's 1%*. Toronto: James Lorimer.

Owen, William F., Richard Carmona, and Claire Pomeroy. 2020. Failing another national stress test on health disparities. *JAMA* 323 (19): 1905–1906.

Paglino, Eugenio, et al. 2022. Excess all-cause mortality across counties in the United States, March 2020 to December 2021. MedRxiv preprint, May 2, p. 9.

Payne, Keith. 2017. *The broken ladder: How inequality affects the way we think, live and die*. New York: Viking.

Piketty, Thomas, Emmanuel Saez, and Gabriel Zucman. 2018. Distributional national accounts: Methods and estimates for the United States. *The Quarterly Journal of Economics* 133 (2): 553–609.

Pinker, Steven. 2018. *Enlightenment now: The case for reason, science, and humanism.* New York: Viking.

Reardon, Sean, and Kendra Bischoff. 2011. *Growth in the residential segregation of families by income, 1970–2009, US2010 project*, November.

Reny, Tyler T., Loren Collingwood, and Ali A. Valenzuela. 2019. Vote switching in the 2016 election: How racial and immigration attitudes, not economics, explain shifts in white voting. *Public Opinion Quarterly* 83 (1): 91–113.

Ruiz, Michele. 2021. Covid-19 and gender equality: Employers can help women from being unfairly punished for challenges they face. *Forbes Magazine*, April 17, 2021. https://www.forbes.com.

Runciman, Walter G. 1966. *Relative deprivation and social justice: A study of attitudes to social inequality in twentieth-century England.* London: Routledge & Kegan Paul.

Saez, Emmanuel, and Gabriel Zucman. 2014. Wealth inequality in the United States since 1913: Evidence from capitalized income tax data. NBER Working Paper No. 20625, October.

Saez, Emmanuel, and Gabriel Zucman. 2020. Trends in US income and wealth inequality: Revising after the revisionists. NBER Working Paper No. 27921, October.

Saez, Emmanuel, and Gabriel Zucman. 2019. *The triumph of injustice: How the rich dodge taxes and how to make them pay.* New York: Norton.

Saez, Emmanuel. 2019. *Striking it richer: The evolution of top incomes in the United States*, March 2.

Sandel, Michael J. 2020. *The tyranny of merit: What's become of the common good?* New York: Farrar, Straus and Giroux.

Saville, Christopher W.N.., and Daniel Rhys Thomas. 2022. Social capital and geographical variation in the incidence of Covid-19: An ecological study. *Journal of Epidemiology and Community Health* 1: 1–6.

Semega, Jessica, et al. 2020. *Income and poverty in the United States: 2019.* Washington D.C.: US Census Bureau, September.

Sharfstein, Joshua M., and Christopher C. Morphew. 2020. The urgency and challenge of opening K-12 schools in the fall of 2020. *JAMA*, June 1.

Shaw, Kate M., et al. 2016. Chronic disease disparities by county economic status and metropolitan classification, behavioral risk factor surveillance system. *Preventing Chronic Disease Public Health Research, Practice, and Policy* 13 (E119).

Singh, Gopal K., and Mohammad Siahpush. 2006. Widening socioeconomic inequalities in US life expectancy, 1980–2000. *International Journal of Epidemiology* 35: 969–979.

Sitaraman, Ganesh. 2017. *The crisis of the middle-class constitution: Why economic inequality threatens our republic.* New York: Knopf.

Stiglitz, Joseph E. 2013. *The price of inequality: How today's divided society endangers our future.* New York: Norton.

Stiglitz, Joseph E. 2015. The origins of inequality, and policies to contain it. *National Tax Journal* 68 (2): 425–448.

Streedhar, Anita, and Gopal Anand. 2021. Behind low vaccination rates lurks a more profound social weakness. *New York Times*, December 3.

Szreter, Simon, and Michael Woolcock. 2004. Health by association? Social capital, social theory, and the political economy of public health. *International Journal of Epidemiology* 33 (4): 650–667.

Taylor, Paul, and Richard Fry. 2012. *The rise of residential segregation by income: Social & demographic trends.* Pew Research Center, August 1.

Trounstine, Jessica. 2018. *Segregation by design: Local politics and inequality in American cities.* New York: University Press.

Wilkinson, Richard G. 1992. Income distribution and life expectancy. *British Medical Journal* 304 (6820): 165–168.

Wilkinson, Richard G., and Kate Pickett. 2011. *The spirit level: Why greater equality makes societies stronger*. New York: Bloomsbury.
Woolhandler, Steffie, et al. 2021. Public policy and health in the trump era, report of the lancet commission on public policy and health in the trump era. *The Lancet* 397 (102275): 705–753.

Chapter 4
The Covid-19 Pandemic and "Rising Deaths of Despair" in the United States

Thomas F. Remington

Abstract Rising rates of age-specific mortality fatal drug overdoses, suicides, and poisonings and accidents involving alcohol in the United States, particularly for Caucasian American males in their prime working years, have attracted a good deal of attention in recent years. The rising numbers of "deaths of despair" are all the more striking in view of the decline in mortality rates from other major causes of mortality, including cancer and heart disease, as well as the fact that they are not seen in other advanced economies. Since the beginning of the Covid-19 pandemic, the effects of the pandemic have exacerbated the longer-term trend toward rising deaths of despair. The social and psychological stresses associated with the pandemic, from isolation and loss of employment, are a clear contributing factor to this sharp increase. In this chapter, I outline two channels through which the pandemic and the rising rates of drug overdoses could be related. These are, first, individual-level factors, including the high rate of employment losses in the lowest-paid occupations in the lowest-paid industries. The higher rate of labor force non-participation, not only among workers at or nearing retirement age, but also among those in younger age groups, and among workers in leisure and hospitality sectors, suggest that wage levels and working conditions continue to deter a return to employment. Second are effects associated with place of residence. These include the loss of social cohesion (rising "anomie," in Durkheim's term) in communities that have been affected most by the loss of opportunity. One measure of the importance of place-based effects is the fact that county-level rates of vaccination are inversely correlated with rates of drug overdoses and Covid-related mortality.

Keywords Covid-19 pandemic · Deaths of despair · Suicide · Gun violence · Drug overdose · Social and individual level factors

T. F. Remington (✉)
Department of Government, Harvard University, Cambridge, USA
e-mail: tremington@fas.harvard.edu

Political Science Department, Emory University, Atlanta, USA

C. Aspalter (ed.), *Covid-19 Pandemic*,
https://doi.org/10.1007/978-981-99-2497-4_4

Introduction

Rising rates of age-specific mortality fatal drug overdoses, suicides, and poisonings and accidents involving alcohol in the United States, particularly for Caucasian American males in their prime working years, have attracted a good deal of attention in recent years. The rising numbers of "deaths of despair," as Case and Deaton (2020) have termed them, are all the more striking in view of the decline in mortality rates from other major causes of mortality, including cancer and heart disease, as well as the fact that they are not seen in other advanced economies (Case and Deaton 2020; Graham and Pinto 2019, 2021). Although suicides, deaths from chronic liver disease, and deaths from alcohol poisoning are among the categories classified as "deaths of despair," it is drug overdose deaths that have risen the fastest in the last twenty years. Between 1999 and 2017, the rate of deaths from drug overdoses rose 3.6-fold, with the highest rates recorded in the Appalachian region as well as several counties in other states. Drug deaths rose at a still faster rate after 2013, when synthetic opioids such as fentanyl became widely available and frequently prescribed (Shiels et al. 2020).

Analysis of the uneven demographic and geographic distribution of deaths of despair reveals the complex interconnections between economic inequality and the social-psychological factors that contribute to the sharp increase in these deaths, and indicate that the Covid-19 Pandemic has exacerbated them. Death rates from opioid overdoses have risen during the pandemic.

According to the CDC, after levelling off in 2018 and 2019, during the 12-month period from December 2019 to December 2020, as the virus and its dislocations spread, the number of drug-related deaths rose from 71,130 to 92,478. Then between December 2020 and December 2021, the number rose again, to 103,598 (CDC 2022a). This was the highest number of deaths from drug overdoses ever recorded in a one-year span. The Covid-19 has burdened the most vulnerable members of society with still heavier economic and psychological stress. Figure 4.1 shows the surge in deaths from drug overdoses during 2020 and 2021 (CDC 2022b).

The social and psychological stresses associated with the pandemic, from isolation and loss of employment, are a clear contributing factor to this sharp increase. As to suicides, although age-adjusted suicide rates declined slightly in 2020 from their peak in 2018, data for 2021 and 2022 are not yet available. It may therefore yet turn out that suicide rates have risen in 2021 along with deaths from drug overdoses.

Social and Individual-Level Factors

In this chapter, I outline two channels through which the pandemic is contributing to the rising rates of drug overdoses and gun homicides. These are, first, individual-level factors, including the high rate of employment losses in the lowest-paid occupations in the lowest-paid industries. The higher rate of labor force non-participation, not

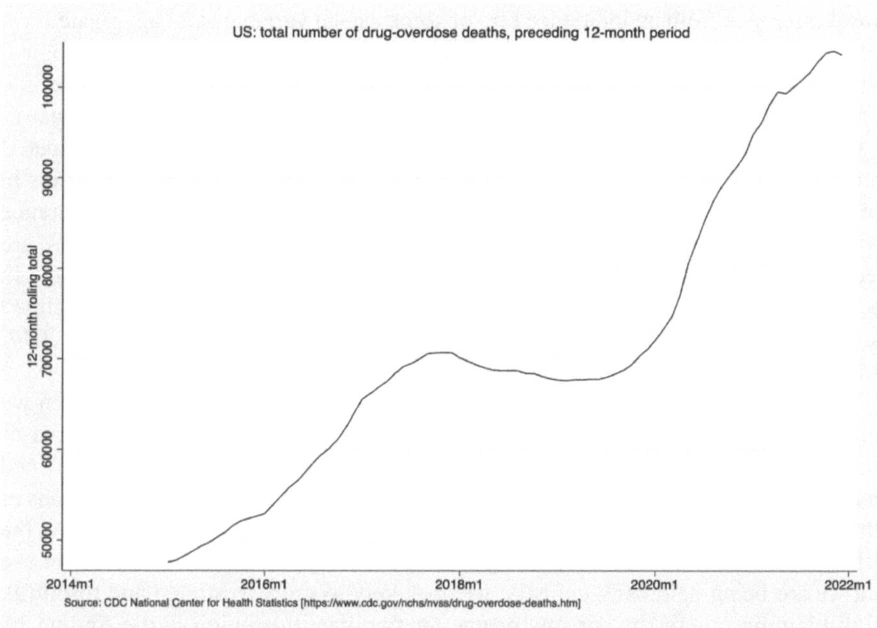

Fig. 4.1 Drug overdose deaths, rolling 12-month totals, United States

only among workers at or nearing retirement age, but also among those in younger age groups, and among workers in leisure and hospitality sectors, suggest that wage levels and working conditions continue to deter a return to employment. Second are environmental effects associated with place of residence. These include the fabric of social networks and milieu in communities that have been affected most by the loss of opportunity. That these societal or community-level effects are operating is indicated by the fact that at the county level, rates of vaccination are inversely correlated with rates of drug overdoses.

Public health statistics broken down by place of residence, at the county and state levels, confirm the existence of these relationships, although of course they do not explain them. An extensive literature from the fields of sociology and public health linking social and psychological conditions to behavioral outcomes, including the self-destructive behavior associated with fatal drug overdoses, suicides and alcohol abuse, helps in interpreting the causal effects at work.

Therefore, we can treat these aggregate-level statistics as evidence of both individual-level and social factors. County- or state-level rates of drug overdoses, vaccinations, Covid-related mortality, gun homicides and so on, suggest that variation in the incidence of particular factors such as poverty and unemployment is correlated with variation in individual-level behaviors outcomes such as drug overdoses, violence, and so on. In that sense, we treat place names as no more than stand-ins for variables affecting individuals. To be sure, we cannot draw a direct causal inference from an incidence rate of some causal variable at an aggregate level such as a state or county to individual behavior—that is known as the ecological fallacy (i.e. we cannot suppose, for example, that the fact that a majority of people in a given district vote Republican means that any given individual is Republican).

On the other hand, it is equally erroneous to isolate individuals from their spatial and temporal setting. Our actions are influenced by our relationships with others in our social context, such as people who constitute our reference groups. Reference groups serve as a point of comparison; one's peers, or one's family members, are frequently the basis on which individuals develop their sense of how they stand in society relative to others who are comparable to themselves. Evolution has inclined us to see ourselves in relation to others, according to psychologists (Payne 2017; Marmot 2014; Wilkinson and Pickett 2009; Runciman 1966).

We judge ourselves by the expectations we form by observing others whom we regard as like us and with whom we identify. We are likely to see ourselves as relatively better or worse off than they, or to have more or less opportunity to succeed than they; to consider ourselves treated fairly or unfairly, based on our perceptions of others in a similar situation to ours. As inequality in a society widens, therefore, the differences in income, social standing and opportunity to rise widen. If we believe that we are being held back unjustly, we are likely to grow frustrated and resentful, often blaming others for our misfortune. A familiar illustration is the finding by Hochschild (2016) that low-income workers living in environmentally despoiled parts of Louisiana were more likely to blame the federal government than the oil companies for ruining their livelihoods, and to consider their chances stymied by those "cutting in line" ahead of them—among whom they were apt to name women, African Americans, and immigrants.

It follows from this idea that people living in a particular region are more likely to compare themselves and assess their own place in society through comparison with others living in the same region; reference groups are more likely to be local than distant. And even apart from those in one's immediate environment who serve as a reference point, many judge the prospects for improving their conditions by pragmatically observing the kinds of jobs and housing available to them in their areas. Moreover, as a great deal of recent research about the impact of local neighborhood conditions on social mobility proves, some neighborhoods are powerful brakes on upward mobility across generations, while others afford wide opportunity for advancement (Chetty et al. 2017, 2014). The place where one grows up and lives has a powerful effect on one's prospects for mobility, both social and geographic. Growing up in a community with higher median income, lower income inequality, a higher number of two-parent families, better primary schools, greater social capital, and lower residential segregation, is significantly related to the likelihood of earning a higher income than one's parents later in life. Place-based effects have to do with more than simply job opportunity; they also include the effects of social milieu, including opportunities for human capital development (Chetty 2021; Putnam 2016).

These considerations help us in interpreting the strong geographic effects observed in rates of deaths of despair during the pandemic. For example, the data shows a significant association between the level of economic insecurity prevailing in a county and the rate of deaths of despair: counties classified as being at the highest level of economic insecurity had rates of deaths from drug and alcohol poisoning, liver disease, and suicide that are 60% higher than rates in counties with the lowest levels of insecurity (Knapp et al. 2019)[1]. The evidence strongly indicates, therefore, that in addition to individual-level risk factors, community-level influences also contribute to the heightened number of deaths of despair.

As Fig. 4.2 shows, some parts of the country have particularly suffered from drug overdose deaths. The figure shows the trend for the United States and three states that have been particularly affected, Tennessee, Kentucky and West Virginia. Two states in the Deep South—Mississippi and Louisiana—saw extremely sharp increases in the rate of drug overdose deaths as well, as did Alaska, Montana, Vermont and the state of Washington. The figure normalizes the data by calculating deaths per million population.

Figure 4.3 maps the growth rate in 12-month totals from January 2020 through November 2021 by state. Again, as it shows, several states in the Appalachian region saw substantial increases over this period, as did California, Colorado, Minnesota, Louisiana and New Jersey.

Another manifestation of the destructive effects of the pandemic, as mediated by the strong spatial inequalities of the society, is violence involving firearms, which has risen sharply since the pandemic began. Again, the three-way relationship among inequalities by place and socio-economic status, the impact of the pandemic, and deaths of despair is particularly clear. CDC researchers found that the poorest counties

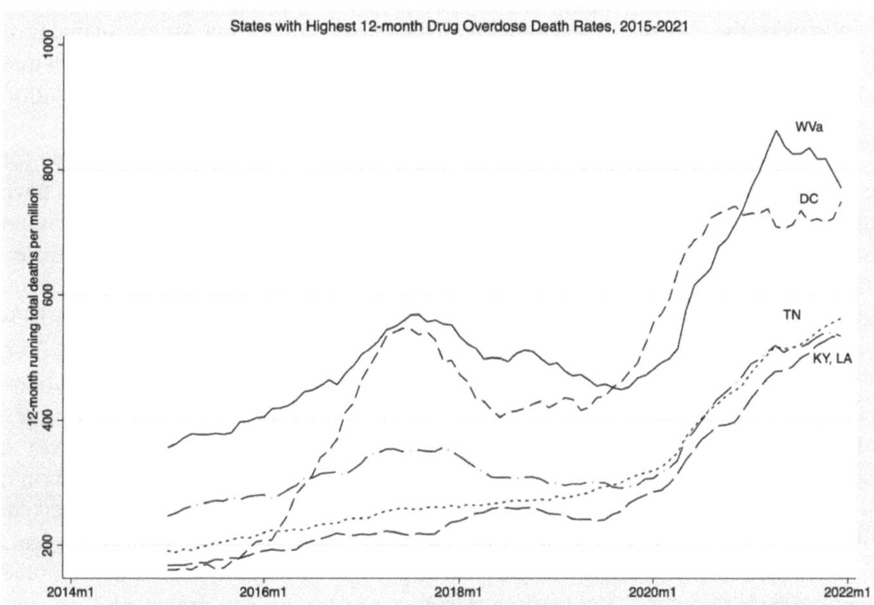

Fig. 4.2 Drug overdose deaths per million population, 2015–2021

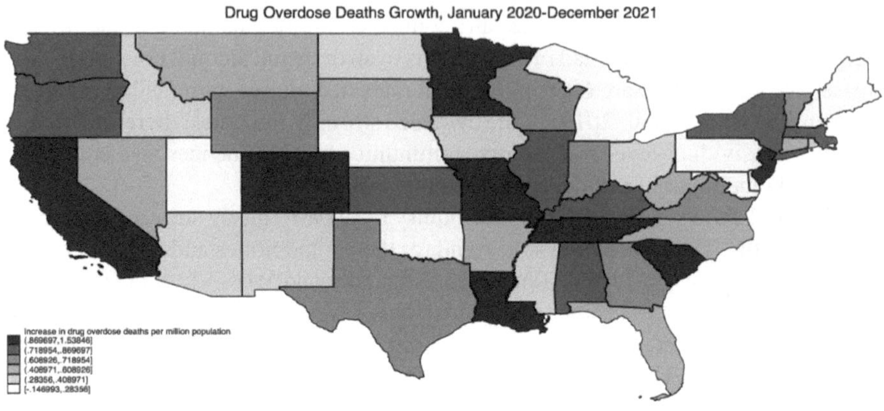

Fig. 4.3 Drug overdose deaths increase, January 2020–December 2021, by state

experienced levels of gun-related homicides that were 4.5 times higher than counties with the lowest poverty rate (CDC 2022a). They cite several sources of stress, some underlying factors associated with deep inequalities in opportunity, as well as more immediate sources associated with the pandemic, such as job losses, disruptions to familiar routines, social isolation and anxiety.

The highest rates of gun violence, and the highest increases, were recorded among young men, and particularly African American and American Indian youth. Young African American males (ages 10–24) experienced a rate of gun-related homicide that was more than twenty times higher than the rate for Caucasian American males of the same age. In 2020, the total level of homicides using firearms reached a level that had not been experienced since 1994, rising from 4.6 deaths per 100,000 population to 6.1 (Kegler et al. 2022).

The influence of the gun lobby on federal legislation has made it impossible for the government to collect comprehensive figures on gun ownership, but surveys have managed to collect some data on gun purchases. A survey conducted in 2021 found that about 7.5 million Americans bought a firearm for the first time some time between January 1, 2020, and April 26, 2021. About half were women, 20% African American, and a similar number Hispanic American (Miller et al. 2022). Overall, around 19% of all American adults who bought a firearm in that period did so as first-time gun owners. The rate of purchases of new firearms roughly quadrupled by comparison to the 2010–2015 period. Even more telling is the fact that gun purchases surged in January 2021—the month of President Biden's inauguration and the January 6 insurrection at the Capitol—with a smaller spike occurring in June 2020, the month after George Floyd's murder at the hands of the police in Minneapolis, Minnesota. Coinciding with the effects of the Covid pandemic, these politically charged events evidently incited a response on the part of a large number of Americans that prompted them to acquire firearms. Evidently a related set of forces also provoked a wave of aggressive violence channeled into self-destructive or homicidal behavior.

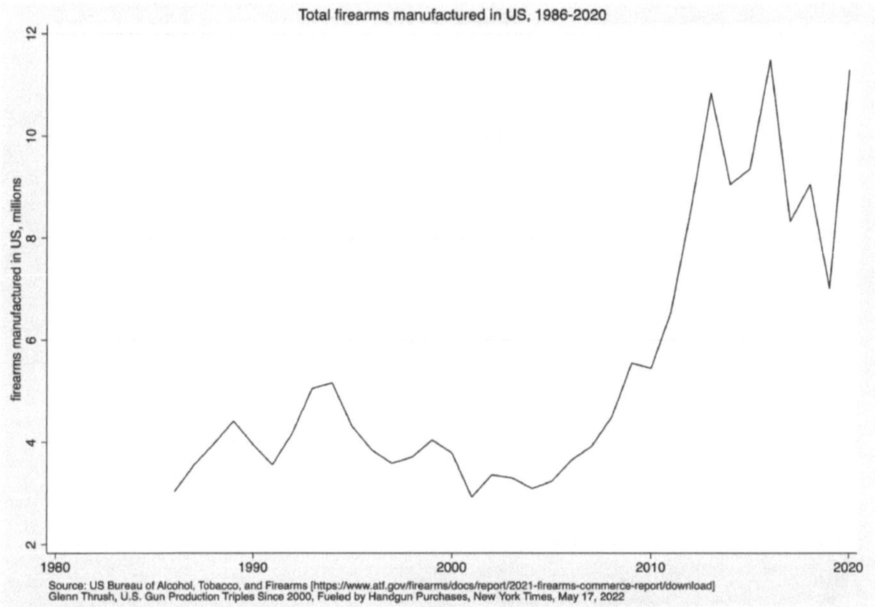

Fig. 4.4 Total firearms manufactured in US, 1986–2020 (in millions)

We also have figures on gun manufacturing (although these do not include the rapid growth in "ghost guns" which are produced from kits or made using additive manufacturing [3-D printers]), and therefore not registered and not traceable when used to commit a crime). These figures show that gun production in the US rose rapidly after the mid-2000s, from three million in 2004 to over 11 million in 2020 (cf. Fig. 4.4).

Similar trends are visible in the suicide data, as Fig. 4.5 indicates. Although suicide rates rose steadily from 2000 through 2018 before declining slightly, the rate for males using firearms to commit suicide continued to rise.

The increased rates of drug overdose deaths and of gun purchases, production, and homicide are fueled by the combination of fear, anxiety, helplessness, anger and despair experienced by those already facing rising obstacles to well-being as inequality in economic condition and opportunity rises.

The opioid overdose epidemic reflects the interaction of physical and emotional pain, which operates both as cause and effect of not working. Krueger (2017) found that as of 2017, nearly half of men who were not in the workforce were taking pain medications daily, of which nearly two thirds were prescription medications. 57% of Caucasian American men out of the labor force and with less than a college education reported living with pain. These rates are higher in counties where there are more people not in the labor force, suggesting that there is a social and geographic factor involved.

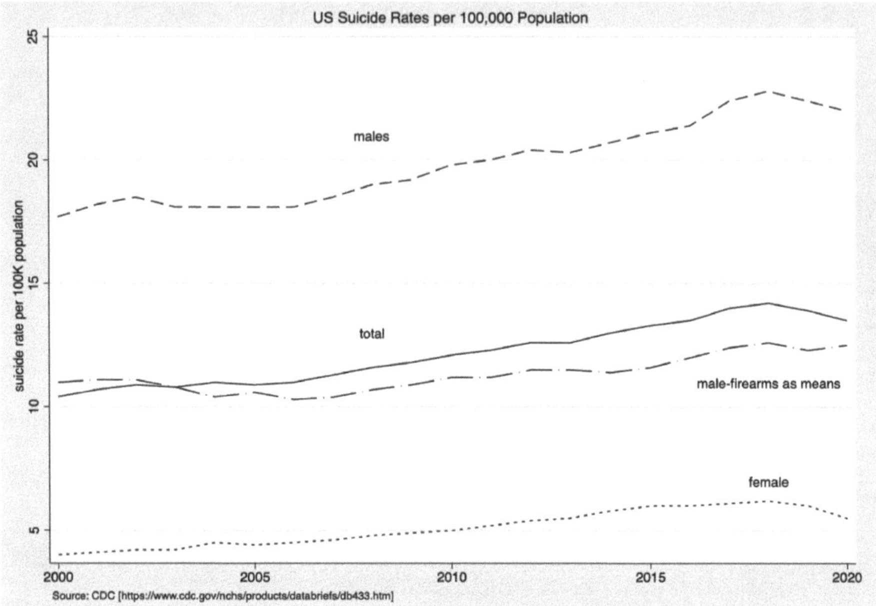

Fig. 4.5 US suicide rates, 2000–2020 (per 100,000 population)

One effect of inequality is greater insecurity at the individual and household level. That is, more than was the case several decades ago household incomes, fluctuate widely across individual lifetimes, as a result of lay-offs, severe illness or disability, or changes in family circumstances—the three biggest contributors to sudden income losses. These circumstances are often related. In what Hacker (2008) terms "the great risk shift," the public policies of retrenchment and privatization of social insurance provision have transferred the risks of the sudden loss of a significant portion of individual income to individuals, individual and household (Hacker and Rehm 2022; Hacker 2008, 2004).

As a result, individual and household well-being have become more vulnerable to employment, health and personal shocks that leave people without the means to replace their income. The erosion of public provision of social insurance in tandem with the polarization of the labor force—that is, the tendency for employment in jobs paying middle-level wages to shrink at the expense of employment in higher- and lower-wage jobs (Autor et al. 2020; Goldin and Katz 2008, 1998)—has driven higher insecurity; one response to which has been greater use and abuse drugs or alcohol to relieve stress, pain, and hopelessness, or even to commit suicide. The drug companies targeted those groups in the population who were most susceptible to being offered a supposedly non-addictive form of relief from pain; these were the segments of society most likely to become addicted to the painkillers (Graham and Pinto 2021). Deaths of despair are most concentrated among individuals who have low educational levels (and are therefore often marginal in the labor force), in rural areas, and in areas where manufacturing and mining employment has declined. As Graham and Pinto (2020) emphasize, deaths of despair are a response to the loss of hope. Another response, particularly as the Covid-19 pandemic spread, has been to direct violent aggression at others.

For these reasons, it is not surprising that the county-by-county distribution of drug deaths is closely related to the spatial incidence of deaths from the Covid virus. When median household income and percent of the population classified as urban are included in an OLS model regressing drug overdose deaths on registered Covid deaths, nearly half the variation in the rate of drug overdose deaths is explained by the three variables. Figure 4.6 indicates the strength of the relationship.

Inequality, we can reasonably conclude from the data, manifests itself in the closely interconnected dimensions of space and time: spatial inequality rises, reinforcing inequalities of economic opportunity and well-being and social status and connectedness. These together have shaped the course of the Covid-19 Pandemic, bringing about sharp differences in mortality rates by race and ethnicity, income and education, and location of residence and employment. Moreover, because inequality in access to health care has deepened, vulnerability to more severe illness is also unequally distributed by social class, race, ethnicity, and location. Inequality by social and economic status and by location also influences the behavioral responses of individuals and communities. There is a strong geographic gradient in the trajectories of deaths of despair. Suicides and deaths from alcohol poisoning are more

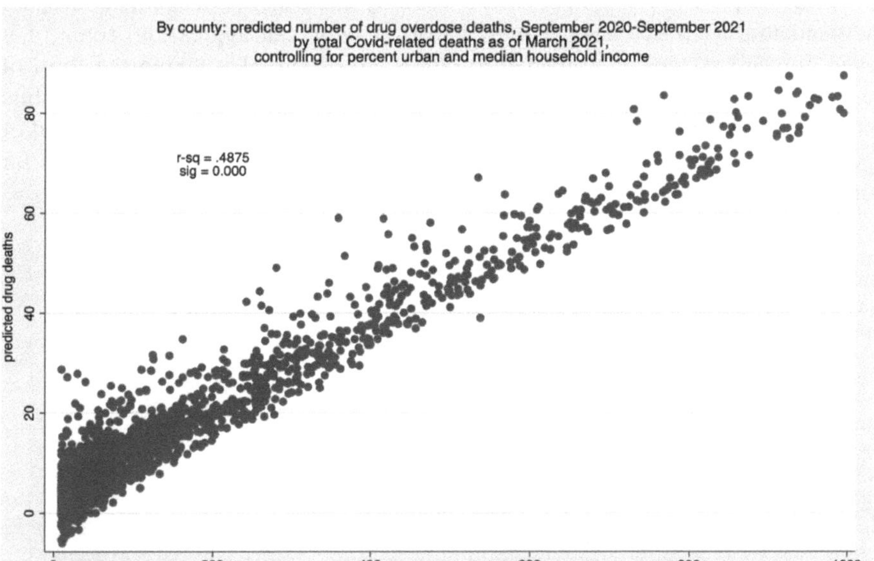

Fig. 4.6 Drug overdose deaths predicted rate, by registered covid deaths, by county

common in western states; deaths from drug overdoses are more frequent in the Appalachian Belt—West Virginia, Kentucky, Tennessee, and parts of Indiana, Pennsylvania, North Carolina, Ohio and Virginia. These deaths are also highly unequal as between men and women, across age groups, and initially between Caucasian and African American populations. Since 2015–16, however, all ethnic and ethnic groups experienced similar rates of increase in deaths of despair (Shiels et al. 2020).

Similarly, the rapid increase in gun purchases and homicides using firearms is distributed unequally across Caucasian and African American populations, age groups, and region. Among all gun owners, 63% are male. However, among new purchases of guns after the start of the pandemic, half the purchases were made by women, 20% by African Americans and an equal number by Hispanic Americans (Miller et al. 2022). Firearm ownership varies widely by region. Among adults who own guns, more than 43% are in the South, about 22% each are in the Midwest and West, and only 11.5% are in the Northeast. Although about 27% each of gun-owners live in cities and in the country, almost 45% live in suburbs. 42% of them have annual incomes of at least US$100,000, whereas fewer than a quarter receive incomes under US$50,000.

Homicides using guns have a similar regional skew, with the Appalachian states again distinctive for their high rates, as Table 4.1 shows.

These figures support the argument in this chapter that there are complex reciprocal causal pathways linking aggregate-level inequalities to individual-level behavior, and that these effects have been exacerbated by the pandemic. It is reasonable to claim that rising inequality affects both Covid mortality and patterns of deaths of despair. The pandemic itself has also increased fear, anxiety, and aggression, some of it turned outward as violence directed at others, and some of it taking the form of the abuse of drugs and alcohol, often leading to death one's own death. The public health literature has demonstrated powerful correlations, but a full causal model of the interaction among inequality, Covid, and deaths of despair would require a far more comprehensive theory.

Table 4.1 Homicides using firearms, per 100,000 population (2020)[2]

New England	2.0
Mid Atlantic	4.1
East North Central	7.7
West North Central	5.7
South Atlantic	7.5
East South Central	11.3
West South Central	7.5
Mountain	4.4
Pacific	4.0

Note that ethnic difference distinguishes the victims of gun homicides far more than does region: the rate of homicides using firearms for African Americans is 26.6 per 100,000 and 2.2 among Caucasian Americans

Still, we can posit that there is a strong role for societal-level influences on deaths of despair that cannot be reduced to individual-level factors such as poverty, insecurity, poor education, and poor health. The fabric of communities, from the immediate neighborhood through the county and state, also shapes people's sense of self-worth and aspiration. This fact is well demonstrated in the literature on the ways people respond to comparisons of their current situations to what they think possible in the future, what they experienced in the past, and what they observe among others who serve as reference groups for them. Consequently, the standards for assessing their own situations are culturally-bound. Those who consider their lot in life to have been determined by God or by fate or nature tend to respond to a sense of relative deprivation differently than do those considering that others are to blame for their circumstances (Dittmann et al. 2020; Stephens et al. 2019; Buttrick et al. 2017; Dittmann and Stephens 2017; Cheung and Lucas 2016; Delhey and Dragolov 2014). We seek to make sense of our position relative to others. If we believe that our status is all part of God's plan, or fair, or that we can achieve a more satisfactory status, we are more likely to be content. If we consider our position unfair or that we are looked down upon by others, we are more likely to be dissatisfied.

Evangelical Christianity

Religion, for many, can offer an outlet for affirmation and a source of hope. Religious beliefs and values are strongly shaped by family and social milieu. In the Bible Belt, for example, people are much more likely to consider themselves born-again or evangelical Christians. Whereas in Mormon-dominated Utah, only 17% of the population considers themselves born again, and only 19% in Massachusetts, in states in the Deep South and in Appalachia, rates range from 60 to 70% in the Carolinas to as high as 75% in Mississippi (PRC 2014).

This strong geographic skew invites us to consider whether the same cultural forces conducive to these high rates of evangelical religious identity may also be driving the responses to the Covid pandemic and to the abuse of drugs. Indeed, the share of born-again identifiers by state is strongly and positively related to the rates of drug overdose deaths, as Fig. 4.7 shows.

By the same token, since rates of (registered) Covid deaths are also strongly correlated with drug overdose deaths, it is not surprising that Covid deaths by state, per 100,000 population, are also positively correlated with the percent born again or that vaccination rates are also strongly correlated with percent born again (Figs. 4.8 and 4.9).

In both cases, Bible Belt—the Deep South and Appalachia—again stand out as strongly affected by Covid mortality. Percent born again explains 24.66% of the variation in (registered) Covid death rates in a simple OLS model. Likewise, evangelical Christian identification is strongly related to vaccination rates, as Fig. 4.9 indicates.

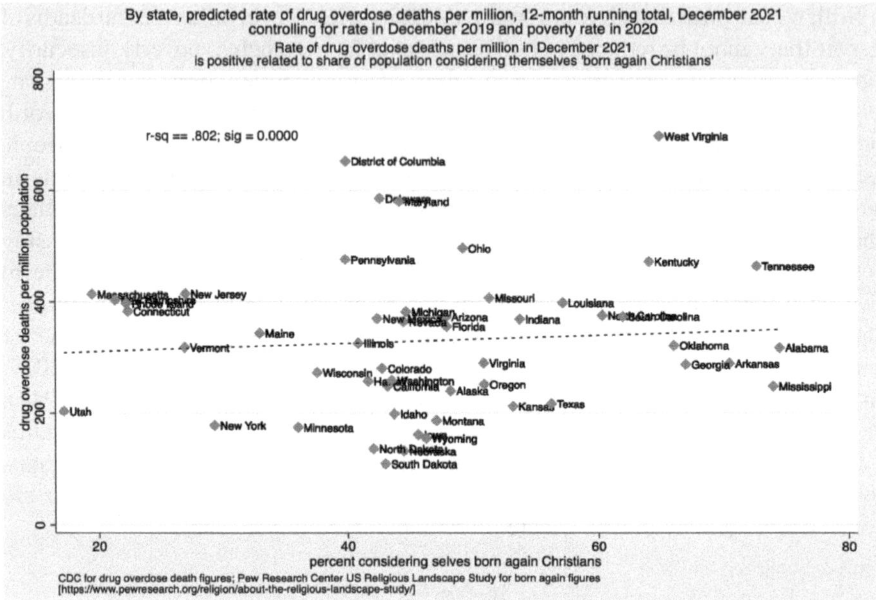

Fig. 4.7 Drug overdose deaths per million population, by state, for December 2021, and percent calling selves born again Christians

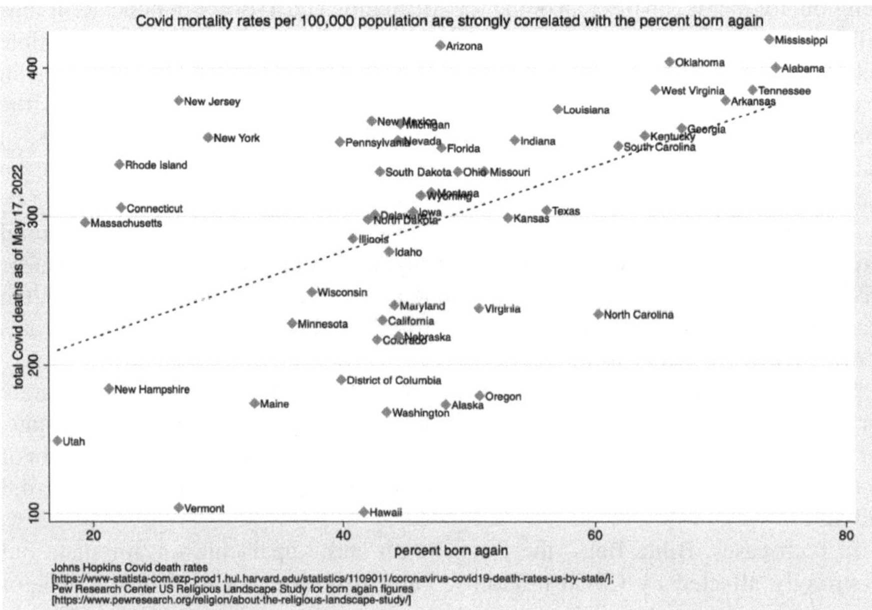

Fig. 4.8 Covid-related total mortality per 100,000 population, by state, as of May 17, 2022, and percent calling selves born again Christians

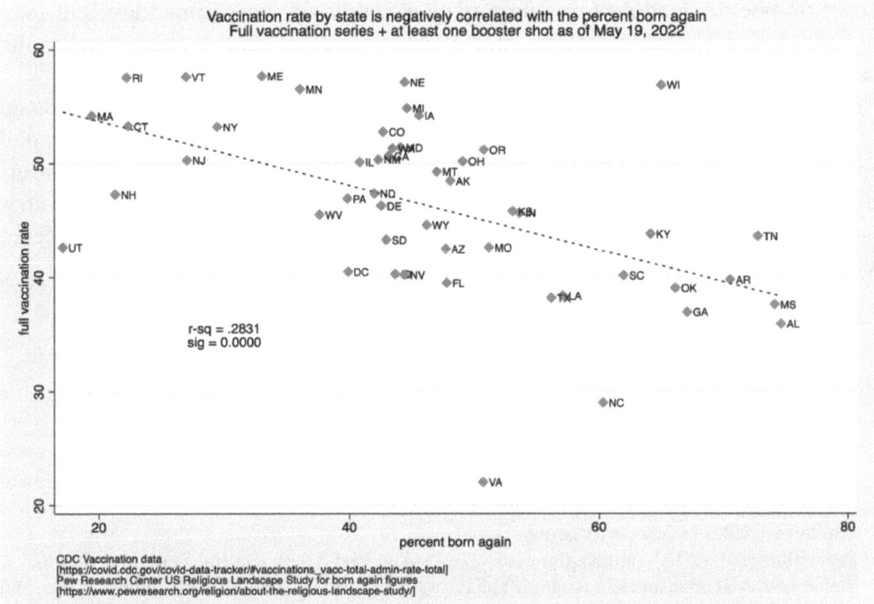

Fig. 4.9 Percent fully vaccinated by state by percent born again

In a simple regression of vaccination rates against born again percentages, the slope would imply that in a state with a 10% higher level of born-again Christians, there would be 2.8% fewer people fully vaccinated.

Concluding, we can sum up the findings by making three observations about the way rising economic inequality and spatial inequality is related to the Covid-19 Pandemic and the rising rates of deaths of despair.

Conclusions

Concluding, we can sum up the findings by making three observations. First, in addition to the effects of variables operating at the individual level, such as poverty and low education, inequality has affected the circumstances of the social environments in which people live, work, and raise families. It significantly shapes both the opportunities that individuals have to move socially and spatially, and the likelihood that their children will be able to move up the social ladder. Because the pandemic has reinforced these economic and spatial differences, widening the gap between rich and poor individuals and rich and poor regions, opportunities have been further narrowed.

Second, the narrowing of opportunity through the widening of differentials across space and economic-social circumstances has had a strong social-psychological impact on people, leading to a surge of gun purchases, gun homicides, and fatal drug overdoses. Theses surges are most concentrated among the groups and in the places where the loss of hope is most keenly felt.

Finally, the confluence of these social-psychological influences has contributed to the deepening of the political and cultural polarization across social strata and geographic regions. Individuals and places that identify deeply with the most conservative evangelical strains of Christianity have been the most likely to resist vaccination against Covid; they are at the same time the people and places who have suffered the greatest losses to Covid-related deaths.

Notes

1. See Knapp et al. (2019). Knapp et al. calculated an index of overall insecurity based on labor force participation rates; unemployment; share of income spent on rent payments; employment in service jobs; and percentage of adults with a subprime credit rating. They divided counties into three tertiles of insecurity levels.
2. See Miller et al. (2022) and Kegler et al. (2022). The East-South-Central States are: Kentucky, Tennessee, Alabama, and Mississippi. The East-North-Central States include Indiana, Ohio, and Illinois in addition to Michigan and Wisconsin. The Mid-Atlantic and South Atlantic region contains other states with regions that are commonly considered part the Appalachian region, including Pennsylvania, West Virginia and Virginia. The Appalachian Belt is therefore divided among different census-designated regional zones.

References

Autor, David, Claudia Goldin, and Lawrence Katz. 2020. Extending the race between education and technology. SEII Discussion Paper, No. 2020/01, January

Buttrick, Nicholas, Samantha Heintzelman, and Shigehiro Oishi. 2017. Inequality and well-being. *Current Opinion in Psychology* 18: 15–20.

Case, Anne, and Angus Deaton. 2020. *Deaths of despair and the future of capitalism*. Princeton University Press: Princeton.

CDC. 2022a. Firearm deaths grow, disparities widen: Comprehensive strategies can prevent violence and help reduce racial and ethnic disparities. https://www.cdc.gov.

CDC. 2022b. Website. National Center for Health Statistics. https://www.cdc.gov/nchs/nvss/drug-overdose-deaths.htm.

Chetty, Raj. 2021. Improving equality of opportunity: New insights from big data. *Contemporary Economic Policy* 39 (1): 7–41.

Chetty, Raj, et al. 2014. Where is the land of opportunity? The geography of intergenerational mobility in the United States. *Quarterly Journal of Economics* 129 (4): 1553–1623.

Chetty, Raj, et al. 2017. The fading American Dream: Trends in absolute income mobility since 1940. *Science* 35 (6): 398–406.

Cheung, Felix, and Richard E. Lucas. 2016. Income inequality is associated with stronger social comparison effects: The effect of relative income on life satisfaction. *Journal of Personality and Social Psychology* 110 (2): 332–341.

Delhey, Jan, and Georgi Dragolov. 2014. Why inequality makes Europeans less happy: The role of distrust, status anxiety, and perceived conflict. *European Sociological Review* 30 (2): 151–165.

Dittmann, Andrea G., and Nicole M. Stephens. 2017. Interventions aimed at closing the social class achievement gap: Changing individuals, structures, and construals. *Current Opinions in Psychology* 18: 111–116.

Dittmann, Andrea G., Nicole M. Stephens, and Sarah S.M. Townsend. 2020. Achievement is not class-neutral: Working together benefits people from working-class contexts. *Journal of Personality and Social Psychology* 119 (3): 517–539.

Goldin, Claudia, and Lawrence F. Katz. 1998. The origins of technology-skill complementarity. *The Quarterly Journal of Economics* 113 (3): 693–732.

Goldin, Claudia, and Lawrence F. Katz. 2008. *The race between education and technology.* Cambridge: Harvard University Press.

Graham, Carol, and Sergio Pinto. 2019. Unequal hopes and lives in the USA: Optimism, race, place, and premature mortality. *Journal of Population Economics* 32: 665–733.

Graham, Carol, and Sergio Pinto. 2020. *Despair is hurting American's labor markets.* Brookings, December 19.

Graham, Carol, and Sergio Pinto. 2021. The geography of desperation in America: Labor force participation, mobility, place, and well-being. *Social Science & Medicine* 270: 113612.

Hacker, Jacob S. 2004. Privatizing risk without privatizing the welfare state: The hidden politics of social policy retrenchment in the United States. *American Political Science Review* 98 (2): 243–260.

Hacker, Jacob S. 2008. *The great risk shift: The new economic insecurity and the decline of the American Dream.* New York: Oxford University Press.

Hacker, Jacob S., and Philipp Rehm. 2022. Reducing risk as well as inequality: Assessing the welfare state's insurance effects. *British Journal of Political Science* 52: 456–466.

Hochshild, Arlie. 2016. *Strangers in their own land: Anger and mourning on the American Right.* New York: The New Press.

Kegler, Scott R., et al. 2022. Vital signs: Changes in rirearm homicide and suicide rates—United States, 2019–2020. *CDC Morbidity and Mortality Weekly Report*, May 10.

Knapp, Emily A., et al. 2019. Economic insecurity and deaths of despair in US counties. *American Journal of Epidemiology* 188 (12): 2131–2139.

Krueger, Alan B. 2017. Where have all the workers gone?: An inquiry into the decline of the U.S. labor force participation rate. *Brookings Papers on Economic Activity*, Fall: 1–87.

Marmot, Michael. 2014. *The status syndrome: How social standing affects our health and longevity.* New York: Henry Holt.

Miller, Matthew, Wilson Zhang, and Deborah Azrael. 2022. Firearm purchasing during the Covid-19 pandemic: Results from the 2021 national firearms survey. *Annals of Internal Medicine* 175: 219–225.

Payne, Keith. 2017. *The broken ladder: How inequality affects the way we think, live and die.* Penguin, New York.

PRC, Pew Research Center. 2014. US religious landscape study. https://www.pewresearch.org.

Putnam, Robert. 2016. *Our kids: The American Dream in crisis.* New York: Simon & Schuster.

Runciman, Walter G. 1966. *Relative deprivation and social justice: A study of attitudes to social inequality in twentieth-century England.* London: Routledge & Kegan Paul.

Shiels, Meredith S., et al. 2020. Trends in mortality from drug poisonings, suicide, and alcohol-induced deaths in the United States from 2000 to 2017. *JAMA Open* 3 (9): 1–13.

Stephens, Nicole M., Sarah S.M. Townsend, and Andrea G. Dittmann. 2019. Social-class disparities in higher education and professional workplaces: The role of cultural mismatch. *Current Directions in Psychological Science* 28 (1): 67–73.

Wilkinson, Richard G., and Kate Pickett. 2009. *The spirit level: Why more equal societies almost always do better*. London: Allen Lane.

Chapter 5
Aging and Long-Term Care Problems During the Covid-19 Pandemic

Franca Maino and Marco Betti

Abstract The Covid-19 Pandemic, while disrupting many aspects of life, has had an enormous effect on the health care system in all countries, with long-term care (LTC) facilities being disproportionately affected. Nursing homes and senior living communities were in the difficult position of keeping older people safe while providing care and mitigating infection risks for patients and staff. At the same time, the pandemic brought into question the capacity of LTC systems' to efficiently respond to nontraditional societal needs: Older adults living at home experienced enormous consequences in their daily lives, such as loneliness, scarcity, and inadequate health care and LTC services and assistance. Beginning with a brief description of the welfare systems' characteristics, in this chapter we investigate the impact of the Covid-19 Pandemic on older adults across a selection of European countries during the past 3 years, including how care changed for LTC residents and older people living at home, and identify the main weaknesses of the LTC systems. We also identify facilitating factors of the difficulties and policy tools to help reform this sector by looking at the Pandemic as a possible window of opportunity to overcome the obstacles to building sustainable LTC systems. In fact, the European population over-80 is expected to more than double by 2050, leading to significantly increased demand for LTC. This demographic challenge has been accompanied by changing social patterns, such as smaller families, different residential patterns, and increased female labor force participation, all of which are contributing to an increased need for paid care and innovative services.

Keywords Covid-19 Pandemic · Long-term care problems · Long-term care systems · Social changes · Social policy · Long-term care policy

F. Maino (✉)
Dipartimento di Scienze Sociali e Politiche, Università degli Studi di Milano, Via Conservatorio 7, Milano, Italy
e-mail: franca.maino@unimi.it

M. Betti
Dipartimento di Scienze della Comunicazione, Università degli Studi di Teramo, Via Renato Balzarini 1, Teramo, Italy

C. Aspalter (ed.), *Covid-19 Pandemic*,
https://doi.org/10.1007/978-981-99-2497-4_5

Introduction

The Covid-19 Pandemic disrupted many aspects of life and has had an enormous effect on the health care delivery system in many countries, with long-term care (LTC) facilities being disproportionately affected. Nursing homes and senior living communities were in the difficult position of keeping older people safe while providing care and mitigating infection risks for patients and staff. At the same time, the pandemic called into question the capacity of LTC systems to respond efficiently to nontraditional societal needs: Older adults living at home faced enormous consequences in their daily lives, such as loneliness, scarcity, and inadequate health care and LTC services.

In this context, in this chapter we focus on the impact of the pandemic in a selection of European countries that belong to different "welfare regimes" (Ferrera, 1996; Castle et al., 2010; Greve, 2013): Denmark, representing the Nordic tradition or the Scandinavian regime; Germany, representing the Continental European or the Continental regime; Spain and Italy, representing the Southern European regime and two different trajectories from the original Mediterranean model; and the United Kingdom, representing the liberal or the Anglo-Saxon regime (Ranci and Pavolini 2013; Greve 2017; Daly et al. 2022). Our approach is characterized by an institutional perspective (Streeck and Thelen 2005) and focuses on institutional change in LTC policies during the past 30 years. The reforms implemented in the various countries contribute to the identification of different trajectories that conditioned the countries' response to the challenges posed by the Covid-19 Pandemic.

In general terms, LTC is one of the most rapidly developing policy areas, experiencing significant institutional change and innovation over the past few decades throughout the European continent. In contrast to the mainstream welfare policy (e.g., health care, education, and social security), LTC has seen a broader scope of transformations, ranging from retrenchment and cost containment to a growth in public financing and an expansion of coverage (Ranci and Pavolini, 2013).

Indeed, LTC policies have historically been less institutionalized because the need for care was considered a relatively new social risk compared with old social risks, such as poverty or unemployment (Taylor-Gooby, 2004; Ranci, 2010). Moreover, caring was considered a moral obligation to be shared by families and society and was constructed as women's responsibility rather than men's. Finally, these responsibilities have not been adequately recognized as formal social rights, such as paid leave, income support, or pension contributions (Ranci and Pavolini, 2013).

The institutional context changed, and debate in the public discussion did not emerge until the 1990s, when population aging became a more widespread and growing problem. Before then, the rights of people whose care was dependent on others had not been recognized (Leira and Saraceno, 2004). Thus, in the following decades, LTC policies became characterized by the recognition of social rights on the one hand and increased social responsibilities on the other (Morel, 2006).

The chapter is divided into three parts. In the first part, we describe the main trends and challenges that existed in the LTC sector before the Covid-19 outbreak, including how care changed for residents and older people living at home and identifying the main weaknesses of the different LTC regimes. In the second section, we describe the main trajectories of institutional change over the past 30 years and then focus on the main characteristics of LTC systems before the pandemic. According to our reading, the characteristics and evolutions of the various LTC regimes have helped condition the responses of individual governments. In the third section, we identify measures and policies that were introduced in the LTC sector as a response to the pandemic crisis. We conclude the chapter by focusing on what we have learned from the pandemic crisis and on policy tools to overcome the obstacles to reforming this sector by looking at the pandemic as a possible window of opportunity.

Trends and Challenges in the Long-Term Care Sector

In the paragraphs that follow, we provide a concise description of some trends in the countries under analysis. Using recent OECD data, we examine demographic changes, the role of informal carers, the characteristics of LTC workers and settings, and the financial dimension.

In regard to demographic trends (Fig. 5.1), in recent decades the share of the population age 65 years and over has nearly doubled, on average, across OECD countries, from less than 9% in 1960 to more than 17% in 2019, and today older people make up an increasing proportion of the population. In Italy, this share of the population will exceed one third by 2050. Similar values are observed in Spain, whereas in Denmark and the United Kingdom older adults will represent less than 25% of the population (in OECD countries, in the same period, this proportion will rise from 17.3% in 2019 to 26.7%).

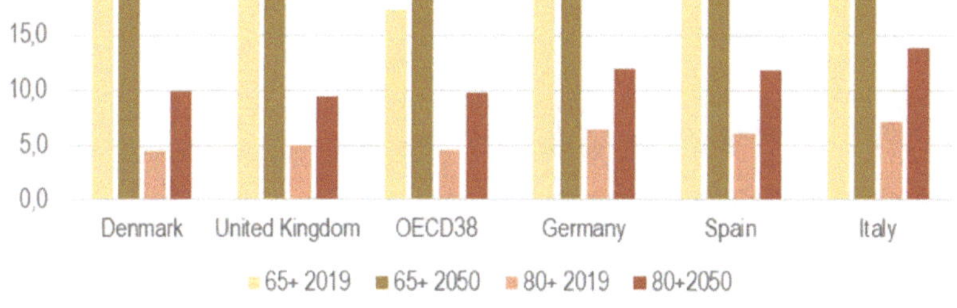

Fig. 5.1 Share of the Population Age 65 + and 80 +, 2019 and 2050. *Source* (OECD, 2022)

As is well known, family is one of the most crucial sources of care for people with LTC needs. However, because of the informal nature of the care they provide it is not easy to obtain accurate data on the number of people caring for family and friends across countries, or on the frequency of their caregiving. In Germany, 18% of people age 50 and over reported providing informal care at least weekly in 2019 (in OECD countries, this value is around 13%). On the other hand, Italy and Spain (Fig. 5.2) report much lower values. On average, across OECD countries, 62% of those providing daily informal care were women (Fig. 5.3). Spain had the most significant gender imbalance (76%), but other countries showed similar results, ranging from 62% in the United Kingdom to 65% in Italy.

LTC is also a labor-intensive service, and formal care (defined as paid staff, typically nurses and personal carers who provide care and/or assistance to people limited in their daily activities at home or in institutions, excluding hospitals) is in many cases a necessary complement to informal, unpaid family work. In regard to the education level of these workers, across OECD countries, less than one quarter held tertiary education (Fig. 5.4).[1] This value is higher in the United Kingdom than in Germany. Italy and Denmark, on the other hand, have similar values.

Moreover, nonstandard employment (including part-time and temporary work) is observed in the LTC sector (Fig. 5.5) as affecting women disproportionately. For instance, 47% of LTC workers in Germany work part-time, and a lower level is observed in Spain (where the share of temporary work is around 34%, contributing to job insecurity). The other countries, excluding the United Kingdom, show similar

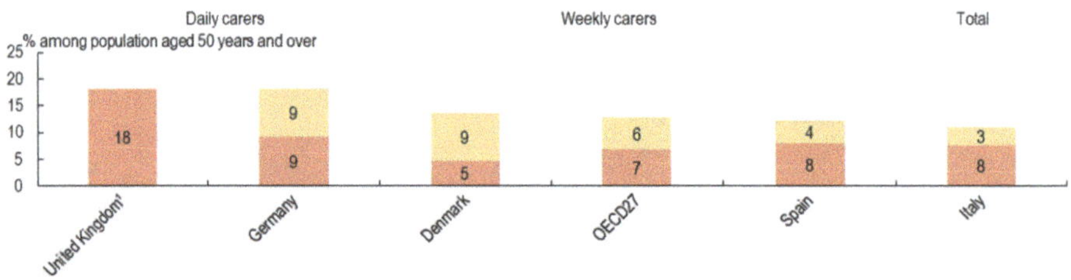

Fig. 5.2 Percentages of informal carers among the population age 50 +, 2019 (or nearest year). *Source* OECD (2022)

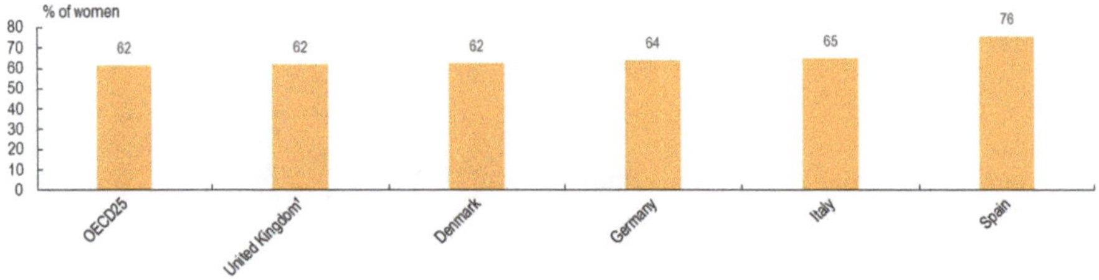

Fig. 5.3 Percentages of women among informal daily carers Age 50 +, 2019 (or nearest year). *Source* OECD (2022)

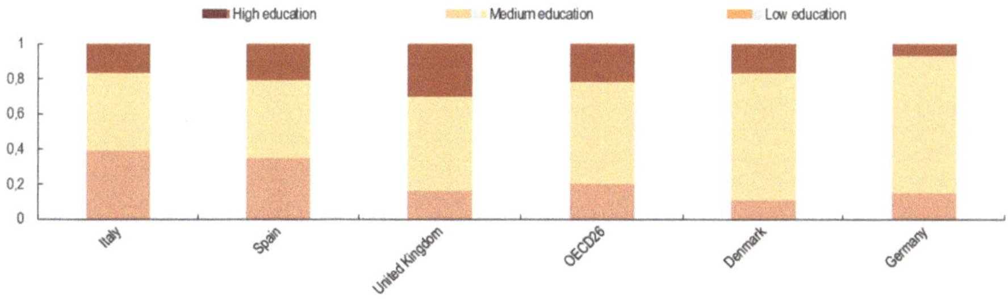

Fig. 5.4 Long-term care workers by level of education, 2019 (or nearest year). *Source* OECD (2022)

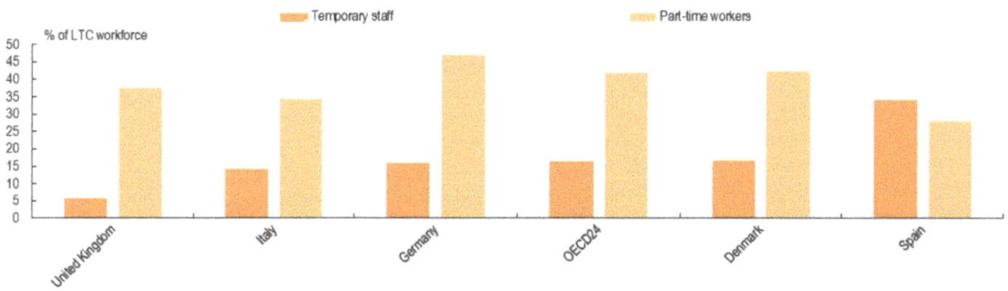

Fig. 5.5 Percentages of long-term care workers who work part time or on temporary contracts, 2019 (or nearest year). *Source* OECD (2022)

trends. Workers under this type of contract typically have less access to training and do not always have benefits (e.g., paid annual leave, low job security, and less access to social protection). In addition, a lack of continuity in staffing could affect the quality of care.

In regard to setting, although countries have increasingly taken steps to ensure that people in need of LTC services who wish to live in their homes for as long as possible can do so, many people will at some point require services that cannot be delivered at home. In this case, the number of beds in LTC facilities and LTC departments in hospitals offer a measure of the resources available to provide LTC services to individuals outside their homes. In 2019, across OECD countries, there were 46 beds per 1,000 people age 65 and over (Fig. 5.6), mainly located (43) in LTC facilities, with just three beds in hospitals. The number of beds varies enormously among the countries, ranging from 19 in Italy to 54 in Germany. More generally, between 2009 and 2019, OECD countries reduced the number of LTC beds in facilities by an average of 3 beds per 1,000 people age 65 and over (Fig. 5.7). The number of beds changed most significantly between Denmark (-22) and Spain (+13).

Finally, in regard to care spending and unit costs, LTC has seen the highest growth in recent years. In 2019, across OECD countries, 1.5% of GDP was allocated to LTC, including the health and social components (Fig. 5.8). The highest spender was Denmark, with a 3.6% GDP. Farther away, we noted that the United Kingdom and Germany have similar values, whereas Spain and Italy do not reach 1% GDP.

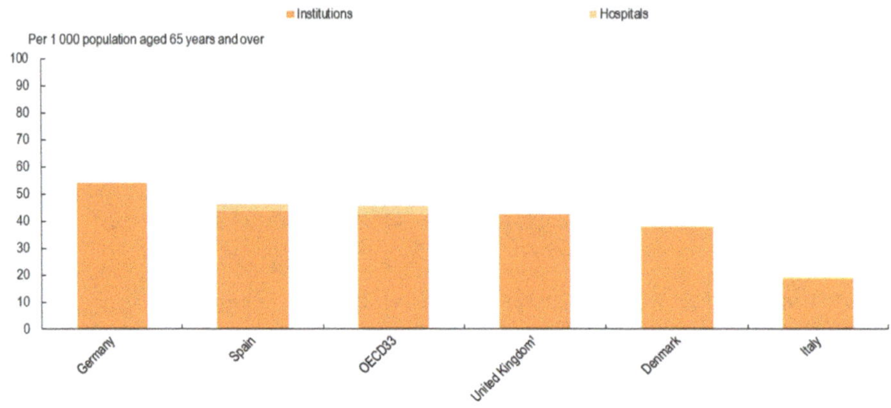

Fig. 5.6 Long-term care beds in institutions and hospitals, 2019 (or nearest year). *Source* (OECD, 2022)

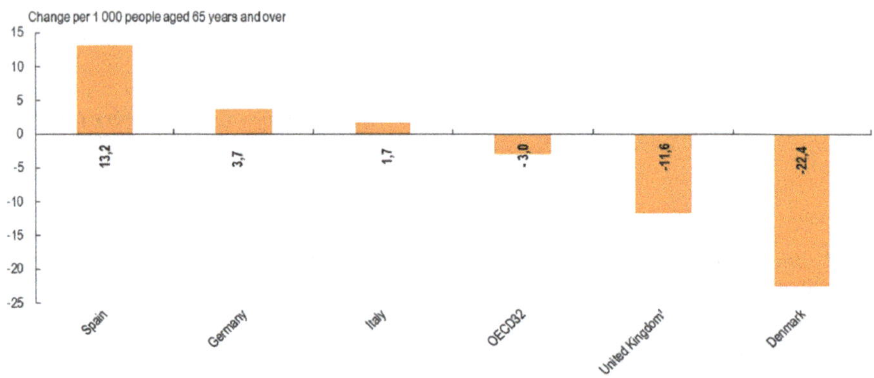

Fig. 5.7 Trends in long-term care beds in institutions and hospitals, 2009–2019 (or nearest year). *Source* (OECD, 2022)

In general, this variation partly mirrors differences in the population structure but mainly reflects the stage of development of formal LTC systems.

Pre-Pandemic Long-Term Care Reforms in Denmark, the United Kingdom, Germany, Spain, and Italy

Until the early 1990s, there were only two models of LTC in Europe: (a) a universalistic model, with levels of coverage above 20%, and (b) a residual model, with relatively lower coverage levels (usually below 10%) and higher reliance on family

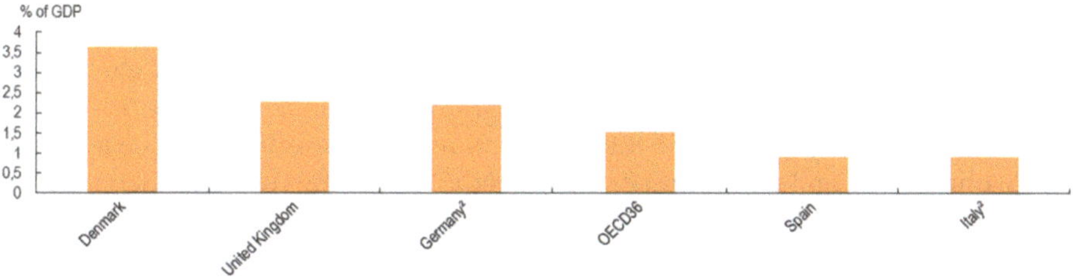

Fig. 5.8 Total long-term care spending as a share of GDP, 2019 (or nearest year). *Source* (OECD, 2022)

care and informal use of health services. The first model was composed of Scandinavian countries, whereas the Continental and Southern European ones belonged to the second. In this context, there was also a sub-model, represented by England and Italy. The two countries, although belonging respectively to the universal model and the residual one, shared a specificity: A large part of the coverage was obtained not through services but through cash/care allowances (the "Attendance Allowance" in England and the "Companion Allowance" in Italy; Pavolini and Ranci 2015).

Starting in the 1990s, the field of LTC policy changed radically. At the base of this transformation were two assumptions: (a) the population of older people who are not self-sufficient had grown a lot, and its needs had become more and more complex, and (b) the welfare responses designed for the previous context were inadequate to meet current needs. We briefly recall three factors: sociodemographic trends, financial costs, and cultural pressures (Pavolini and Ranci 2015). This phenomenon was simultaneously experienced in all our countries, with only slight differences.

In regard to sociodemographic pressures, the aging of the population contributed to a significant increase in the number of dependent people in need of care (Lafortune and Balestat, 2007). Moreover, the participation of women in the labor market grew, with negative effects on the supply of family care and an increase in demand for formal care services (Sarasa and Mestres, 2007; Saraceno, 2008). In this context, dependence—concentrated in the older population—emerged as a "new social risk" (Taylor-Gooby, 2004; Costa and Ranci, 2010; Maino, 2013).

The second source of pressure relates to cost containment, also linked to the fact that the older population often is entitled to other welfare services (such as pension). Therefore, the LTC reforms need to be framed as part of a broader trade-off between retrenchment and restructuring trends in traditional welfare policies (e.g., pensions, education, or health care) and expansion in newer forms of social risk coverage. As we have seen, these trends are linked with the sociodemographic pressures referred to earlier, leading to increased pensions and national health care systems costs due to the aging population. Meanwhile, social assistance systems, often financed by national or local social assistance programs, have been stressed under the push of a considerable mass of dependent older people seeking care services (Österle, 2001).

The third relevant pressure is related to cultural attitude towards care. Although demand for professional care services dominated the 1970s and the 1980s, a new orientation, toward efficiency and flexibility, predominated in the 1990s (Daly and Lewis, 1998). This change was also the result of a twofold convergence: On the one hand, the role of New Public Management, seeking a formalization and marketization of service provision (Ascoli and Ranci, 2002), and on the other, new ideas about self-determination and empowerment. Influential groups representing people with disabilities started calling for freedom of choice, welfare pluralism, and cash-for-care measures (Da Roit and Le Bihan, 2010).

Given this context, the characteristics of the LTC reforms introduced in the last three decades and the institutional change brought about by these reforms before the pandemic are described in the following two sections.

Long-Term Care Reforms: Main Characteristics and Achievements

These pressures led to a profound rethinking of the model of care. The countries with a previous universalistic LTC model—England and Denmark—did not explicitly introduce significant changes. Despite that, market rules were introduced in terms of free choice and greater competition among providers (Ranci and Pavolini, 2015).

In England, publicly funded adult social care coverage has shrunk significantly, and intensive home care services are provided only to those with the highest levels of need. As a consequence, many people are excluded from publicly funded residential or domiciliary care because of modest assets and/or income levels. In addition, with the introduction of quasi-markets, care services have become more fragmented. At the same time, personal budgets are shifting responsibilities for managing resources and risks onto individual older people and their families. Further instabilities arise from the division of responsibility for social care between the central government and local authorities. Research has shown how these reforms were introduced not to exercise tighter control over public spending on social care but to alter how existing limited resources are allocated and used (Glendinning, 2013: 196–197).

In Denmark, changes did not touch either coverage levels or accessibility criteria. Reform of LTC policies can be seen as a case of substantial change through restructuring—originating from cost containment related to the dominant discourse of New Public Management—rather than retrenchment. Reforms introduced control and flexibility elements that gradually yet substantially changed the organization of LTC. More specifically, the existing institutions of universality, localism, the home helper, and the principle of "at home as long as possible" have been redefined with new elements, including free choice, standards, and centralism.

New tensions between control and flexibility emerged in response to this change, especially in the relations between central and local levels and the interactions between users and professionals. On the one hand, free choice encapsulates a radical form of decentralization and focuses on individual service providers rather than the local authorities. Conversely, the flexibility inherent in micro-level market interactions is severely limited by public control of the emerging market (Burau and Dahl 2013: 92–93). In addition, the central government also regulates the activities of local authorities in an increasingly detailed way (Dahl 2011). Denmark recently reduced spending on LTC but also increased the focus on rehabilitation and welfare technology. The balance between these issues seems to be a central aspect of the LTC welfare state's development in the coming years (Greve 2018: 26).

In contrast, all the countries except Italy, characterized at the beginning of the 1990s by a residual LTC model, have gradually introduced significant paradigmatic policy changes aimed at expanding LTC coverage and generosity and establishing a principle of universalism. The reforms introduced share a common approach to care support, differentiated according to the level of dependence of the beneficiaries and provided through three or four different levels of provision. However, only Germany adopted a strictly "social insurance model" (Ranci and Pavolini 2015).

With the introduction of LTC, Germany established a social support system related to LTC needs. The scheme aimed to combine new social risk with the cost-containment efforts and created a new type of universalism, characterized by comparatively high thresholds, a medium level of support, and cash benefits to maintain family care provision on a lower level. Because the scheme fundamentally restructured both funding—social and mandatory private insurance—and social care rights and defined the principles for the reorganization of care provision, the mechanism for change can be described as both *radical change* (in terms of the restructuring of care rights and funding) and *incremental transformation* (related to the reorganization of care provision). This reform also expanded formal care work on different qualification levels and impetuses for the professionalization of care work even though this occurred in a context of gradual deterioration of employment conditions.

The LTC was widely supported in Germany. The basic principles of the scheme, including free choice and the emphasis on family care, correspond with traditional societal values. However, despite increasing public support, various aspects of the scheme—such as the design of social rights, the mix of private and public funding, and the organization of care provision—have resulted in care gaps for specific groups and emerging inequalities among beneficiaries (Theobald and Hampel, 2013: 132–133). Moreover, private for-profit ownership as well as the market logic should be reconsidered, because competition leads to cost reduction and rationalization that affect workers and residents and thus the quality of care (Müller, 2018: 46). The most recent reforms, adopted between 2015 and 2019, were aimed at extending eligibility by reforming the definition and assessment method of "in need of care." The greatest challenge today is the recruitment of sufficient numbers of professional LTC staff (EC, 2021b: 70).

In Spain, the Dependency Act came into force in January 2007, aiming to create a universalistic LTC system. First, the Spanish model is one of shared responsibility among the dependent persons, families, and the public sector, and it favors the freedom to choose from among a limited set of different care arrangements. In other words, it seems to foster a new ethos of joint responsibility. Second, the system for autonomy and care for dependency is the outcome of converging social and demographic changes and the mobilization of social and institutional actors in favor of the reform (in particular, the third sector and social partners through social dialogue). Third, it is also a care model, which replaces the social assistance logic with a universal approach built around an institutional setup in which state and autonomous regions are obliged to cooperate. Despite this, this situation has often caused territorial heterogeneity and inequalities in terms of coverage, benefit types, and the social impact of the reform. Finally, the coverage was continually increased, but more because of cash benefits than services. This circumstance is mainly the result of the continued existence of a social structure of informal care (which the 2008 economic crisis partly reinforced); the limited supply of social services; and public spending conservatism, which has diminished investment in social service infrastructures. Care recipients' preference for cash benefits is backed up by the offer of relatively cheap migrant labor, to which frail older people and their families often resort (Cabrero and Gallego, 2013: 218).

The greatest challenge for the Spanish LTC system is improving its effectiveness. This will require reducing high waiting lists for access to services, expanding the supply of home and community services, making community care benefits more flexible and compatible, further developing the system for autonomy and care for dependency in rural areas, standardizing the criteria for copayments in autonomous communities, strengthening the reconciliation between informal care and working life, and improving coordination between the central and regional administrations (EC, 2021b: 134).

Among the countries that have adopted the residual LTC model we must also consider Italy, which, unlike what has been observed in Germany and Spain, has not undergone any reform in recent decades. In other words, no relevant LTC policy changes have taken place in the past 30 years, and the only intervention has been related to the regularization of migrants (Costa, 2013).[2] Therefore, the system seems to be shaped mainly around informal and migrant care work as a cheap way to deal with LTC issues, thus limiting public investment (Van Hooren, 2012). As Maino and Razetti (2020) pointed out, the peculiarity of the Italy case consists of a polarization in the supply of LTC interventions between two poles: (a) informal family-based home care solutions and (b) full institutionalization. This situation is linked to the shortcomings (in some cases, the full absence) of intermediate solutions that in other countries have been established to bridge the gap between pure informal home care assistance provided by families and residential health care-driven assistance. Recently, the context has shifted and, as we will see below, space is opening up for reform, the outcome of which, however, remains uncertain.

This institutional inertia has paradoxically contributed to a significant transformation in Italy's care regime that, following a path of incremental institutional change, has ultimately resulted in a largely unintended extension of the public provision through the main cash allowance program. From a cash benefit primarily used to cover an adult dependent's additional income needs, the main cash allowance program has become a financial resource that allows dependent older people to purchase the low-cost care services offered in the private market. The relatively low amount of this benefit has been compensated by the availability of a large number of migrant care workers who are willing to accept low salaries. However, this change has produced numerous inequalities while the ambiguity of public regulation of migration has fueled an illegal labor market (Pavolini, Ranci and Lamura 2017). Moreover, there are no national standards guiding home care and residential care, and many decisions and evaluation criteria are delegated to the regional and municipal levels. This situation produces extreme heterogeneity in evaluation conditions and access criteria (EC, 2021b: 182).

Long-Term Care Reforms and Pre-Pandemic Institutional Change

While all European LTC systems have faced a similar trade-off since the 1990s, between the emergence of a new social risk—dependency—and cost-containment pressures, they diverged in how this policy dilemma was institutionally filtered and framed. Denmark, considered one of the Scandinavian universalistic countries, faced more severe financial constraints, given the country's already-developed LTC system. As a consequence, cost-containment measures were adopted that were not presented as a paradigmatic challenge; on the contrary, in countries with a residual LTC model, demand-side and financial pressures from other welfare sectors were strong, and existing services could not manage the rising social demand. It thus was necessary for a paradigmatic change and the introduction of national programs defining new entitlements and the corresponding financial constraints. In Italy and England, nationwide cash-based measures that were already in place—even with limited resources to beneficiaries—offered an institutional buffer against the need for radical reforms. In other words, the limited expansion of services (or even their cutbacks) was partially compensated by the diffusion of cash programs (Pavolini and Ranci 2015).

Adopting the typology proposed by Streeck and Thelen (2005), which uses the concepts of *gradual transformation*, *reproduction by adaptation*, and *breakdown and replacement*, we can describe how institutional change has taken place in five countries (Denmark, the United Kingdom, Germany, Spain, and Italy) up to the pandemic crisis. In Table 1 we summarize this brief historical reconstruction, focusing on reforms from the 1970s to 2012, the type of institutional change, and the effects on public financing. The institutional change approach also appears particularly useful for understanding the trajectory of the LTC in various countries and its current configuration at the dawn of the pandemic.

In Denmark, change was characterized by "reproduction by adaptation." Market rules and consumerist approaches were introduced, but rationing did not come into the picture. The regulation was concerned with both securing and extending the welfare rights of citizens and, as a consequence, encompassed both measures of control and standards of choice/flexibility. England showed a gradual transformation process by altering the access to and generosity of LTC programs and adding new care measures. This trend could be seen as an implicit attack on universalism, focusing attention on a more targeted use of public care services (Glendinning, 2013). Despite that, the evaluation of the reform is more complicated; the decrease in services' coverage was, in fact, numerically compensated by the increase in the attendance allowance.

On the contrary, in residual LTC models, the role of users' associations was less relevant and mainly directed at maintaining the existing system, based on nationally organized neo-corporatist actors that saw LTC reforms as part of a broader restructuring/dismantling of the welfare state. In Germany, the reform introduced in 1995 was proposed by a coalition government between the Christian Democratic Party and the Liberal Party, with the agreement of the Social Democratic Party and trade unions. Similar coalitions were active in Spain. In terms of institutional mechanisms, the change was characterized by a breakdown-and-replacement process. The capacity to build a general political agreement around a specific reform project was not present in Italy, where the fragmentation of the policy field, the territorial inequalities, and the preference for cash programs—already in place—dissuaded any attempt at reform. Despite that, a process of institutional change took place, and the recalibration of the whole LTC system made the existing national cash-based allowance the type of LTC provision used by an increasing number of dependent people.

In Italy, although no reform has been introduced since the 1980s, a process of institutional change nonetheless took place. The failure to provide adequate welfare despite external changes resulted in slippages in institutional practice (Hacker, 2004). In other words, this institutional inertia without recalibration of the whole LTC system made the existing national cash-based allowance the type of provision used by an increasing number of severely dependent older people. From this point of view, Italy shared a path of change similar to England (Ranci and Pavolini 2015).

The Pandemic and Its Consequences: Measures and Policy in the Long-Term Care Sector

The Covid-19 Pandemic—from the first wave to the subsequent ones—has had a substantial impact on LTC systems, and European countries have had to take measures to urgently protect care recipients and caregivers. Different sources[3] have shown that LTC systems have been significantly affected by the pandemic because of their users' high vulnerability to Covid-19. High mortality rates in care homes in the first wave of the pandemic raised severe concerns about the capacity of LTC systems to cope with emergencies. In most member states, residential care providers were largely unprepared for the epidemiological threat, including in regard to insufficient sanitary procedures related to the isolation of potentially infected people, shortages of personal protective equipment, inadequate testing, and staff shortages. In Table 5.2 we provide an overview of the emergency preparedness systems in our five countries at the time of the Covid-19 outbreak.

The pandemic amplified the existing structural challenges caused by the aging population and affected access, affordability, quality, workforce, informal carers,

Table 5.1 Long-term care reforms, types of institutional change, and effects on public financing (1970–2020)

Country	Reforms from 1970s to 2020			Types of institutional change (Streeck and Thelen 2005)	The effects on public financing
	Situation in 1970–1980	Main reform since the 1990s	Other reforms following the main one (if present)		
Denmark	Universalistic	None	Re-centralization (1990s) Restructuring • "Common Language" (1998) • "Free choice" in homecare (2002)	Reproduction by adaptation	Restructuring
Great Britain	Semi-universalistic	None	Community care reforms (1990s)	Gradual transformation: layering and displacement (services), drift (allowance)	Retrenchment risks/responsibilities shifting from LAs to individual older people and their families
Germany	Residual	The Care Insurance Reform (1994)	• Cost-containment policies (since 2000s) with an increase in benefits in 2008 • Complementary Nursing Act (2002)	Breakdown and Replacement	Expansion (in the 1990s) with some retrenchment in the 2000s (cost-containment considerations have continuously worked as a limiting factor)
Spain	Residual	Dependency Law (2006)	Slow and fragmented implementation of the new care system	Breakdown and Replacement	Expansion
Italy	Residual	None	Piecemeal regularization of migrant care work (since 1990s)	Gradual transformation, Drift	Unplanned (partial) expansion

Source Authors' elaboration on Ranci and Pavolini (2013, 2015) and sustainability of LTC. Therefore, countries have implemented several policy measures to counter the negative consequences of Covid-19 in the LTC sector.

During the first wave of the pandemic (March-July 2020), ad hoc measures were promptly introduced. The nature of LTC services, which implies close physical contact, made service delivery increasingly challenging in times of social distancing measures. Member states have limited access to LTC services to reduce the risk of spreading Covid-19: day care centers were subject to restricted access or temporarily closed, and home care access was reduced or limited to strictly necessary visits. In addition, residential care has been more difficult to access, and the placement of new residents in residential care was temporarily restricted. To ensure access to LTC, in many countries caregiving via telecommunication has been reinforced, and the use of telephone communications and teleconsultations between caregivers, patients, and health professionals has increased.

In addition, informal care compensated for a significant share of previously provided care professionals and, in some cases, also for the higher costs related to measures against Covid-19. At the same time, people in need of LTC preferred to reduce or not use informal or formal LTC, to minimize their risk of contracting Covid-19; however, the number of those less able to afford LTC increased because of the economic downturn. For this reason, some member states have introduced temporary support or even reinforced financing. Germany, for example, increased the monthly allowance for personal hygiene equipment for people in need of care. The overall picture suggests that unmet LTC needs have increased during the pandemic, and the challenge of LTC affordability became a severe problem (EC, 2021b).

In regard to the first weeks and months of the pandemic, Daly et al. (2022) analyzed the major responses to the virus in our case study countries, where quite a significant variation emerged (Table 5.3). In general, in regard to lockdown, Germany and Denmark introduced precautionary measures regarding access and isolation early on, but in England, Spain and Italy the care homes were not prioritized. Moreover, in regard to testing and monitoring, in England, Italy, and Spain testing was heavily rationed, with supplies mainly concentrated in hospitals. This meant that infection and mortality rates in care homes were probably hidden. Denmark encountered a shortage of testing equipment, too; however, care homes were neither ignored nor downgraded vis-à-vis hospitals because they were already included in national prevention guidelines. Also in Germany, from the first week onward, care homes were recognized as legitimate targets for the testing strategy adopted as part of the country's integrated approach.

Protecting LTC recipients and carers from Covid-19 was and is essential and required innovative solutions. Covid-19, in fact, brought into focus the need to balance patient well-being with patient survival, challenging the capacity of LTC systems to provide adequate and high-quality care. Member states have taken several measures to limit the adverse effects of the pandemic on the well-being of care home residents and to protect the most vulnerable older people. In our five countries, soon after the start of the pandemic particular meeting areas were designed; contacts with visitors were carried out using telephones or video tools; or, when visits were allowed,

Table 5.2 Emergency preparedness systems in Denmark, Germany, Italy, Spain, and the United Kingdom in 2020

	Long-Term Care Emergency System: Main Traits
Denmark	• Denmark had guidelines surrounding infection control in the LTC sector before 2020 and has a permanent task force, the National Operational Staff, which includes a plethora of authorities • Other guidelines have been published during the Covid-19 Pandemic, including those relating to the ban of visits to LTC facilities, except for dying patients, as well as infection prevention during external visits, when the ban was lifted • The Danish Health Authority is chairing a "Covid-19 Task Force on Hospital Capacity," with representatives from national authorities and the Danish regions
Germany	• There were pandemic plans in place at the national and local levels before 2020 and, since 2001, the Infection Protection Act, together with laws and ordinances issued at the Länder level, has regulated infection control at the federal level. Nevertheless, the LTC sector was overlooked until 2020, when a task force was created to support LTC institutions facing the pandemic • Germany also has task forces, at the national and subnational levels. As an example, in the federal state of Bavaria, an LTC-specific infectiology task force is required to be mobilized if a Covid-19 outbreak happens in an LTC facility
Italy	• The governmental website of the Department of Civil Protection regularly publishes information on several emergencies and risks, including health emergencies • Both the Ministry of Health and the Higher Institute of Health (Istituto Superiore di Sanità) had developed guidelines on national emergency plans as well as more specific plans for pandemic flu before 2020, without the inclusion of specific measures for the LTC sector • In 2020, the Higher Institute of Health published the first instructions and guidelines for prevention of and control over the spread of infection in LTC facilities. Specific guidelines for the LTC sector were also developed at the regional and local levels • Italy has also organized several task forces both at the national (Scientific Technical Committee, Comitato Tecnico Scientifico) and regional levels
Spain	• Before 2020, the Spanish government had published influenza national plans with some specific measures foreseen for the LTC sector, but the specific training exercises—although foreseen in the plans—had not yet been tested • The national government has authorized the regional governments to take over the management of facilities (both public and private) and rapid response teams have been deployed as part of the National Aged Care Emergency Response
United Kingdom	• Since 2020, the Ministry of Health has devoted a page of its website to older people and LTC • The United Kingdom has paid growing attention to the LTC sector during the Covid-19 Pandemic, through specific guidance on the admission and care of residents in care homes and the creation of a capacity tracker for LTC facilities

Source Authors' elaboration on Rocard et al. (2021: 86–89)

Table 5.3 Policy measures implemented during 2020 to protect long-term care recipients and workers from Covid-19 and to maintain continuity of care during the crisis

Policy measures country	Improve access to PPE (Funding or direct distribution)	Prioritized testing of care home residents and staff	Restrictions withinfacilities (Restricted visits, isolation measures)	Boosting staff numbers (Funding or staff redeployment)	Expanded telehealth services	Coordination between LTC and primary care/ hospital	Change in regulations/ inspections	Prioritized vaccination of care home residents and staff
Denmark	Yes	Yes	Yes	Yes	Yes	Yes	Yes	Yes
Germany	Yes	Yes	Yes	Yes	No	Yes	Yes	Yes
Italy	Yes	Yes	Yes	Yes	Yes	Yes	No	Yes
Spain	Yes	Yes	Yes	Yes	No	No	No	No
United Kingdom	Yes	Yes	Yes	Yes	Yes	No	No	Yes

Source Authors' elaboration on Rocard et al. (2021: 25)

their rules were revised to ensure visitors were not showing any Covid-related symptoms. To stop the infection from spreading through care homes, external visits were banned, residents were often isolated from one another, and visits from carers were limited to attending to their basic needs.

People in need of LTC living at home experienced loneliness and anxiety during the pandemic. To help them, community-based social services were provided by digital technologies. In many cases, civil society organizations and the private sector played an important role. Some local administrations allocated funds to civil society associations to enable them to help counteract loneliness among older people through outreach activities by telephone or digital meetings and to help with food purchases.

Covid-19 has negatively affected the working conditions of the LTC workforce and has led to a more complex situation for informal carers. Although working conditions were already challenging in the LTC sector before the pandemic, Covid-19 has put even more pressure on social workers. Workers have, in many cases, been exposed to higher stress levels because of increased uncertainty regarding the evolution of the situation, pressure to protect their care recipients, and anxiety over getting infected themselves. At the beginning of the crisis, the LTC sector faced shortages in personal protective equipment and tests to adequately protect employees and users. Shortages of workers worsened during the crisis, as infected carers or carers at risk of having been infected had to quarantine and were unavailable to do their job.

Member states have introduced a wide range of measures to support LTC workers during the crisis, ranging from providing personal protective equipment to prioritizing LTC workers for testing and special accommodation and transport for LTC workers. A few member states provided psychological support to LTC workers. Many member states made efforts to increase the pool of available staff in the first part of the pandemic, either by mobilizing workers from other sectors, including the health care sector, or by recruiting volunteers, medical students, and retirees, as in Germany and Italy. Other measures to accommodate the increased pressure on and demand for LTC workers included bans on firing LTC workers (as in the case of Spain) and relaxed working time regulations. Member states with a high number of foreign workers eased the entry of LTC workers and live-in carers from the other Member States. Germany introduced measures to acknowledge the problematic situation of LTC staff by providing bonus payments for LTC workers or live-in caregivers. Covid-19 put additional strain on informal carers, too. Reductions in the availability of formal care services, in particular day care centers, would lead to more people having to step in to provide informal care to someone in their family and an increasing workload for people already providing informal care. Several member states have reported increased reliance on informal care during the pandemic. Member states introduced support measures for informal carers during the pandemic, including special care leave. Germany introduced the right to receive a caregiver allowance as a wage replacement benefit for an extended period of up to 20 working days (instead of 10 days) to provide or organize care in situations caused by the pandemic.

Member states have provided financial support to strengthen LTC systems during the pandemic and to implement measures to protect LTC beneficiaries. The additional costs for LTC systems have been mainly caused by introducing new hygiene measures (e.g., purchasing personal protective equipment, providing tests, and making adaptations to buildings) and by premiums for staff working during the crisis. Member states have made additional funding available to support LTC systems during the pandemic, as in the case of Germany and Denmark. In systems with subnational competencies, such as Denmark, Germany, Spain, and Italy, the state, in most cases, made grants available to regions and municipalities to finance the extraordinary burden of care.

Covid-19 affected LTC reforms beyond the ad hoc measures taken during the crisis. The crisis spurred a public debate on the shortcomings and weaknesses in the system in most of the member states and may influence planned or ongoing reforms. Some member states started to introduce structural changes to the LTC system in response to Covid-19 that remained in place after the crisis. In France, the law of 7 August 2020 on social debt and autonomy created a fifth sector of the National Health System, dedicated to the loss of autonomy of older people and people with disabilities, with €1 billion funding. It is the first step in a global reform of the French organization. The Netherlands intends to strengthen the connection and collaboration between LTC and health care and to focus research on pandemic-related issues. Germany planned to present further measures relating to the efficiency, financing, and staffing of LTC.

Health and LTC services reform entered the political agenda in Italy and is at the core of the Resilience and Recovery National Plan. The Draghi government, formed in February 2021, has created two Ministerial commissions to examine care and support for older people. The government's priorities included learning from and mitigating the impact of Covid-19 on the delivery of care and accelerating the introduction of a structural LTC reform. In October 2021 the Draghi government approved a Delegated Act that the Parliament approved in March 2023 under the new center-right government led by the Prime Minister Giorgia Meloni. Italy's new LTC act aims to facilitate and ensure the implementation of LTC as the new pillar of care assistance for older people: This will take the form of integrated activities, allowing people to enjoy independence and security for as long as possible. The Italian government has committed itself to a comprehensive reform of LTC, that now needs the Legislative Decrees to fully entered into force and to be implemented. The main aim of the proposed reform is to strengthen the integration of social care and health care, which is a prerequisite for ensuring quality and affordable LTC for all age groups. The Italian LTC is centered on the cash-for-care, unconditional and universalistic measure, the Companion Allowance. In the last 30 years, none of the reform proposals have succeeded in passing. From 2021, the long-term care sector, however, has gained ground with an increase in non-self-sufficient people (3.8 million, 5% of the elderly population) and the worsening of older people's condition due to the emergency. The Covid-19 pandemic has marked a "watershed" in the pre-existing scenario. First, it raised public and private actors' awareness of the long-term care sector's shortcomings due to high mortality rates among elderly people in nursing homes and the digression of relational poverty. Second, the Resilience and Recovery National Plan opened a window of opportunity to achieve structural reform, also supported by an advocacy coalition—the Pact for new welfare for non-self-sufficiency—that arose to push for long-term care reform. The reform must be completed by 2024, and the outcome is still uncertain: It can be radical or incremental. However, the path to close the gap between Italy and other European LTC systems seems now open.

The crisis strongly affected LTC systems and made clear structural weaknesses in the five countries we considered. The pandemic has put LTC recipients, a very vulnerable population, at health and loneliness risk, affected their well-being, and limited their access to formal LTC services. The pandemic had strong implications for LTC workers and informal caregivers. Member states have made great efforts to implement measures to protect LTC recipients and support LTC workers and informal caregivers. To do so, they have made significant additional funding available. But the ongoing pandemic crisis has shown that more investment and reforms are needed to tackle the weaknesses in the LTC sector and the lack of financial resources, and the insufficient organization, management, or coordination of LTC services. Although the full effects on LTC systems are not clear and are still changing, the Covid-19 crisis will likely have long-lasting impacts on the LTC sector. The situation may require a review of the provision of LTC services and the organization and financing of LTC policies, influencing choices on the social and financial sustainability of current LTC provision.

Conclusion

It is too early to assess how deep and lasting the effect of the pandemic crisis on LTC will be, as the crisis is still ongoing. As discussed, a few countries have introduced structural changes to their LTC systems that may remain in place after the crisis. Some, such as Italy, are involved in the process of structural reform (that might lead to a "breakdown and replacement" type of institutional change), but the result is still uncertain.[4] In addition, many countries are still in a phase where short-term crisis management is the priority, and it is too premature to evaluate the feasibility of making some temporary measures permanent (EC, 2021b). Although likely to be significant, it is also too early to determine the severe and long-term effects of the Covid-19 crisis on LTC systems and how it may also affect the mindsets of policymakers and public opinion about redesigning LTC policies. It is therefore important to draw lessons from the crisis to improve long-term strategies on a structural basis and make them more resilient in the future.

The LTC sector was heavily touched by the pandemic crisis, as shown by the high number of infections and deaths among older adults. Delays in prioritization of containment and weak mitigation measures, as well as delays in testing LTC workers and recipients, generated delays in the definition and implementation of adequate policies. After the first two waves, older people more broadly, and those in LTC institutions in particular, have been prioritized in the ongoing Covid-19 vaccination plans in many countries. Vaccine effectiveness has made a clear impact on LTC systems. Such positive developments should not jeopardize the urgency of ensuring that LTC is better prepared to face future emergencies.

During the pandemic, models of care were questioned. Most older adults prefer to stay in their homes as long as possible, but many countries have insufficient home care services. Home-based options may limit infection transmission but require adequate personal protective equipment and job quality for LTC workers. Institutional care will still be necessary for older dependent people but must be made safer and more people centered. This means reforming the LTC policies to guarantee residents better living conditions and quality of life.

The pandemic has amplified the need to improve infection control and prevention. Countries have now developed specific Covid-19 infection control protocols and enhanced training for staff. In the future, ensuring relevant training and ways to deploy experts regularly is likely to reduce preventable safety failures. This requires providing access to information and resources in the form of guidelines and procedures on infection prevention to ensure all facilities establish safe routines for care. Several countries are now recommending that LCT facilities should have one or more trained infection control officers as a condition for accreditation and to deploy accredited infection prevention and control experts into residential care homes to provide training and assist with the preparation of outbreak management plans (Rocard et al., 2021).

The LTC sector was ill prepared to face a health emergency. Although many measures were taken during the pandemic to improve the sector's performance, more needs to be done (Rocard et al., 2021). Some countries are now recommending that LTC preparedness for health emergencies requires regular and specific assessments of readiness at the facility level and in home-care settings.[5] The recommendations include having a contingency plan or guidelines for each facility and adapting it. The challenges in making protocols operational depend on the definition of clear responsibilities, infrastructure capacity, and the role of health professionals. Alternative solutions for intermediate care and appropriate coordination channels with health care professionals must be available and implemented for future health emergencies. Response plans for LTC homes must also include using technology and other digitalized means to connect residents with family and friends and for safe visits. A clear communication plan with residents' families and transparency in communications should be part of a new strategy.

The pandemic has reopened the debate on the LTC workforce, care quality, and safety. Several countries highlighted concerns about staff ratios, shortages, and skill mismatches before the pandemic. Solutions for rapidly replacing individuals on sick leave and training new personnel need to be found. Rapid staff recruitment and retention will remain challenging without addressing adequate pay and improving job quality. Promoting social dialogue and collective bargaining can be a tool to enhance the quality of jobs in the sector and provide solutions for professional development. The lack of sufficient, qualified medical staff with skills to deal with complex cases and structural problems involving insufficient coordination with the rest of the health care system also need to be addressed. Covid-19 has also stressed the physical and psychosocial risks associated with LTC jobs pointing out the necessity for a broader mental health approach and a more intensive support.

The pandemic has also revealed the lack of standardized, comprehensive, and timely data collection in the LTC sector. Much data on LTC to provide a complete and accurate analysis of staffing (e.g., hours worked by LTC workers, sickness absence), job quality, care quality, and outcomes, are still missing. Overall, policy experts and policymakers agree on the insufficient evidence of the impact of policies on the sector. In that respect, a good data set will be the first step toward generating a more robust culture of evaluation and evidence-based policymaking in LTC and ensuring that quality standards are appropriately measured and enforced to guarantee minimum standards of care in the future.

As we have discussed, the quality of LTC is affected by funding and related sustainability issues, including workforce conditions, organization, and technology. An adequate workforce is strategic to meeting the rising demand for high-quality services, but difficult working conditions and low salaries may contribute to staff shortages. Moreover, if investment in skills and new technologies is key to improving efficiency, digitalization and ICT technology can have ambiguous effects on both working conditions and organization (EC, 2021a: 59). On the one hand, technology can improve the quality of the services provided. For example, ensuring timely visits, freeing up carers to spend more time socializing with users, making services more personalized, and increasing users' independence. Remote care management—as in the case of innovative home applications and virtual medical visits - can also improve health outcomes and can be particularly beneficial for older people in their homes and in residential care. On the other hand, there are several challenges, such as the risk of reduced human contact—which could increase loneliness—issues related to practical usage and malfunctioning of technical solutions, which could negatively affect the level of users' trust, insufficient digital skills among both older people and their caregivers, access and organization, and data protection.

Notes

1. OECD define tertiary education as a level or stage of studies beyond secondary education. Such studies are undertaken in tertiary education institutions, such as public and private universities, colleges, and polytechnics, and also in a wide range of other settings, such as secondary schools, worksites, and vocational courses. It includes undergraduate and graduate credentials that encompass certificates, diplomas or academic degrees.
2. Regularization is a State's policy response to the presence of irregular migrants residing in a given country. Each country has its own regularization procedures. Italy had long been a country of emigration, and a comprehensive migrant policy was absent until the 1980s. Since 2000, large-scale regularizations and the enlargement of the EU have changed the migration flow into Italy (Bettio et al., 2006). In 2013, the number of foreign nationals in Italy exceeded 4.4 million, and the share of the foreign-born population accounted for 9.4% (Miyazaki 2019). Italy has thus become one of the largest host countries for migrant workers in Europe.
3. See the OECD Observatory on Policy Responses to the Covid-19 Crisis (https://www.oecd.org/els/health-systems) and, among others, European Commission (2021a,b).
4. The uncertainty is also due to the Draghi government crisis in July and the early elections scheduled for fall 2022.

5. Such assessments would include evaluation of infrastructure, resident characteristics, human resources, material resources, protocols for different scenarios, and evaluation for the revision and actualizations of protocols.

References

Ascoli, U., and C. Ranci, eds. 2002. *Dilemmas of the welfare mix: The new structure of welfare in an era of privatization.* New York: Springer.

Bettio, F., A.M. Simonazzi, and P. Villa. 2006. Change in care regimes and female migration: The 'care drain' in the Mediterranean. *Journal of European Social Policy* 16 (3): 271–285.

Burau, V., and H.M. Dahl. 2013. Trajectories of change in Danish long-term care policies: Reproduction by adaptation through top-down and bottom-up reforms, In: *Reforms in long-term care policies in Europe: Investigating institutional change and social impacts*, eds. C. Ranci and E. Pavolini, New York: Springer.

Cabrero, G.R., and V.-M. Gallego. 2013. Long-term care in Spain: Between family care tradition and the public recognition of social risks, In: *Reforms in long-term care policies in Europe: Investigating institutional change and social impacts*, eds. C. Ranci and E. Pavolini, New York: Springer.

Castles, F.G., S. Leibfried, J. Lewis, H. Obinger, and C. Pierson, eds. 2010. *The Oxford handbook of the welfare state.* Oxford: Oxford University Press.

Costa, G. 2013. Long-term care Italian policies: A case of inertial institutional change, In: *Reforms in long-term care policies in Europe: Investigating institutional change and social impacts*, eds. C. Ranci and E. Pavolini, New York: Springer.

Costa, G. and C. Ranci. 2010. Disability and caregiving: A step toward social vulnerability, In: *Social vulnerability in Europe: The new configuration of social risks*, ed. C. Ranci, Basingstoke: Macmillan.

Dahl, H.M. 2011. Who can be against quality?, In: *Home, care and practices—Critical perspectives on frailty*, eds. C. Ceci, K. Björnsdottir and M. E. Purkis, London: Routledge.

Daly, M., M. León, B. Pfau-Effinger, C. Ranci, and T. Rostgaard. 2022. Covid-19 and policies for care homes in the first wave of the pandemic in European welfare states: Too little, too late? *Journal of European Social Policy* 32 (1): 48–59.

Daly, M., and J. Lewis. 1998. Introduction: Conceptualizing social care in the context of welfare state restructuring, In: *Gender, social care and welfare state restructuring in Europe*, ed. J. Lewis, Aldershot: Ashgate.

Da Roit, B., and B. Le Bihan. 2010. Similar and yet so different: Cash-for-care in six European countries' long-term care policies. *The Milbank Quarterly* 88 (3): 286–309.

EC, European Commission, Directorate-General for Employment, Social Affairs and Inclusion. 2021a. *Long-term care report: Trends, challenges and opportunities in an ageing society*, vol. 1, country profiles, Brussels: European Commission.

EC, European Commission, Directorate-General for Employment, Social Affairs and Inclusion. 2021b. *Long-term care report: Trends, challenges and opportunities in an ageing society*, vol. 2, country profiles, Brussels: European Commission.

Ferrera, M. 1996. Il modello sud-europeo di welfare state. *Rivista Italiana Di Scienza Politica* 1: 67–101.

Glendinning, C. 2013. Long-term care reforms in England: A long and unfinished story, In: *Reforms in long-term care policies in Europe: Investigating institutional change and social impacts*, eds. C. Ranci and E. Pavolini, New York: Springer.

Greve, B., ed. 2013. *Routledge handbook of the welfare state.* London: Routledge.

Greve, B., ed. 2017. *Long-term care for the elderly in Europe.* Oxon: Routledge.

Greve, B. 2018. Long-term care: Universality withering away in Nordic welfare state? *Politiche Sociali/social Policies* 1: 15–28.

Hacker, J. 2004. Privatizing risk without privatizing the welfare state. *American Political Science Review* 98 (2): 243–260.

Leira, A., and C. Saraceno. 2004. Care: Actors, relationships and contexts—The multidimensional concept of care, In: *Contested concepts in gender and social politics*, eds. B. Hobson, J. Lewis and B. Siim, Cheltenham: Elgar.

Maino, F. 2013. Tra nuovi bisogni e vincoli di bilancio: Protagonisti, risorse, innovazione sociale, In: *Primo rapporto sul secondo welfare in Italia 2013*, eds. M. Ferrera and F. Maino, Torino: Centro di Ricerca e Documentazione Luigi Einaudi.

Maino, F., and F. Razetti. 2020. *Superare l'immobilismo: Alla ricerca dell'innovazione nelle politiche di LTC*, Biblioteca della Libertà, Anno LV, No. 229.

Miyazaki, R. 2019. Migrant care workers and care-migration policies: A comparison between Italy and Japan. *Asia Europe Journal* 17: 161–177.

Morel, N. 2006. Providing coverage against new social risks in Bismarckian welfare states: The case of long-term care, In: *The politics of post-industrial welfare states*, eds. K. Armingeon and G. Bonoli, London: Routledge.

Müller, B. 2018. Privatization and marketization of long-term residential care in Germany: Effects on care and care work. *Politiche Sociali/social Policies* 1: 29–50.

Österle, A. 2001. *Equity choices and long-term-care policies in Europe.* Aldershot: Ashgate.

OECD. 2022. *Health at a glance 2021.* Paris: OECD.

Pavolini, E.; C. Ranci, and G. Lamura. 2017. Long-term care in Italy, In: *Long-term care for the elderly in Europe: Development and prospects*, ed. B. Greve, Oxon: Routledge.

Ranci, C. (ed.). 2010. *Social vulnerability in Europe: The new configuration of social risks*, Basingstoke: Palgrave.

Ranci, C., and E. Pavolini, eds. 2013. *Reforms in long-term care policies in Europe: Investigating institutional change and social impacts.* New York: Springer.

Ranci, C., and E. Pavolini. 2015. Not all that glitters is gold: Long-term care reforms in the last two decades in Europe. *Journal of European Social Policy* 25 (3): 270–285.

Rocard, E., P. Sillitti, and A. Llena-Nozal. 2021. Covid-19 in long-term care: Impact, policy responses and challenges, *OECD Health Working Papers*, No. 131, Paris: OECD.

Streeck, W., and K. Thelen, eds. 2005. *Beyond continuity: Institutional change in advanced political economies.* Oxford: Oxford University Press.

Taylor-Gooby, P. 2004. *New risks, new welfare,* Oxford: Oxford University Press.

Theobald, H., and S. Hampel. 2013. Radical institutional change and incremental transformation: Long-term care insurance in Germany, In: *Reforms in long-term care policies in Europe: Investigating institutional change and social impacts*, eds. C. Ranci and E. Pavolini, New York: Springer.

Van Hooren, F. 2012. Varieties of migrant care work: Comparing patterns of migrant labour in social care. *Journal of European Social Policy* 22: 133–147.

Chapter 6
Older People During the Covid-19 Pandemic: An International Comparison of Four Cities

Johnston H. C. Wong and Ghee W. Ho

Abstract The fate of older people living in cities during the Covid-19 Pandemic was miserable. In America, for instance, the CDC confirmed that patients above 65 years of age are composed more than 90% of deaths. This paper examined the fatalistic effects of the Pandemic on older people living in four cities, two in Europe and two in Asia. Older people in Milan and Wuhan were more reliant on close family relationships whereas public services played a bigger role in older people's care in Hong Kong and London. A case study approach was employed to describe the responses of the government in these four cities and their eventual health outcomes. Official reports and statistics, stories commentaries, and stories from the press and non-governmental organizations were used to examine the contexts older people faced. Interactions of social culture, healthcare systems and government responses to the pandemic were discussed in light of theoretical health welfare regimes. Results showed that unprepared, underestimated and under-prioritized government responses were the major reasons for many preventable deaths.

Keywords Covid-19 pandemic · Older people · Preventable deaths · Health welfare regimes · Comparative health and social policy

Introduction

In their 2020 policy brief titled "The Impact of Covid-19 on older persons," the United Nations Sustainable Development Group (UNSDG) reported that across the world 66% of people aged 70 and over had at least one underlying health condition,

---

J. H. C. Wong (✉)
Department of Social Sciences, Beijing Normal University-Hong Kong Baptist University United International College, Zhuhai, China
e-mail: johnstonhuang@uic.edu.cn

G. W. Ho
Department of Life Sciences, Beijing Normal University-Hong Kong Baptist University United International College, Zhuhai, China

C. Aspalter (ed.), *Covid-19 Pandemic*,
https://doi.org/10.1007/978-981-99-2497-4_6

which exposed them to an increased risk of severe complications from Covid-19 (UNSDG 2020). In the same report, António Guterres, the Secretary-General of the United Nations, also stated that:

> The fatality rate for older people is higher overall, and for those over 80, it is five times the global average. Beyond its immediate health impact, the pandemic is putting older people at greater risk of poverty, discrimination and isolation. …. Let's not treat older people as invisible or powerless.

Guterres (2020) was concerned most about older people lacking accessibility and capability and being disadvantaged in all aspects of social determinants of health.

Schmidt-Sane et al. (2020) proposed that shielding should be implemented. Shielding is achieved by separating high-risk people from the general population. Unfortunately, "shielding" or protection for older people was not decisively and effectively implemented. The *total* number of confirmed/registered Covid-19 cases according to the WHO (2022b) as of December 12, 2022, was 649,753,806. The *total* number of deaths was 6,648,457. Furthermore, 74.96% of Covid-19 deaths were people aged 65 or above (see Table 6.1).

Shielding protection is not a standalone measure. It should be supplemented by a comprehensive plan for income maintenance, food supply, health service access and psycho-social comfort. In other words, governments should develop an emergency response plan to protect their older people if they pay attention to these early warnings from the United Nations. Unfortunately, after three years of these UN policy briefs, the world still failed to save its older people from many preventable deaths.

Table 6.1 Covid-19 confirmed/registered cases and deaths by age, for thoses cases where age had been registered, up to Dec 12, 2022

Age range	Confirmed/ registered cases	Confirmed/ registered deaths	Case fatality rate (%)	% Among all deaths
80+	13,364,057	1,269,828	9.50	41.98
75–79	7,071,870	363,735	5.14	12.03
70–74	9,940,145	344,918	3.47	11.40
65–69	12,440,469	288,784	2.32	9.55
<64	320,915,167	757,463	0.24	25.04
Total	363,731,708	3,024,728	0.83	100.00

Notes The total number of confirmed/registered cases with age information provided by WHO is only 363,731,708. The total of confirmed/registered cases with or without age is 649,753,806 up to Dec 12, 2022
Source WHO (2022b)

Emergency and Disaster Risk Management for Health (Health-EDRM)

Health-EDRM Framework

The WHO has fought many public health crises. In the last twenty years, the healthcare sectors have been continuously challenged by SARS, Avian Influenza (H7N9), Influenza A (H1N1), Ebola and Middle East Respiratory Syndrome (MERS-CoV). Supported by the United Nations Office of Disaster Risk Reduction, WHO released the Public Health Emergency and Disaster Risk Reduction Framework (Health-EDRM) in May 2019. It pointed out that a community-centered approach, with a comprehensive plan to mobilize multi-sectoral and multidisciplinary collaborations, is essential (Kayano et al. 2019).

Dr. Tedros Adhanom Ghebreyesus, Director-General of the WHO, emphasized "the critical importance of prevention, preparedness and readiness, together with response and recovery, to save lives and protect health", in the foreword of this framework (WHO 2019: 15).

Concerns for the Vulnerable

Four major processes of "Preparedness, Response, Recovery and Mitigation" form the structure of the Disaster Management Cycle which are applied to public health incidents. Disasters affect disproportionately the vulnerable namely people in poverty, disabled persons, migrants, refugees and displaced persons, women and children, people with chronic diseases and older people.

Health-EDRM involves many disciplines, including government officials, emergency and disaster management, rescue responders, healthcare experts, social and psychological professionals and epidemic preparedness and response people. Health-EDRM stresses the need for the Whole-of-Government and Whole-of-Society strategy. Disaster management is regarded as a responsibility of governments (WHO 2019: 15).

Protecting the Most Vulnerable

Policymakers have to identify those factors that may contribute to containing Covid-19 as vaccines take time to produce and distribute. Natural and social scientists, volunteers and interested persons all over the world are collaborating to provide information and share research findings for that purpose. The UN-Hbitat aims to help local authorities by identifying successful policies, legal measures and governance approaches to protect the most vulnerable in response to the COVID-19 Pandemic.

Older People in Cities

In the Covid-19 Response Plan published by the UN-Habitat in April 2020, it was predicted that: "Crowded cities would be hardest hit by this "urban humanitarian crisis" in which tens of thousands of lives were already lost in over two hundred countries (UNH 2020). The WHO also stated that megacities connected by international flights were hit by the early transmissions of the Pandemic (WHO 2022c).

Social vulnerability in cities when there is a crisis of public health has become a major international concern. Marvel et al. (2020) constructed a vulnerability map to guide public health responses in the United States. In May 2020, Gonzalez (2020), from the UCLA Center for Neighborhood Knowledge, also developed a Vulnerability Index of the Residents in Rental Housing in Los Angeles. These were attempts after the impact of Covid-19 to identify the vulnerable people who needed public and communal attention.

One of the aims of this paper was to explore the Covid-19 impact on older people chronologically to cover the whole period of the outbreak from January 2020 to August 2022. Another dimension of interest was social culture. Older people in Milan and Wuhan have close family relationships during times of crisis. Meanwhile, older people in Hong Kong and London were more dependent on public health and social care. Older people were not able to fight global health crises by themselves without government leadership and community responses. Their likelihood to survive Covid-19 was significantly dependent on government protections, treatments and support.

Focusing on cities, this paper also aimed to study how government responses mediated the negative impact of Covid-19 on older people in four cities namely Wuhan, Milan, London and Hong Kong. Official statistics and reports, w facts and stories reported by the press and journal papers were used to examine how older people survived Covid-19 when it hit their cities hardest.

The study was based on secondary data and there are only four sample cities therefore the findings are illustrative rather than conclusive.

Literature Review

Concept of Health Welfare Regime

Saraceno et al. (2021) found that childless households had a higher risk of poverty than households with children in Denmark (8.3 against 15.9%) while in Italy the reverse was true (24.8 against 16.2%). They also found that adults aged under 65 who lived alone had the highest poverty risk (33.4%) in Denmark, but in Italy, the risk was only 25.9%. They noticed that different countries structured their welfare policies according to cultural preferences. However, people may or may not change their cultural behaviors to capitalize on the welfare benefits provided by the system.

The concept of *welfare regime* refers to the interactions between social policies, that govern access to public goods and social cultures, that shape help-seeking behaviors, which eventually determine the consumption patterns of social services. Health welfare regime, therefore, refers to the consumption of health services which is determined by the provision of health benefits and the cultural perceptions towards those benefits.

Health Welfare Regime explains how older people, examining governmental health practices with self-perceived social and cultural norms, eventually adopted "acceptance" or "resistance" health behaviors. Opposite behavior modes in turn created different outcomes under the impact of Covid-19. A health-protecting regime means specific interactions of public health measures and individual health actions, based on the societal understanding of the division between public and private (family) responsibilities that creates a buffer against the Covid-19 health threats. Studying the effect of the Covid-19 Pandemic under the construct of a health welfare regime involves government responses, social and psychological reactions of the people, health behaviors shaped by people's reactions and the final health outcomes, which are the result of the interactions of the former three factors.

Government Responses

Health Preparedness. Social isolation or distancing is one of the standard practices and in fact kind of public health textbook suggestion for the control of the communicable disease. This approach was called the Venetian Model. It is because the first permanent lazaretto, or plague hospital, was opened by the Republic of Venice, in the year 1423 on the small island of Santa Maria di Nazareth. Tognotti (2013) found that isolation was first introduced as early as 1377 in Dubrovnik on Croatia's Dalmatian Coast.

The John Hopkins University (JHU), in collaboration with the Nuclear Threat Initiative (NTI) and the Economist Intelligence Unit (EIU), announced on October 24, 2019, a Global Health Security Index (GHSI). GHSI is composed of six categories of indicators grouped under the themes of Risks, Prevention, Detection, Response, International public health Norms and Health System capacities and accessibility. There are altogether 37 indicators and 170 questions.

Government responses included health, social and economic measures. Oxford University developed a Covid-19 Government Response Index (UO 2022). The Index included Containment, Stringency and Economic Assistance sub-indices in its initial version when it was first published in early 2020. On 27 July 2022, the vaccination rate was added to the list.

On April 2020, the WHO recommended governments take 6 types of action to contain the spread of Covid-19 (WHO 2020). They included:

1. Controlling transmission within sporadic and clusters of cases;
2. Ensuring sufficient public health manpower and facilities;

3. Minimizing outbreaks in high-vulnerability settings like workplaces and schools;
4. Containing the spreading of cases from high-risk communities; and
5. Engaging the whole communities in the control of Covid-19.

Health Policy Responses. Public Health responses are concerned with the determination and capacity of the government in providing universal acid testing, providing facilities for centralized quarantine, providing medical diagnosis and treatment for people developing Pneumonitis and providing intensive care medical services to save lives. It also involves the country's capacity to develop vaccines and medicines scientifically to prevent and treat the contraction of Covid-19.

Social Policy Responses. For this study, the stringency of social distancing was measured using the Government Response Stringency Index (GSRI) developed by the University of Oxford. This index has 17 indicators, among which the following are related to social distancing (UO 2020). These measures follow the recommendations of WHO by quantifying the scale, duration and frequency of school, dining places, pubs and workplace closures, cancellations of public events and restrictions on local transportation and international travel.

Older People's Reactions

Osborne (2020), speaking on Covid-19, referred to the concept of social cohesion proposed by Emile Durkheim in his famous studies of suicide back in 1987. Santini et al. (2021) have found correlations between social disconnectedness, isolation and mental health among Danish youths.

The effects of social disconnectedness and isolation were well-documented before the Covid-19 outbreak. Morgan et al. (2007), conducted a thorough review of the evolution of the concept of social exclusions and respective methods of measurement. Physical distancing and loss of usual social opportunities for older people, in general, are associated with a greater risk of anxiety and depression (Santini et al. 2020).

Yet there is no common definition among psychologists for social inclusion. Wright and Stickley (2013) after a systematic review of 36 peer-reviewed journal papers concluded that there was no common understanding of social isolation in these studies.

The concept of social isolation is further complicated by the advancement of digital technology. With interactive social media, older people can engage with family members and friends at a negligible cost. Light (2013) considered that "mediated" social networking could greatly promote social connectedness.

Torres et al. (2022) confirmed similar problems of anxiety and depression caused by disconnectedness during Covid-19 among Brazilians. However, upon a further survey among 4,431 participants aged 50 years and older in Brazil, they found that virtual talking connectedness could diminish loneliness despite steep outside-home disconnectedness.

Psychological Reactions. A lot of evidence has shown that isolation during Covid-19 is related to anxiety and depression (Robb et al. 2020), social trust and stress (Jiang et al. 2022), and even suicide Calati et al. (2021, 2023). During a social lockdown, through a heightened sense of disconnectedness suicide risks of older people might have increased (Wand et al. 2020). Several Covid-19-related suicide cases were reported in the US, UK, Italy, Germany, Bangladesh, India and other countries through mass media and psychiatric literature (Sher 2020). Excess suicide as compared to previous years was not yet confirmed.

Health Behaviors of Older People. The psychological reactions of older people, as described above, were shaped by social and cultural norms. Their social, cultural and psychological considerations eventually explained their health behavior towards Covid-19, notably in their willingness in accepting social isolation, testing, vaccinating and hospitalizing.

First of all, there were abundant news reports on Covid-19, particularly about the number of confirmed/registered cases and deaths. Awareness of the high chances of dying and overcrowded situations in hospitals might have led to treatment avoidance among older people when they did not feel well.

There were also reports on mental health consequences caused by social isolation. Older people might react positively to these reports by doing more exercise regularly at home, or surrendering to non-actions. Too many choices of vaccination left older people confused and hesitant to get vaccinated.

If social distancing was relaxed early, then older people would have no desire to get vaccinated. Meanwhile, if social distancing was not relaxed, there was no immediate need to take the vaccination as well. All these factors have led to "vaccination resistance," which was detrimental to older people (Lobinska et al. 2022).

Methodology

This paper focused on the ultimate health outcomes due to the pandemic among older people in the selected four cities, after the mediation of government responses.

Selection of Cities

Several criteria were adopted in the selection of sample cities. In particular:

1. the city should be an international flight center, to reflect the spread of the Pandemic;
2. they should have a substantially large number of older people, such that they can provide insights for other cities;

Table 6.2 Aging rates in the four cities (2021)

City	Older population (over 65) (M)	Population (M)	Aging rate (%)
Wuhan	0.975	8.4	11.61
Milan	2.419	10.8	22.4
London	1.071	9.0	11.9
Hong Kong	1.482	7.8	19

Sources World Bank; Office for National Statistics (UK) and Institute of Statistics of Italy (Istat)

3. they should have a relatively developed healthcare system or similar capacity in "public health crisis preparedness". It allows us to compare non-health or social determinants;
4. their governments have adopted different strategies in responding to Covid-19; and
5. selected cities should cover a variety of different social cultures.

Table 6.2 shows the population and aging rate in Wuhan, Milan, London and Hong Kong. These cities were selected in this study. Due to the limitation in time and manpower, only four cities were chosen. The findings, therefore, are only illustrative not conclusive.

Older people in Wuhan have very close ties with their sons and daughters. They were dependent on their children socially, emotionally and financially to a certain extent as most of them, who worked previously in state enterprises, enjoyed retirement benefits. The Wuhan government provided social subsistence only to the neediest older people without family support. In China, the government's spending on social services for older people was confined to basic protection.

Italy witnessed continuous budget cuts for health and social care since 2004, weakening its universal health coverage and basic social welfare. The Milan government has tried to implement social distancing policies but was unsuccessful. Living together with family members was quite common for Italian older people regardless of their income background. Extended families in Italy are attached socially and emotionally though not financially (Fonseca et al. 2019).

London, and the entire United Kingdom, is often praised for their National Health Services. However, nearly free health care services relying on government funding meant long waiting times and limited supplies. British health services were seriously over-stretched even before the Pandemic. In this welfare state, older people seldom rely on the next generation for financial support. Most of them lived in the community until they became incapable of self-care, whereupon they joined old age homes.

Hong Kong, following the British model, provided the general public with near-free public hospital services while the wealthy has the choice of private care. Property prices were extremely high in Hong Kong and more than 40% of the residents lived in public rental housing. Older people therefore could only stay in private residential care homes as their children's tiny public housing flats were not able to accommodate them. It is worth pointing out that older people living in old-aged homes had much higher Covid-19 health risks.

Timeframe of Study

To account for the severity of Covid-19, the actual number of confirmed/registered cases and the crude death rates were extracted from the WHO Covid-19 Explorer (WHO 2022a). Country statistics were employed instead of city statistics to reflect the larger national contexts and social psychological environments. Figure 6.1 shows the trends of cases and deaths in China. The first wave that occurred in early 2020 was due to the initial outbreak in Wuhan, whereas the second wave in the spring of 2022, was due to the Omicron outbreak in the HKSAR. Therefore, the Covid-19 attacks on Wuhan in early 2020 and on HKSAR in early 2022, would be examined.

The first wave of Covid-19 occurred mainly in Lombardy, including Milan and the northern part of Italy (see Fig. 6.2) appeared in the spring of 2020. The second wave was recorded in the spring of 2021 as Covid-19 spread from northern Italy to the southern part. This paper studied the situation of Milan under the first wave in early 2020.

For the United Kingdom, there were altogether three waves of Covid-19 impact stretching from 2020 to 2022 (see Fig. 6.3). The highest number of deaths was recorded during the second wave. Accordingly, the time frame of study for London began in March 2020 and ended in March 2021. To summarize, the timeframe of this study on the four cities is detailed in Table 6.3.

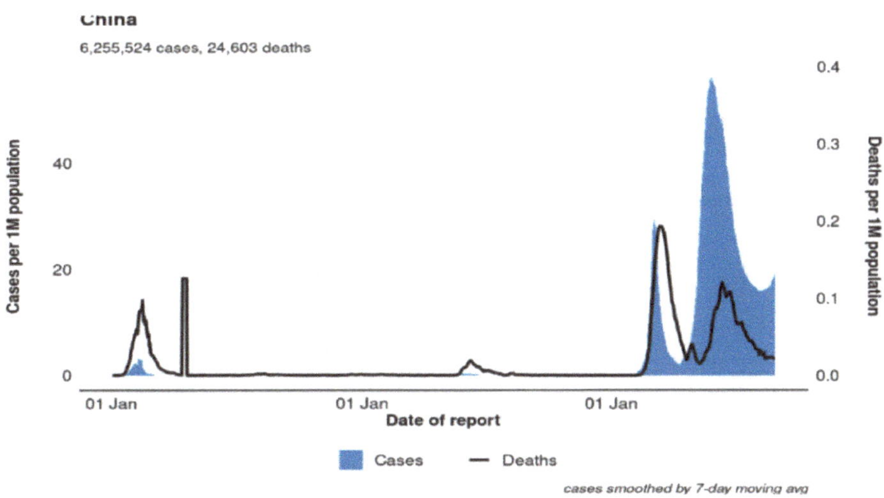

Fig. 6.1 Covid-19 confirmed/registered cases and deaths in China

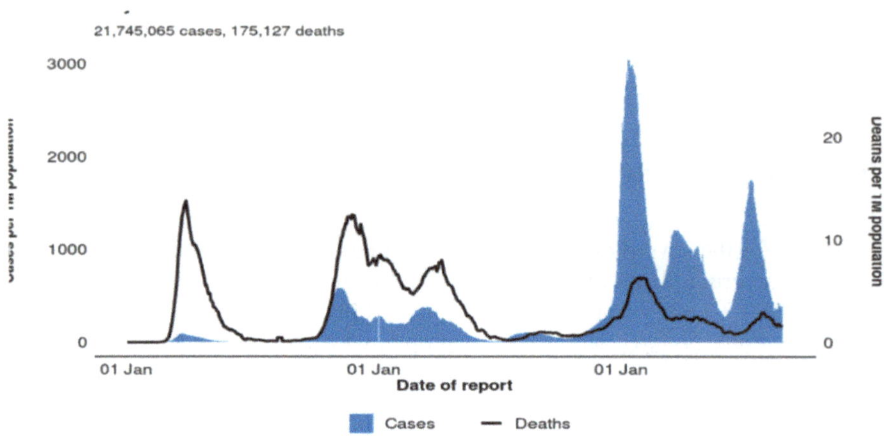

Fig. 6.2 Covid-19 confirmed/registered cases and deaths in Italy

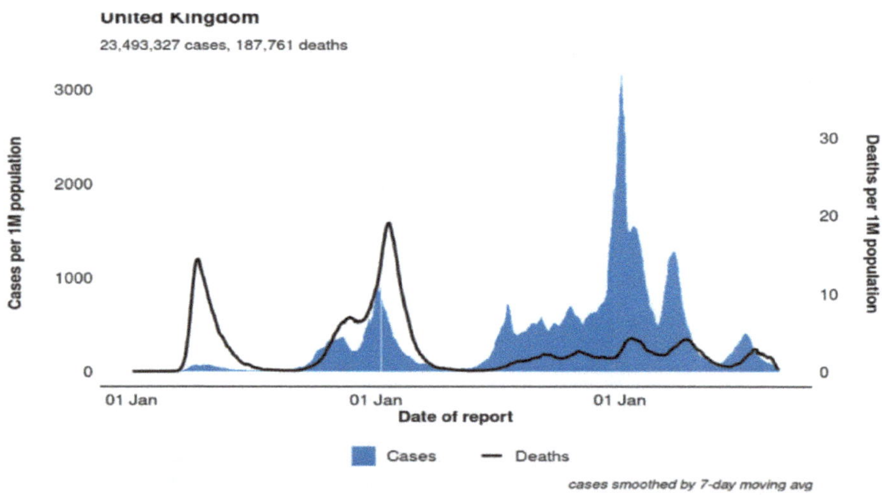

Fig. 6.3 Covid-19 confirmed/registered cases and deaths in the UK

Table 6.3 Period of study for the four cities

City	Beginning	Ending
Wuhan	January 2020	May 2020
Milan	February 2020	May 2020
London	March 2020	March 2021
Hong Kong	January 2022	June 2022

Framework of Case Study

To compare the situations of older people under the impact of Covid-19 in the four cities, a framework of analysis was adopted to establish consistency. This framework was composed of the following themes:

(1) The Impact, or negative health outcomes of Covid-19. Notably, the number of confirmed (registered) cases, the number of deaths and respective attack rates and death rates were studied. It would be difficult to collect data on lower levels of health data like testing rates and hospitalization rates.
(2) Government policy responses, such as whether there were explicit government measures to protect the physical and mental health of older people.
(3) Social and Psychological reactions of people, in particular older people of the city towards the Covid-19 impact.
(4) Consequential health behavior of older people to abide by government containment policies and develop self-care in physical and mental health prevention.

Findings

Case One: Older People in Wuhan (January to May 2020)

Mortality and Case Fatality Rate. The first confirmed/registered case was reported on December 1, 2019. A full analysis of the epidemiological characteristics (see Fig. 6.4) was comprehensively reported by China CDC (2020).

In the following, Fig. 6.5 shows the number of daily deaths in Wuhan. On April 17, 2020, to capture deaths that occurred outside of hospitals, 1,290 deaths were

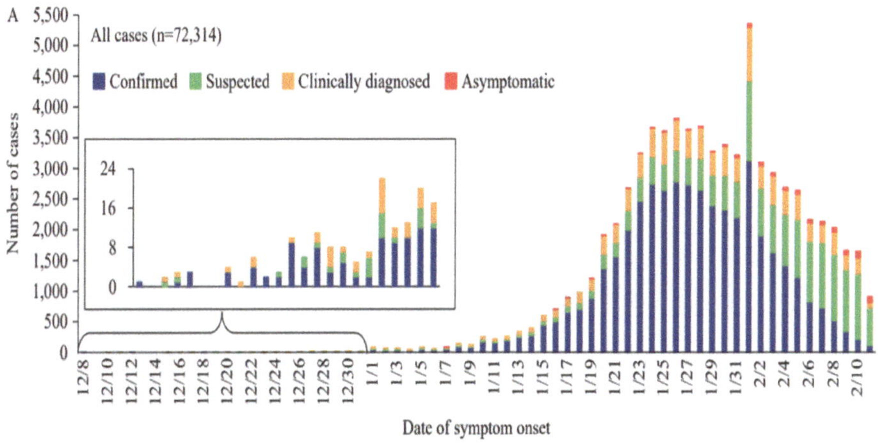

Fig. 6.4 2020 confirmed/registered cases in Wuhan

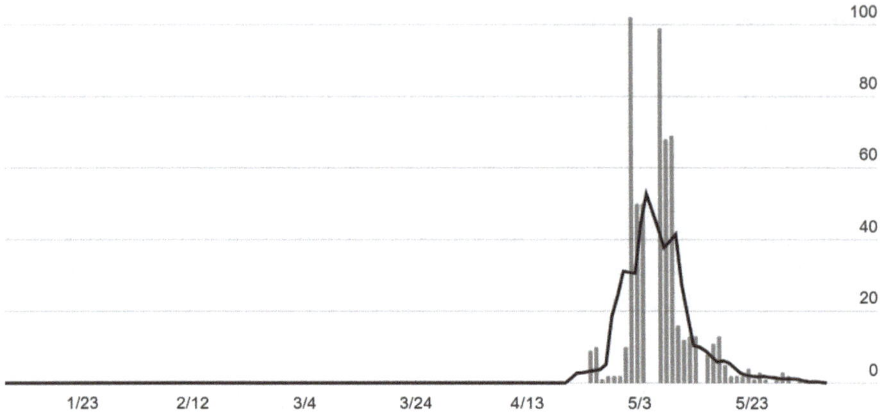

Fig. 6.5 2020 Covid-19 deaths in Wuhan (Wuhan CDC)

added to earlier reported figures, leading to a total of 3,869 deaths reported by the government (XH 2020).

The foreign press has challenged the figure of deaths as under-reported (NYT 2020). However, it is fair to say that under-reporting happened in most cities, as another report by the Economist (2021) showed that there were excess deaths in Wuhan, New York and London. It is difficult to judge whether excess deaths can be attributed to the lethality of the coronavirus or the failure of government responses.

According to Yang et al. (2020), the mortality rate of people older than 60 in Wuhan was 216.8 per 100,000 and between 40 and 59 was 18.9 per 100,000, averaging a rate for all ages 36.2 per 100,000.

The mortality rate for adults ≥60 was 5 times higher than the rate for all ages, 10 times higher than the rate for older adults (40–59 years of age) and almost 100 times higher than the rate for younger adults (20–39 years of age). The Symptomatic Case Fatality Rate (sCFR) of Covid-19 in Wuhan was also higher (9.09% vs. 0.36–1.97%) for people over 60 years of age than for the other age groups. For older people who were diagnosed as having COVID-19 in hospitals, nearly 1 out of 10 died (see Fig. 6.6).

Fig. 6.6 Covid-19 mortality rate by age in Wuhan

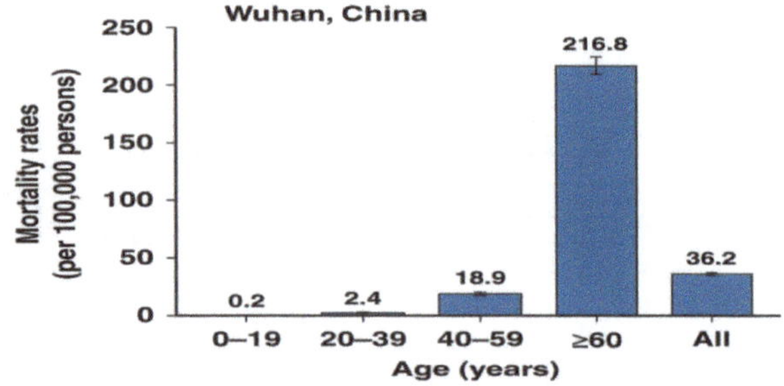

Wuhan Government's Responses to the Crisis. Wuhan deserved special attention because it provided "Guinea pig" demonstrations for all the other cities in the world. It took medical teams 7 days to identify the DNA structures of the coronavirus.

Announced by the Wuhan Epidemic Prevention and Control Headquarters on January 23, 2020, a city lockdown, during which citizens were not supposed to leave the city by land, water, or air, took immediate effect. This marked the sudden beginning of the impact stage of the epidemic amidst the festive air of the Chinese Lunar year. The severe measure of locking a major city with 11 million residents and a national stay-at-home order, was unprecedented. To support Wuhan, the central government of China started to build cabin hospitals and deploy medical staff from all over the country to man the additional facilities.

Pan et al. (2020) pointed out that not until February 2, 2020, when centralized quarantine and treatment were adopted, was the rise of confirmed (registered) cases slowed down. From February 17 onwards, the Wuhan government was able to provide universal acid tests to all residents. The city lockdown was lifted on April 18, 2020, after 76 days.

Social and Psychological Reactions Among Older People. Covid-19, like any other communicable disease, spread among social circles. A choir, composed of mainly older singers, went for a picnic and cross-infected, then many of them died. The loss of acquaintances was very depressing. In January 2020, Wuhan was celebrating the Chinese Lunar New Year, a time of family gatherings and feasts. If older people caught the disease via their younger family members and passed away, their sons and daughters suffered from guilt and loss for a long time.

Covid-19 deaths were painful. It attacked the lungs of people and created difficulties in breathing. People sent their seniors to hospitals and were physically separated from them thereafter. Some of them were only informed to pick up the ashes and remains of their loved ones from the Crematorium, even without the chance to say farewell. This was unbearable to most surviving sons and daughters.

Kong G. Y. of Hua Zhong University pointed out that "Final accompaniment" with seniors of families through their last periods of life, is important in many cultures (qq.com 2020). Condolence is important for the relief of grief and sadness. However, the final accompaniment was not possible during the chaotic situation of Covid-19. From January 23, 2020, the city was locked down until April 8, for a total of 77 days. Kong admitted that it was difficult to account for the psychological impacts of Covid-19 because never were so many people, nearly 11 million, "locked down" for so long.

Those who fortunately managed to recover were rejected by their neighbors when returning home, due to the misbelief that the discharged patients were still contagious. Starting in late February, the Centers for Disease Control and Prevention to provide psychosocial support to Wuhan mobilized 300 psychiatrists and psychological staff from all over China. Dr. Wang Z., a psychiatrist, talked about an old male patient who refused to be discharged because he worried that his son might reject his return to their house (qq.com 2020).

During the pandemic, the Psychological Association of Hubei Province (PsyA-Hubei) provided a 24-h hotline to answer Covid-related inquiries. The president of the association, Mr. Xiao J. X., pointed out that other than young people in the identity development stage, older people need special attention most during the pandemic (163.com 2020). However, only 19% of their inquiries came from older people who were not used to seeking help.

In the beginning, most inquiries were about information seeking, according to Li Meng a counselor at PsyA-Hubei. After mid-February 2022, psychological depression and pessimism began to dominate the consultations. One day she received 5 calls, all from older people who were living alone while their sons or daughters worked in other cities. The left-alone older people were worrying about the disease in fear and helplessness.

Health Self-Protecting Behaviors Among Wuhan Residents. Dr. Wang Z. found that people react to the coronavirus disease differently from that earthquakes or fires. The communicable disease had no definite time to end and fortunate people it could not kill (qq.com 2020). A prolonged impact stage was regarded as the main challenge of Covid-19 among many psychological counselors. It created anxiety and fear (ifeng.com 2020), and induced shame and sense of guilt, and deep grief among the Wuhan residents.

Hospital rush did occur in the early stage of outbreaks. People in horror and anxiety flocked to hospitals leading to cross-infection and resource and labor strains on inadequate medical facilities (China CDC 2020).

Nevertheless, as little was known about this newly discovered coronavirus, people had to rely on their immune systems and the doctors could only treat symptoms. Patients with morbidities had the highest risks. Among the Covid-19 deaths, there were doctors and nurses. This news certainly spread pessimism and hopelessness. Furthermore, since hospitalization meant total cut-off from family communication, avoidance of medical care, the reluctance to hospitalization and preference to die at home were common.

With the availability of cabin hospitals, patients having less severe symptoms were taken care of. The people of Wuhan adjusted well to these facilities. Treatment with Chinese medicines and organization of physical activities were introduced and reported openly on social media. People, more confident in managing the disease, became more dutiful in following social distancing regulations.

However, for the same reason of self-protection, community fear and hate towards the discharged patients were irrationally developed. It has been suggested large-scale epidemics like Covid-19 can cause survivors to feel shame and self-criticism (Gilbert 2009). Unfortunately, Chinese people having mental health problems seldom seek help.

Case Two: Older People in Milan (February to May 2020)

Mortality and Case Fatality Rate. The WHO warned world governments against the coronavirus outbreak as an international public health emergency on January 30, 2020. Italy became the first European country attacked by the coronavirus after reporting a confirmed case in Lombardy on February 20, 2020.

The Istat and the Istituto Superiore di Sanità (ISS), quickly explained the characteristics of the epidemic and its effects on total mortality in Italy. Later they also distinguished the different medical conditions between the first (February–May 2020) and the second (October–January 2021) epidemic waves (Istat 2021a).

Milan, having a population in 2020 of 1,236,837, being the capital of Lombardy and the second largest city in Italy after Rome (Worldmeters 2023) was hardest hit in the first wave.

On March 27, Italy recorded more than 9,100 new Covid-19 deaths, higher than the daily rate in Wuhan (Worldometers 2020). While the global average Covid-19 fatality rate was 3.4% (WHO 2022a), Milan's rate was 10% (see Fig. 6.7).

Gallaratese, having 33% of inhabitants aged over 65, was the 'oldest' urban neighborhood in Milan and Europe. (Arup 2018). The large size of older people made Milan very fragile in front of Covid-19. In Lombardy, people aged 70 and older, made up 37% of confirmed/registered cases. There were only 12% of cases in Wuhan for the same age group. Out of all registered cases, 47% were hospitalized, among them again 17% required intensive care (Cereda et al. 2021). Soon, hospital beds were fully

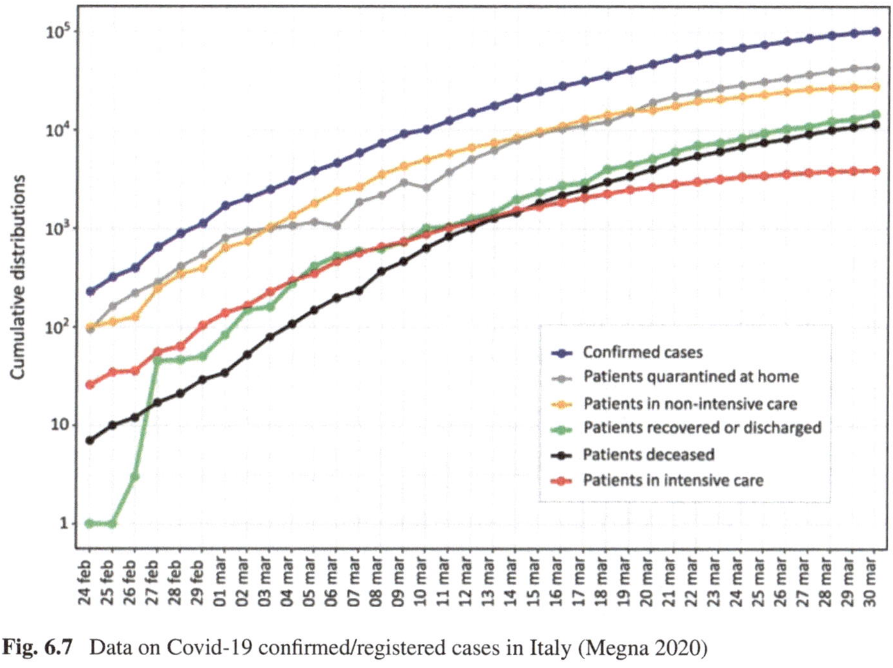

Fig. 6.7 Data on Covid-19 confirmed/registered cases in Italy (Megna 2020)

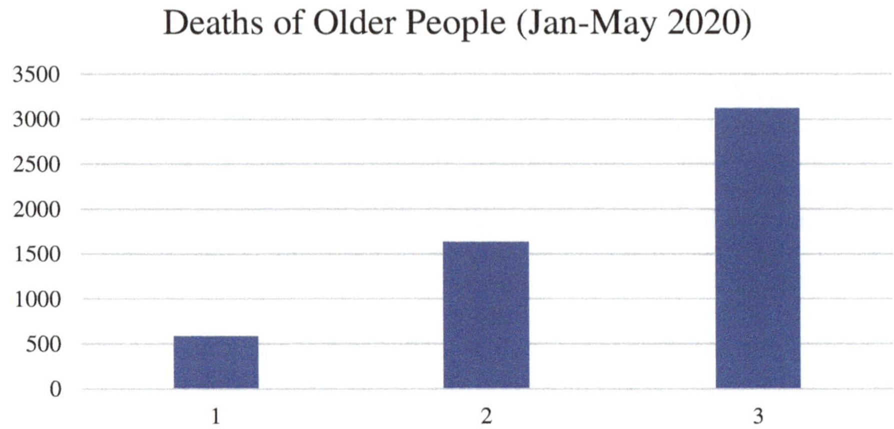

Fig. 6.8 2020 Covid-19 deaths in Milan, older people by age group (1 = Age 65–74, 2 = 75–84, 3 = over 85)

exhausted in Northern Italy, particularly for intensive care. Megna (2020), opined that workloads in hospitals, the entire Italian public health system, and the country's economic decline, were worrisome.

Fabio et al. (2020) studying admission data of the San Raffaele Scientific Institute of Milan from February 25 to March 24, 2020, found that the median age was 65 (IQR 56–75) and 72.9% of them were males, among 410 registered cases (see Fig. 6.8). Almost 75% of patients were reported of Obesity and 56.3% had comorbidities, with hypertension, coronary heart disease, diabetes and chronic kidney failure being the most common. Furthermore, 4.2% were under treatment for cancer. As of May 1, 2020, 23.1% (95) of patients had died, 5.9% (24) were still hospitalized and the rest 71% (291) had been discharged.

The total number of deaths among older people in Milan from January to May 2020, was 19,921 (Odone et al. 2020). The average same-period figures from 2015 to 2020 were only 3,091 (Istat 2022) (Fig. 6.8). The increase in mortality for all causes was 85% for subjects above 85 years of age, 56% for ages between 75 and 84, and 35% for ages between 65 and 74. The overall increase was 68.6%. Statistics confirmed that age over 65, with a history of coronary artery disease, active cancer, low lymphocyte count and high Radiographic Assessment of Lung Edema score, was related to the highest mortality rate.

Between March and April 2020, 29,000 deaths were caused directly by to Covid-19, and 5,000 more deaths were attributed to pneumonia and influenza caused indirectly by Covid-19 (Istat 2021b). There were over 100,000 more deaths than the average for the previous five years. The sharpest increase happened to people over 80, registering 77,000 more deaths than the average of the previous five years (2015–2019). These were the highest number of excess deaths since the Second World War. Male life expectancy at birth fell by 1.4 years to 79 and female life expectancy fell by one year to 84.4. Overall life expectancy at birth in 2020 decreased by 1.2 years from 2019.

Government Responses to Handle the First Wave of Covid-19. Months before the first reported case back at the end of November 2019, Mario C. Raviglione from the Global Health Department of the University of Milan reported that a four-year-old boy in Milan might have already contracted the disease, reported (UM 2020). If this was the case and Covid-19 was already widespread in the entire region, an explosion of the epidemic in Lombardy was understandable.

In other words, the Italian government neglected some early warnings and missed the opportunity to intervene early. The Italian government then had no choice but to impose a complete lockdown from March to May 2020, prohibiting all non-essential activities and halting almost all commercial business (Ortenzi et al. 2020).

Discontinuity of public services victimized the older people who were incapable of adapting, for example when public transportation was unavailable. Physical activity during the lockdown, especially among already inactive people, notably decreased (Füzéki et al. 2021).

According to the Bloomberg Health Efficiency Index 2019 (Bloomberg 2019), the top scores were awarded to Hong Kong (92.6), Singapore (81.9) and Japan (74.1). Italy (66.1) ranked 6th place. However, when challenged by Covid-19, the "efficient" Italian healthcare system was surprisingly ineffective. Stefano Centani, Professor of respiratory illnesses at Milan University, attributed the reason to prolonged underfunding and constant cuts of health resources. Budget cuts for public hospitals have been going on for almost 30 years in Italy. Prante et al. (2020) revealed that in Italy, public and compulsory healthcare expenditure per capita increased by less than 26.8%, in 18 years from 2000 to 2018. It was the lowest growth among all European countries (Fig. 6.9).

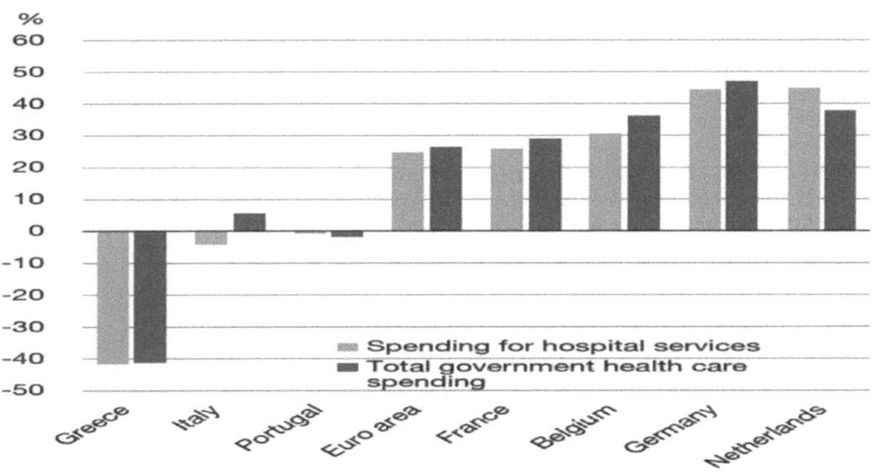

Fig. 6.9 Change in public health spending (2000–2018)

Health Minister Roberto Speranza acknowledged in Italy a limit on hospital personnel spending at 2004 levels minus 1.4%, was imposed to bring down the national debt (Reuters 2020). Under the attack of Covid-19, shortages of medical and nursing staff became a problem almost impossible to solve.

Southern Italian regions, spared by the first wave, did not learn from the lessons of Milan. Thinking, in mid-year 2020, that the epidemic was over, older people in Italy were still unprotected to face the tremendous impacts of Covid-19 in its second and third waves. At the end of 2020, Italy registered 65,011 Covid-19 fatalities since February, while there were deaths of 64,170 in Britain, 57,911 in France and 47,624 in Spain (Worldometers 2020, Dec. 17). When came to August 18, 2022, death figures had climbed to 174,300 (Worldometers 2022, Sept. 2).

The major reasons for such a large number of deaths included the premature government relaxation of lockdown measures in July 2020, a regionalized healthcare system with uncoordinated responses, disparities in regional capacities and inabilities and the failure to scale up medical services.

Psychological Reactions Among Older People. CESVI, an international NGO, launched an assistance program for older people over 65 in Bergamo and Milan to provide home deliveries of groceries, medication, meals and personal protective equipment, as well as transport for scheduled medical visits (CESVI 2020, Mar. 19). In Bergamo, with the help of 450 volunteers, more than 1,000 requests for support have been fulfilled and around 922 elderly people have been assisted. There were also requests for delivering clean clothing to hospitalized patients, collecting medical examination reports and transporting patients for medical visits or examinations. Nicoletta Rossi, who worked on the project, explained,

> Often, those who call us are upset and confused. Behind every person is a story and I feel that it is my responsibility and duty to listen to and understand it to find the correct solution.

A similar project sponsored by CESVI in Milan had a team of 15 social workers who assisted more than 200 over-65 s, called "Veniamo Noi da Te" (We Come To You). In addition to providing deliveries of necessities and carrying out errands, social workers also provided psychological support through helplines for the elderly. Marina Malgeri, a worker on the project, explained,

> We meet people who tend to be alone, who don't see anyone and are afraid. I meet about 4–5 elderly people every day and often at first they don't agree to meet me because fear takes over them. But most of the time I find the front door open and that they want to have a chat and share their fears and hopes to ease the burden of loneliness.

Health Behaviors of older people in Milan. Social distancing is not a part of Italian culture. As the younger generation often lives with the old, older people were easily exposed to the virus (Auriemma and Iannaccone 2020). Therefore, in the beginning, health behavior among older people in Italy could be regarded as having a social distancing reluctance. However, it was mistaken to assume that older people in Milan were not resilient to the challenge.

First of all, in terms of health literacy, Galle et al. (2021), found a satisfactory level of knowledge concerning Covid-19 and related control measures in their sample of the Italian elderly examined. Their data are in line with other studies performed on older people and in the general population in China and the US, but higher than those reported in a sample of the Brazilian elderly affected by diabetes.

However, the study also found a significantly higher risk of unhealthy habits among Italian older people. There were health-defeating behaviors in diet, physical activity and worsening sleep quality. Female respondents were affected more than males except in the categories of weight gain and increased smoking. These types of phenomena can be classified as "compensation unhealthy behavior."

Guida and Carpentieri (2021) used GIS to measure pedestrian flow and confirmed that when the city converted some primary healthcare facilities for Covid-19 purposes and restricted the use of public transportation, older people who needed health services regularly were significantly affected (see Fig. 6.10). However, older people who used to visit hospitals by public transportation have opted for other transport means provided by NGOs.

From a historical point of view, the welfare system in Italy was characterized by its familistic orientation, as the family plays a central role in assisting its senior members (Mazzola et al. 2016). This orientation, legitimizing the traditional definition of roles in the family, with men as the breadwinners and women not participating in the workforce, was fostered by the Catholic Church in Italian society. Care of seniors had limited support from external caregivers and even less from public institutions. Nevertheless, older people in Milan have learned to seek help from NGOs and volunteers, as CESVI's stories have indicated above. It revealed that Italian older people could adapt to crises by sourcing from systems external to families.

Concerning mental health behavior, a study in Milan showed that the number of suicides in 2020 was not higher than that of the previous year in 2019 (Raffaella et al. 2021). Suicides slightly rebounded to higher than 2019 levels in April 2021 (see Fig. 6.11). It might have been due to the delayed effect of post-traumatic

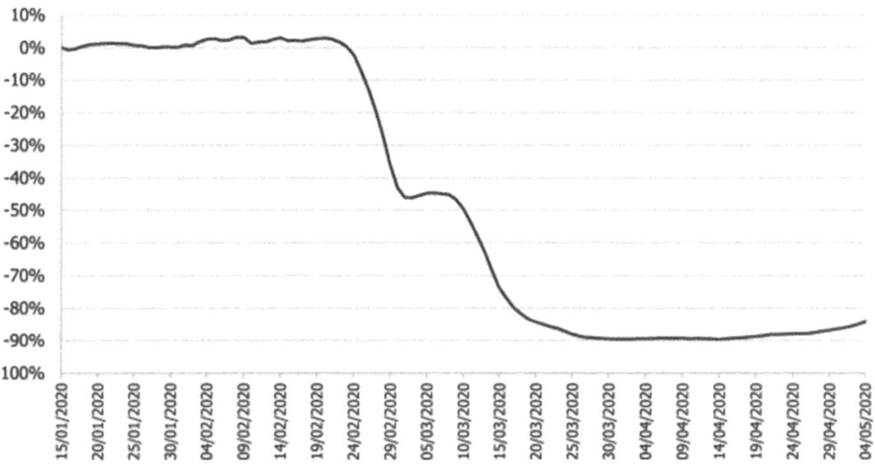

Fig. 6.10 The decline in public transportation use in Milan

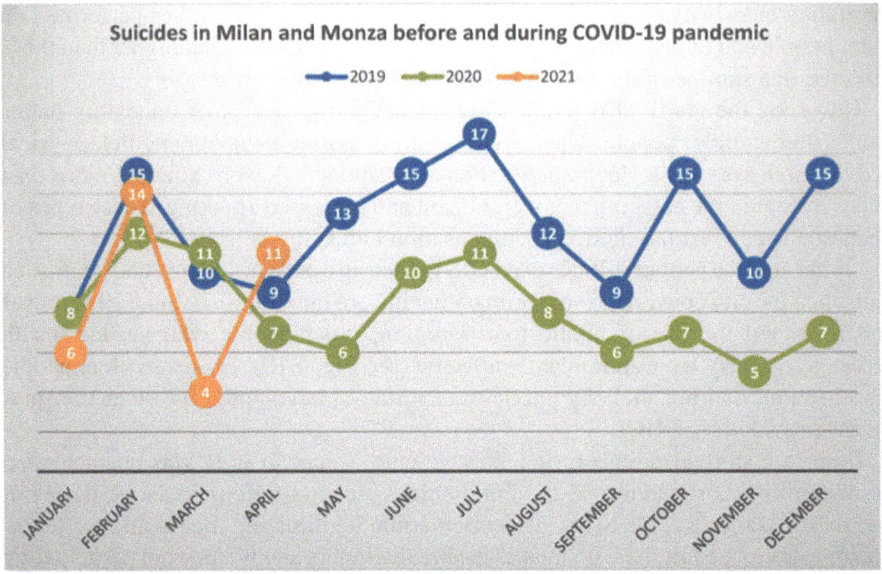

Fig. 6.11 Suicides before and during Covid-19 in Milan

psychological disorder following disasters. Nevertheless, excess suicides could not be confirmed.

Case Three: London and Its Older People (March 2020 to March 2021)

Mortality and Case Fatality Rate. Only 13 days after that of Milan, the outbreak onset of Covid-19 began in London on March 8, 2020. The performance of the United Kingdom was, unfortunately, the worst among western European countries (Fig. 6.12), followed by Italy, France, Germany and Spain. Until the end of August 2022 in the UK there were 23,492,875 confirmed/registered cases and 187,761 deaths. Its case fatality death (CFD) rate was 0.799%. South Korea had a similar number of 23,026,960 cases, but only 26,618 deaths with a CFD rate of only 0.116% (Statista 2022a).

The UK defined a coronavirus death as a person who died within 28 days of a positive test. The highest number of confirmed/registered cases during the first wave was reported in the Southeast region of the UK, including the Metropolitan of London. London's population of over 65 years of age (11.9%) was smaller than in other parts of England as it offered more job opportunities and attracted more young people. Older people were composed of only 10% in Inner London and 13.8% in Outer London. The aging rate was 19.6% in the rest of England (GLA 2022).

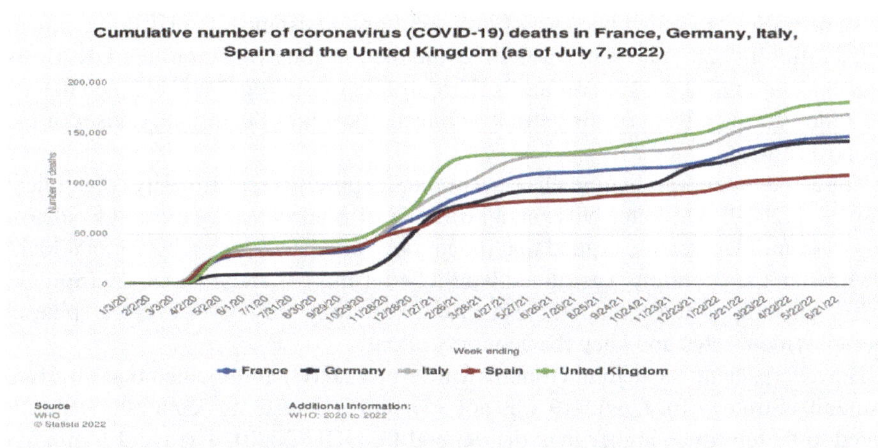

Fig. 6.12 Covid-19 deaths in Western European countries (Statista 2022a)

Up to June 27, 2022, the number of Covid-19 deaths reported in London hospitals was 19,102 (GLA 2022) (Fig. 6.13). As patients who died in hospitals were estimated only at 79% of total deaths by local authorities, the adjusted Covid-19 deaths in London was around 24,000. The crude death rate of Covid-19 was 266.58 per 100,000. The crude death rate for the entire UK was even higher at 275.5 per 100,000, counting up to August 18, 2022. The crude death rate for Lombardy in April 2020 was only 112.9 per 100,000. In other words, London's case fatality rate was 7 times higher than that of South Korea and its crude death rate was more than double of Lombardy.

Government Ambivalent Responses. While China followed the textbook public health theory of social distancing to meet the challenges of Covid-19 and Italy tried to adopt

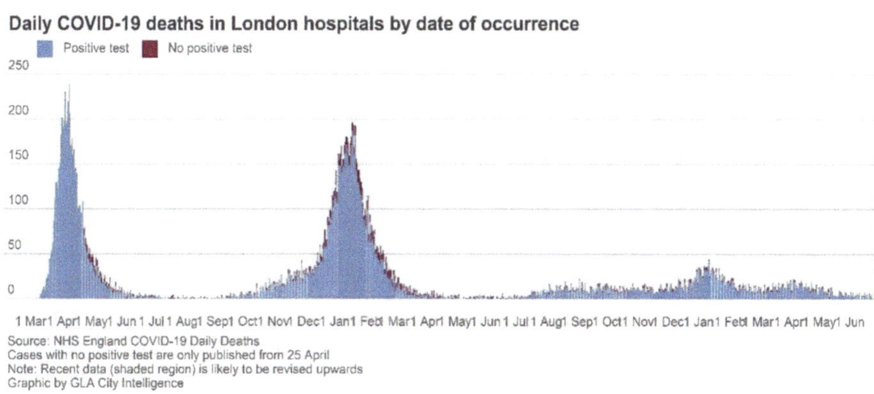

Fig. 6.13 Daily Covid-19 deaths in London

the same policy but failed because of initial cultural resistance, the UK government took a different path. On March 13, 2020, the then Prime Minister of the UK, Boris Johnson, announced the government's "herd immunity strategy" and claimed that he had followed the advice of Sir Patrick Vallance, the Chief Scientific Adviser of the UK government.

The actual intentions behind this herd immunity policy were primarily economical (Yan et al. 2020). Dr. Peter Nilsson, a professor of Internal Medicine and Epidemiology at Lund University, argued that the number of deaths caused by societal lockdown when the economy was ruined would be far more than by Covid-19 (Sputnik 2020). This supported the "flexible restrictive strategy" aimed to avoid a spike in unemployment rates and keep the economy afloat.

However, scientists at John Hopkins University (JHU) commented that the Herd Immunity Strategy for Covid-19 was not advisable because its death rate was estimated to be ten times higher than the general flu (JHU 2020). The Herd Immunity Strategy did not receive full support in the UK either. More than 200 scientists had written to warn about the stress it would create for the UK National Health Service (Macmahon 2020). Herd immunity can only be reached when a critical percentage of the population becomes resistant to an infectious disease either through vaccination or infection, explained Yonatan Grad, an epidemiologist at the Harvard T. H. Chan School of Public Health. He estimated that the required percentage would be around 60% of the world population for Covid-19, according to its infectivity. John Rose at Yale estimated that the soonest date for the availability of a scientifically tested safe vaccine would be January 2021 (Belli 2020).

Boris Johnson aimed to achieve Herd immunity through the direct infection of the British people by the coronavirus. However, the UK government has withdrawn from this herd immunity strategy and imposed closures of pubs, gyms, restaurants and cinemas. This was followed by a premature relaxation of social closures in July 2020.

Government Protection for Older People Was Absent. Of all registered Covid-19 deaths in the UK during the first wave between outbreak onset and June 26, 2020, 17,127 (31%) occurred within care homes (cf. Fig. 6.14). As there were additional deaths in hospitals, care home residents may have represented 21,775 (40%) of deaths. In comparison, deaths in care homes accounted for 47% of all Covid-related deaths in Scotland, 42% in Northern Ireland, 30% in England and 28% in Wales. Including care home residents who died in hospitals as well, care home resident deaths accounted for 51% of all Covid-related deaths in Northern Ireland, 50% in Scotland, 39% in England and 34% in Wales. Excess Death Rates in care homes as compared to previous years were 79% in England, 66% in Wales, 62% in Scotland and only 46% in Northern Ireland (Bell et al. 2020).

Schultze et al. (2022) reported that between February 2019 and March 2021, out of the 4,340,648 people aged 65 years or older, 95,212 (2.2%) were classified as residing in a care or nursing home.

There were 1,914 older people in aged homes in London alone. Even before the pandemic, because most aged home residents were above 80, age-standardized

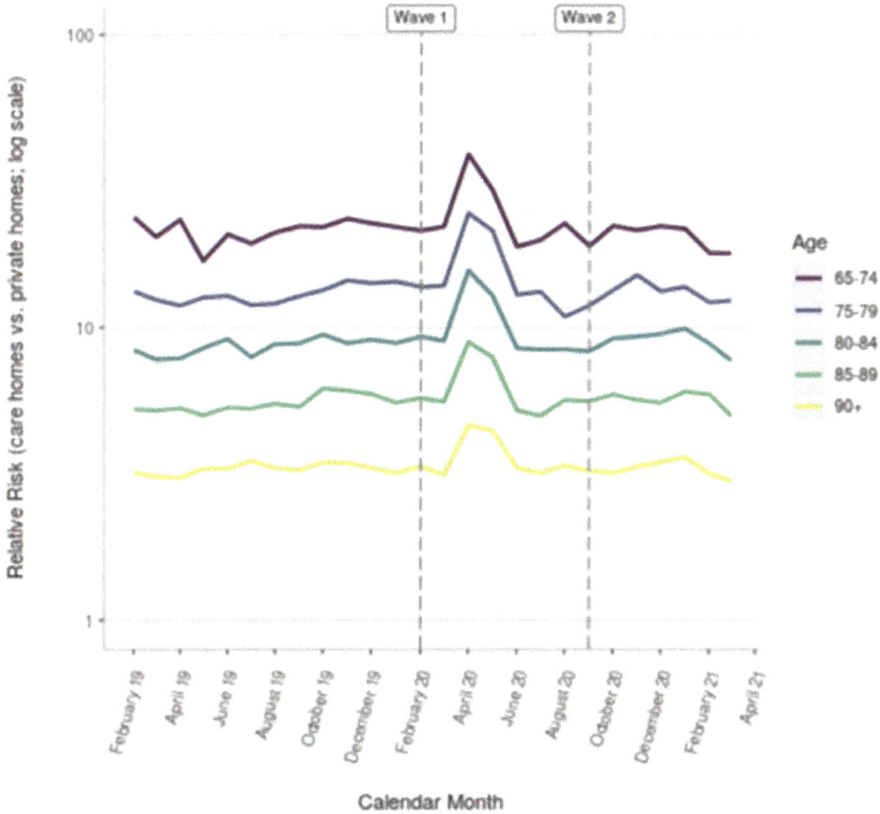

Fig. 6.14 Death risks in UK care homes by the age

mortality risks were approximately 10 times higher among care home residents compared to those in private housing, with a comparative mortality figure (CMF) of 10.59. However, in April 2020, these relative differences had increased to CMFs of 17.57 (16.43, 18.79) among women and 18.17 (17.22, 19.17) among men. Fortunately, CMFs did not increase during the second wave.

In England, guidelines for preventative measures for aged homes focused mainly on testing staff and residents, and were introduced only on March 30, 2020. Family visiting was banned since the national lockdown on March 23, 2020, but reopened after the first wave. However, the UK government's Covid-19 action plan for adult social care was not published until April 15, 2020. There were widespread reports of limited availability of both testing and personal protective equipment (PPE) during the first wave. A policy of regular testing of staff and residents, regardless of symptoms, was not announced until July 3, 2020 (BGS 2022).

All these setbacks may have contributed to the disproportional high risks for older residents in care homes. It is also important to point out that in Fig. 6.14, the highest relative risk happened in the range of 65–74, the youngest of the elderly. These healthier older people would not have died if they were better shielded.

On March 17, four days after the WHO declared Covid-19 a global pandemic, the UK Government ordered the discharge of 25,000 patients from hospitals into care homes, including those infected or possibly infected with Covid-19. Amnesty International (2020) considered the UK Government's decisions "shockingly irresponsible" since they "put tens of thousands of older people's lives at risk."

Care Home residents were also denied access to NHS. The son of one care home resident said that

> From day one, the care home was categorical. ... He only had a cough at that stage. He was only 76 and was in great shape physically. ...The care home called me and said he had symptoms, a bit of a cough and that doctor had assessed him over a mobile phone and he would not be taken to the hospital. Then I spoke to the GP later that day and said he would not be taken to the hospital but would be given morphine if in pain ... He died a week later.

Psychological Reactions Among Older People in London. Robb et al. (2020) and her team at the Imperial College of London conducted a comprehensive survey on older adults in London. Her study explored the associations between social isolation, anxiety and depression. A total of 7,127 voluntary participants (mean age = 70.7 [SD = 7.4]) were recruited from May to July 2020. To measure emotional changes during Covid-19, the Hospital Anxiety Depression Scale (HADS) was used. Sleep and loneliness were measured by the Imperial College Sleep Quality questionnaire adapted from the Pittsburgh Sleep Quality Index and Centre for Epidemiologic Studies of Depression Scale.

12.8% of participants (7.8% men and 17.3% women) reported feeling worse on the depression components of HADS accounted for 12.3% (7.8% men and 16.5% women) reported feeling worse on the anxiety components. Some reported feeling improved (1.5% for depression and 4.9% for anxiety). Social categories including female gender, single, widowed and divorced were more likely to indicate feeling worse in both depression and anxiety.

Health Behaviors of British People. In this study, 24.6% of those who smoked reported that they had smoked more and 14.7% of alcohol consumers reported drinking more. About 40% of participants reported sleep disturbances.

Worry and ruminating thoughts provoking cognitive arousal and disturbing cortisol homeostasis resulted in poorer sleep. Reporting of poor sleep, feelings of loneliness and living alone were also related to worsening anxiety and depression. Furthermore, loneliness and poor sleep have a bi-directional relationship.

A study in Southern Italy carried out from June to August 2021 through a web-based survey found similar results. Of 1041 valid respondents of older people (Mean age 76.6, SD = 6.5), 60% of participants reported decreased physical activity, worsening sleep and weight gain due to improper dietary habits (Galle et al. 2021).

Summary. It is sad to see how British people have lost many lives under their once prestigious healthcare system the National Health Service. Schultze et al.'s report (2022) concluded that the relative mortality of people living in care homes compared to private homes increased during the first wave but not the second. This suggests that the mortality peak observed during the first wave may have been avoidable. Those deaths were preventable.

Other than attributing the high number of preventable deaths to the failure of public responses, it can also be explained from a systemic theory. When older people, particularly those living in aged homes, were dependent on public health and social care, whenever the system failed, there was no alternative or community action. Residents in aged homes were composed of only 2% of the older population in England. They were mostly over 80 years of age and unable to self-care. This vulnerable group should not rely entirely on public protection and there should be an intervention structure for community actions.

Case Four: Older People in Hong Kong, China (January to June 2022)

Omicron Mortality and Case Fatality. In the early stages from Jan 2020 to Jan 2022, Covid-19 impact on Hong Kong was relatively mild. Unfortunately, when the coronavirus mutated into the Omicron variant, Hong Kong recorded its peak of Covid-19 deaths. There was no room for complacency. Omicron had a higher infectivity rate and lower fatality rate and killed as many people as the Delta variant in 2021, Fig. 6.15 (WID 2022) shows the attack rate of Covid-19 from 2020 to 2022.

Hong Kong's definition of a Covid-19 death, similar to the UK's, was the death of a person with a positive SARS-CoV-2 result within 28 days of the first positive specimen collection day. According to the WHO, as of August 31, 2022, Hong Kong has reported 1,283,514 confirmed/registered cases and 9,477 Coronavirus deaths (see Fig. 6.16).

According to the HK government (2022), the median age among the deceased was 86, (R = 0–112), with a male-to-female ratio of 1.42. The number of unvaccinated deaths was 6,697, or 71%. Older people aged over 60 years made up 95% of all Covid-19 death cases. Moreover, 54% of the deaths came from Residential Care Homes (see Fig. 6.17). As a rule, government officials blamed the high fatality rate on the old age and comorbidities of patients.

The high case fatality rate was due to the low vaccination rate. Among all Covid-19 death cases in Hong Kong during this wave of Omicron, 71% of them were unvaccinated. The full vaccination rate for Hong Kong older people aged between 60 and 70 was only 81.24% by March 21, 2022 (He et al. 2022), in contrast to 97% in Singapore. Similarly, the full vaccination rate in Hong Kong for older people over 70 years of age was 56.82%, while it was 95% in Singapore (He et al. 2022). The case fatality rate (CFR) in HK for people over 70 was 4.46% while the CFR in Singapore for the same age group was almost 10 times smaller, being 0.48%.

Government Responses and Non-Actions. The Hong Kong government did not learn from the Covid outbreaks in Wuhan, Milan and London. Older people were still

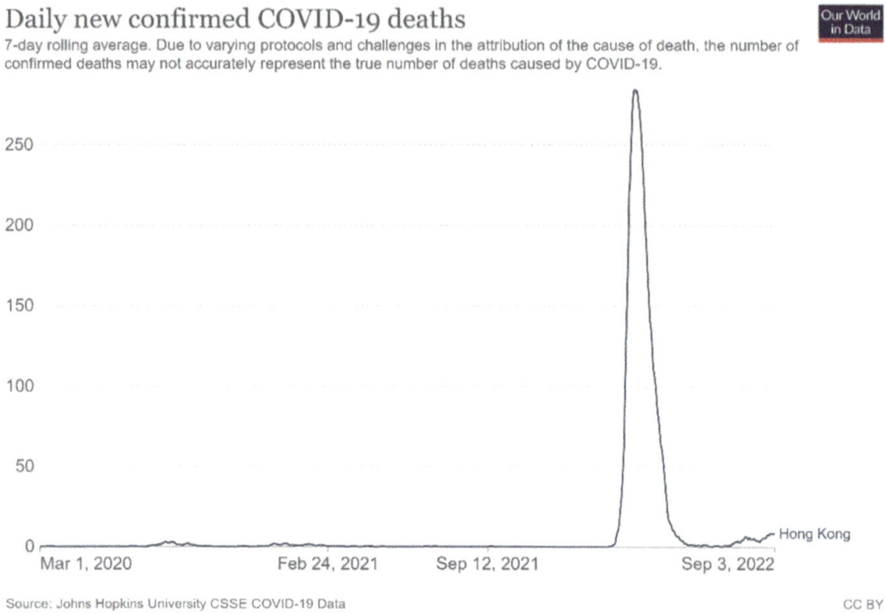

Fig. 6.15 Daily Covid-19 deaths in Hong Kong

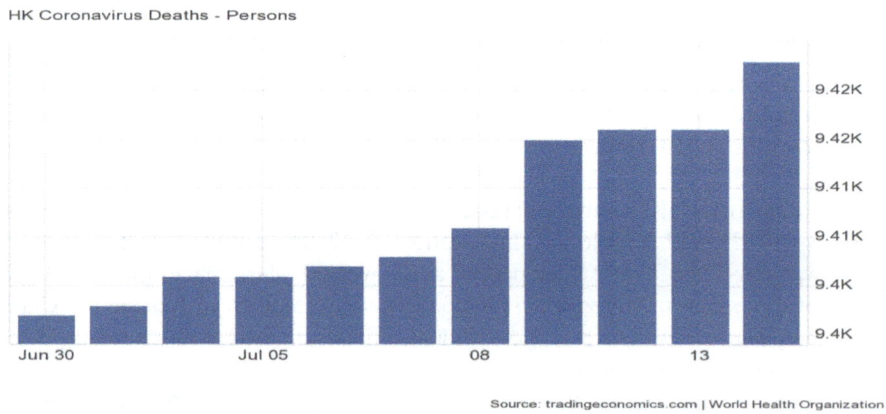

Fig. 6.16 Accumulated registered Covid-19 deaths in Hong Kong (as of July 2022)

not protected properly as care home residents still accounted for more than 50% of Covid-19 deaths.

Carrie Lam, the then Chief Executive of the Hong Kong Special Administrative Region (HKSAR), said on March 23 that control efforts in the ongoing epidemic would be focused on elderly care homes. Such realization came too late. The greatest number of daily new cases, 75,572, was recorded on March 4 and the greatest number

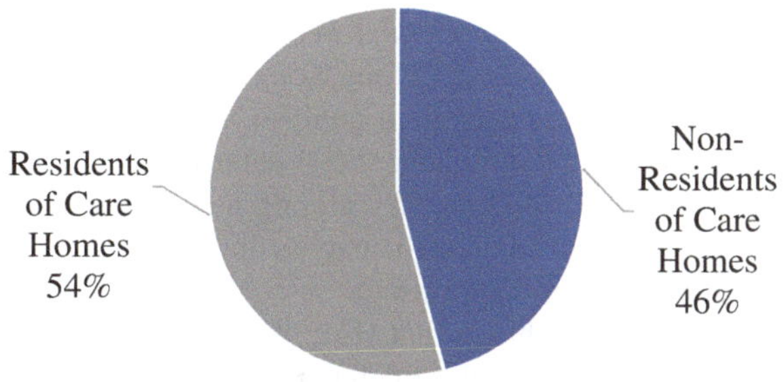

Fig. 6.17 Covid-19 in Hong Kong by residence (N = 9,477)

of daily deaths, 294, was recorded on March 11. The spikes had passed and the damages were done.

During the pandemic, the Social Welfare Department (SWD) of Hong Kong provided social assistance, through the Social Assistance Allowance Scheme (SWD 2022), to residents over 65 to maintain their daily subsistence. Public hospitals and clinics provided free and sufficient services to welfare recipients. However, in 2019, around 44%, or more than 3.3 million residents, lived in public permanent housing (Vetter 2019). The average living space of Hong Kong residents was only 13.5 square meters in 2021 (Statista 2022b). Therefore, married younger generations could not live together with their parents. This was the direct opposite of the social habitation style of the Italians.

These homes were for-profit companies that capitalized on the social security money the government provided to older people. Taxpayers' money was transferred by the market mechanism to the pocket of these private home operators. A few of them were even listed successfully. Due to irresponsible management, these private care homes are generally very crowded and understaffed. Most helpers of the homes did not have dormitories as this would have decreased the incomes of the operators. Quarantine camps set up by the government were unsuitable to private home residents who needed assistance in daily living activities. On-site quarantine was also unfeasible, given the over-crowded conditions in these homes and the limited human resources. In other words, even if the government wanted to impose strict social containment, private elderly homes were actually "*unlockdownable.*"

There were 38,400 persons residing in private elderly homes and 64.2% of them were aged 80 and over, with a median age of 84 (HKCSD 2022). About 15% of older people aged 80 and above lived in care homes, one of the highest proportions in the world. In London, as mentioned above, only 2.2% of older people live in care homes.

Chow (2021) thought that the lessons learned from the SARS epidemic in terms of locking down private homes would still be remembered and that the existing guidelines for Covid-19 protection provided by the elderly services professional association were sufficient because the number of deaths in aged homes in 2020 was mild, but her predictions were wrong. The Hong Kong Government did not scale up protective measures by offering directives, persuasion and onsite services related to vaccination for care homes and their older residents.

Health Behavior Among Older People in Hong Kong. He et al. (2022) compared the case fatality rates between Hong Kong and Singapore to explain the poor performance of the former. However, their analysis was based on a public health perspective that did not consider the broader social determinants of health. The concept of a welfare regime refers to the interplay among health, social, cultural and economic factors. This concept can be used to analyze the difficulties faced by older people during the Omicron attack in Hong Kong.

Research has shown that Hong Kong citizens lack health literacy but have faith in physicians and public media (Kwok et al. 2020). Siu et al. (2022) conducted a qualitative research study where they interviewed 27 older people in Hong Kong. The major reason for vaccine hesitancy and resistance was lacking decisional support from doctors, family and the government and the reliance on the peripheral processing of vaccine-related information.

Weak accessibility to medical consultation and inconvenient vaccination services were other important factors. Patients' illness perceptions and doctor-shopping behavior in severe illnesses can be balanced and moderated (Huang et al. 2022).

Older people in care homes, in both London and Hong Kong, are vulnerable groups who cannot administer self-care and rely on other people's assistance in daily living. They need community interventions if institutional actions fail. Medical professionals have to speak in the same voice loudly and clearly if they want to help these older people. Older people and their family members need direct medical guidance. Social workers can also advocate for the protection of these people.

Discussion

Covid-19 Deaths and Preventable Deaths

As mentioned above, the Bloomberg Healthiest Country Index 2019 ranked Spain and Italy as the best and second-best nations among 169 entries. China ranked 52 in that year. In the 2020 survey, Singapore took first place, followed by Hong Kong, Taiwan, South Korea, Israel, Ireland, Australia, New Zealand, Taiwan and Japan to make up the top 10 (Bloomberg 2020). Rankings of France, Spain and Peru tumbled. Brazil, Russia and the US dropped to the bottom tier because of high Covid-19 mortality and a weakened economy. It demonstrated that Covid-19 has changed the world significantly and in facing its challenges there was no room for complacency. Previous high rankings became meaningless if the government was not responsive to the Covid-19 crisis.

The numbers of Covid-19 deaths of older people during the respective periods of the study were 2,114 in Wuhan, 19,921 in Milan, 19,102 in London and 5,118 in Hong Kong (Table 6.4).

Table 6.4 Covid-19 deaths rate of older people in the four cities

City	Aged population (M)	Registered Covid deaths	Deaths/ 100,000
London	1.071	19,102	1783.57
Milan	2.419	19,921	823.52
Hong Kong	1.482	5118	345.34
Wuhan	0.975	2114	216.8

The major reasons for older people's deaths in the four cities were slightly different. In Wuhan, older people suffered due to cross infections, hospital collapses, comorbidity and inadequate support services.

In Milan, adding to the above problems were familial orientation, cultural resistance to social distancing and inadequate healthcare capacities due to 20 years of budget cuts. These resulted in even higher death rates than Wuhan's.

London's performance was the worst among western European countries counting Spain, Italy, France and Germany. The reasons behind the high case fatality rate in the UK, 7 times higher than South Korea and the high crude death rate, doubling that of Milan, deserved in-depth analysis.

The high case fatality rate in Italy was explained by old age morbidity and hospital rush. However, London only has 11.9% of the aged population while Milan has 22.4%. For UK high crude death rate was related more to the high proportion of the population being infected by Covid-19, rather than a larger older people population.

Both Italy and UK witnessed hospital rush. Italy faced shortages of medical facilities particularly medical manpower and the government tried to introduce stringent social distancing measures at the beginning. For the UK, its hospital rush occurred because its government underestimated the severity of Covid-19. High-infection rate and large numbers of serious patients have brought UK's NHS to its knees.

The ambivalent response strategy of the UK government was a crucial factor as all emergency responses rely heavily on leadership. Its continual and mutual referrals between old age homes and hospitals caused the deaths of many old age home residents. To recall, Schultze et al. (2022) concluded that the relative mortality of people living in care homes compared to private homes increased during the first wave but not the second, and suggested that the mortality peak observed during the first wave was preventable.

While the sustainability of health services for Milan and London was in doubt, the uncoordinated emergency response in Hong Kong was saddening. As stated at the beginning of the Hong Kong case analysis, 54% or 5,118 of the 9,477 deaths came from older people's homes. In other words, 13.33% out of around 38,400 residents of private homes, have died.

Hong Kong had ample time to learn from Wuhan, Milan and London. HK could also draw references to its own experiences from the SARS outbreak in 2003. To everyone's surprise, good practices and traditions in the healthcare and welfare sectors were lost, amidst political debates and public narcissism.

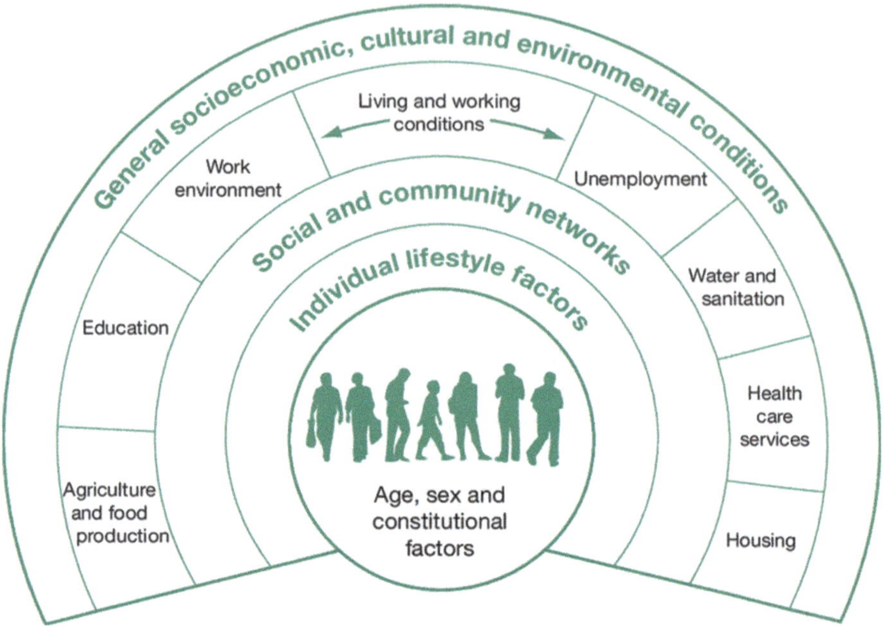

Fig. 6.18 Social determinants of health (WHO)

In a public health crisis, the health sector should not confine itself to medical issues but mobilize the whole government's and whole community's involvement. Public health experts in designing their response plans and actions must take full consideration of the social determinants of health (see Fig. 6.18), as advocated by the WHO. The average living space per capita in rental public housing was only 13.5 square meters. One-fifth of Hong Kong's population was below the territory-defined poverty line. Furthermore, the waiting time for clinical assessment and treatments increased and the needs of older residents in private aged homes were neglected. The public health sector should be aware of these problems.

It means social and psychological responses must be integrated into public health responses. Social, Cultural and Psychological Assessment (SCPA) should be incorporated into the full package of public health emergency assessments. At the least, protection, positive discrimination and scaled-up medical services should be offered to the most vulnerable older residents in private homes.

Older People-Friendly Healthcare

In Wuhan, older people still constituted the major proportion of Covid-19 deaths. Residents of major old age homes which were public were shielded with hospital-like epidemic control measures. A lot of the deaths among old people occurred at home since hospitals were in great shortage. Better healthcare management and quicker response measures could have probably avoided preventable deaths.

In Hong Kong, the ambivalence and non-decisive actions of the government left older people in private homes dependent on the market, at a time when market forces did not work. Public and timely interventions were absent. The older people in private homes were indeed invisible to the busy government leaders.

Auyeung et al. (2020) reported this narrative of a senior geriatrician describing her experience in a surveillance ward caring for older patients:

> I continued to see patients who were critically ill, requiring noninvasive ventilatory support or intubation, but who was declined admission to the intensive care unit due to frailty or advanced diseases. Many of them were over 80. … When the world is focusing on the safety of the masses, the frail, the silent and the old have no voice. When the next epidemic comes, I do hope that we could have some elderly-friendly isolation wards.

Health Welfare Regime

This paper suggested different health outcomes among countries were the result of the interactions between government responses and social and psychological reactions among older people. Differing cultural perceptions of public and private responsibilities in protecting vulnerable older people determined which protective actions were taken.

After reviewing the situations of the four cities, it was obvious that the city government of Wuhan assumed more of a paternalistic role. The government of Milan, though operating under a familistic welfare system, later assumed full responsibility to protect its people. Unfortunately, the familistic welfare culture allowed for continuous budget cuts on its healthcare service to a state where the latter was no longer capable to meet the Covid-19 challenges.

London, under the British welfare system, all older people eventually relied on the mercifulness of the government. The family and the community were not capable of changing the power dynamics. The residents of care homes were the most powerless. Unfortunately, its government set a higher priority on economic recovery than protecting lives.

In the case of Hong Kong, the administration had lost its sensitivity to people's needs and repeatedly failed to carry out healthcare reforms. The Hospital Authority, the Department of Health and the Social Welfare Department were not well coordinated and there was lack of a strong leadership. Administrative negligence regarding the health risks of older people in crowded living conditions, especially in private aged homes, was evident.

The theory of health welfare regime suggested that government welfare provisions and individuals' consumption behaviors of health services, shaped by social and cultural norms, will reach a certain balance during normal times. This mode of balance was upset by the Covid-19 Pandemic. To face the challenges of the Pandemic, both government health policies and individual health behaviors have to change drastically in meeting the challenge.

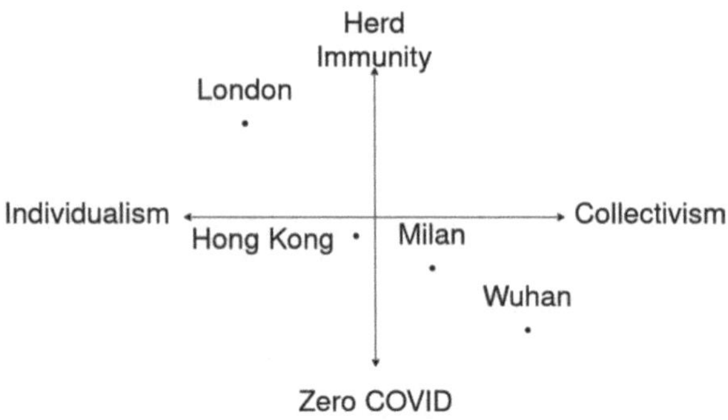

Fig. 6.19 Positioning of the four cities in two contextual factors. *Note* This is a theoretical/proxy representation of the four case studies under scrutiny

Yan et al. (2020) in a comparative study of Sweden, China, France, and Japan, suggested that countries have adopted different strategies during Covid-19 based on two critical contextual factors, i.e. institutional and cultural contexts. Similarly, health behaviors of older people in the four cities of this study were also shaped by two contextual factors. One of them was the government response policies inclined towards Zero-Covid, or Herd Immunity. The other contextual factor refers to cultural inclination towards individualism or collectivism. The positions of the four cities in relation to these two contextual factors are shown in Fig. 6.19.

Older people, especially those over 80, were very reliant on collective public services in most health welfare regimes in the four cities. However, the government of the four cities took different response strategies. If the government took a more cautious and life-protecting strategy like the case of Wuhan, the number of older people's death could be minimized. If the government took a non-decisive strategy, older people have to rely on family and community support, like in the case of Milan. The case of older people in private homes in London was the most powerless, sad to see that happened in a classical welfare state.

In Hong Kong, some older people residents in private homes have families. Did some family members take their seniors away from these homes for better protection and shelter, as a kind of family resurrection when public services failed? This is a proper topic for a follow-up study to understand how individuals change their health behavior as a reaction to nonadaptive public services. Older people did try to adapt to challenging situations, like in the case of Milan. There should be similar adaptive behaviors in the other three cities, pending further research.

Conclusions

This paper is descriptive and exploratory, not deterministic. Both quantitative and qualitative data and information were provided to understand the effects of the Covid pandemic on older people. It explored social factors that explain the high fatality rates among older people, especially those who lived in residential facilities. UN

Secretary-General António Guterres, in May 2020, reminded the public to "not treat older people as invisible or powerless."

In reality, older people were powerless to counteract government decisions. Protection in the UK was reduced to a simple stay-at-home order, with no social or community support. This was considered harmful to mental health (Di Gessa and Price 2022). As mentioned earlier, Amnesty International (2020) considered the UK Government's decision in ordering tens of thousands of older people to leave hospitals and return to aged homes to make room for Covid-19 patients to be a violation of human rights.

Truly older people were hesitant to get vaccinated. They were misled by misinformation and confused by an overflow of information. This is exactly why the community and medical professionals should have intervened more. A major disaster did not only present a test to governments, but it also put all communities to the test of their capacities for mutual help and adaptability to survive.

A successful health welfare regime relies on its people. The people have to learn from the hard lessons of death. We have to become smarter to protect our vulnerable older people, youngsters, brothers and sisters. They should not be treated as invisible and powerless. Developing more community capacities instead of relying on services, will enable better community resilience to future challenges.

References

163.com. 2020. *New problems continued to be reported after an intervention to 14 suicide attempts.* Hubei Psychological Association. https://www.163.com.

AI, Amnesty International. 2020. *Older people in care homes are abandoned to die*, October 4. https://www.amnesty.org.

Arup. 2018. *Shaping ageing neighbourhoods: Milan Gallaratese.* https://www.arup.com.

Auriemma, Vincenzo, and Chiara Iannaccone. 2020. Covid-19 pandemic: Socio-economic consequences of social distancing measures in Italy. *Frontier Sociology* 5. https://doi.org/10.3389/fsoc.2020.575791.

Auyeung, Tung Wai, et al. 2020. Covid-19 and older adults: Experience in Hong Kong. *Asian Journal of Gerontology and Geriatrics* 15 (2): 54–59.

Bell, David et al. 2020. *Covid-19 mortality and long-term care: A UK comparison.* International Long Term Care Policy Network, August. https://ltcCovid.org.

Belli, Brita. 2020. Yale researchers pursuing Covid-19 vaccine based on powerful Yale platform. *YaleNews*, April 29. https://news.yale.edu.

BGS, British Geriatric Society. 2022. *Managing the Covid-19 pandemic in care homes for older people.* https://www.bgs.org.uk.

Bloomberg. 2019. *Bloomberg health efficiency index.* https://Bloomberg.org.

Bloomberg. 2020. *Bloomberg healthiest country index.* https://Bloomberg.org.

Calati, Raffaella, Guendalina Gentile, Michele Fornaro, Stefano Tambuzzi, and Riccardo Zoja. 2021. Preliminary suicide trends during the Covid-19 pandemic in Milan Italy. *Journal of Psychiatric Research* 143: 21–22. https://doi.org/10.1016/j.jpsychires.2021.08.029. Epub 2021 Aug 21. PMID: 34438199; PMCID: PMC9272275.

Calati, Raffaella, Guendalina Gentile, Michele Fornaro, Fabio Madeddu, Stefano Tambuzzi, and Riccardo Zoja. 2023. Suicide and homicide before and during the Covid-19 pandemic in Milan

Italy. *Journal of Affective Disorders Reports* 12: 100510. https://doi.org/10.1016/j.jadr.2023.100510. Epub 2023 Feb 23. PMID: 36852089; PMCID: PMC9946781.

Cereda, Dalina et al. 2021. The early phase of the Covid-19 outbreak in Lombardy, Italy. *Epidemics* 37: 100528. https://www.sciencedirect.com.

CESVI. 2020. *United against coronavirus to protect the elderly people*, CESVI.EU, March 19. https://www.cesvi.eu.

China CDC. 2020. The epidemiological characteristics of an outbreak of 2019 Novel Coronavirus Diseases (Covid-19). *CDC Weekly*. https://weekly.chinacdc.cn.

Chow, Lina. 2021. Care homes and Covid-19 in Hong Kong: How the lessons from SARS were used to good effect. *Age and Ageing* 50 (1): 21–24.

Di Gessa, Giorgio, and Debora Price. 2022. The Impact of shielding during the Covid-19 pandemic on mental health: Evidence from the English longitudinal study of ageing. *The British Journal of Psychiatry,* 1–7. https://doi.org/10.1192/bjp.2022.44.

Economist. 2021. Covid-19 deaths in Wuhan seem far higher than the official count, May 30. https://www.economist.com.

Fabio Ciceri et al. 2020. Early predictors of clinical outcomes of Covid-19 outbreak in Milan, Italy. *Clinical Immunology* 217: 108509. https://doi.org/10.1016/j.clim.2020.108509.

Fonseca, Xavier, Stephan Lukosch, and Frances Brazier. 2019. Social cohesion revisited: A new definition and how to characterize it, *Innovation, The European Journal of Social Science Research* 32 (2): 231–253.

Füzéki, Eszter, Jan Schröder, Nicolò Carraro, Laura Merlo, and Winfried Banzer. 2021. Physical activity during the first Covid-19-related lockdown in Italy. *International Journal of Environmental Research and Public Health* 18: 2511.

Gallè, Francesca, et al. 2021. Knowledge and lifestyle behaviors related to Covid-19 pandemic in people over 65 years old from southern Italy. *International Journal of Environmental Research and Public Health* 18 (20): 10872. https://doi.org/10.3390/ijerph182010872.

Gilbert, Paul. 2009. Introducing compassion-focused therapy. *Advances in Psychiatric Treatment* 15 (3): 199–208.

GLA, Greater London Authority. 2022. *Coronavirus (Covid-19) deaths*. https://data.london.gov.uk.

Gonzalez, Silvia. 2020. L.A.'s *Covid-19 economic crisis: Renter vulnerability index*. UCLA, Center for Neighborhood Knowledge, May 6. https://knowledge.luskin.ucla.edu.

Guida, Carmen, and Gerardo Carpentieri. 2021. Quality of life in the urban environment and primary health services for the elderly during the Covid-19 pandemic: An application to the city of Milan (Italy). *Cities* 110: 101038. https://doi.org/10.1016/j.cities.2020.103038.

Guterres, António. 2020. *Our response to Covid-19 must respect the rights and dignity of older people*, United Nations, May 1. https://www.un.org.

He, Guan Ho, et al. 2022. Association between Covid-19 vaccination coverage and case fatality ratio: A comparative study-Hong Kong SAR, China, and Singapore, December 2021-March 2022. *China CDC Weekly* 4 (30): 649–654.

HKCSD, HK Census and Statistics Department. 2022. *The profile of persons residing in private elderly homes, 2021*. https://www.censtatd.gov.hk.

HKSAR. 2022. *Archive of statistics on provisional analysis on reported death cases*. https://www.coronavirus.gov.hk.

Huang, Fengfeng, Pengfei Guo, and Yulan Wang. 2022. Modeling patients' illness perception and equilibrium analysis of their doctor shopping behavior. *Production and operations management* 31 (3): 1216–1234.

Ifeng.com. 2020. *Much more effort is required to treat PTSD for the Wuhan survivors, than in the case of the Wenchuan Earthquake*. https://news.ifeng.com.

Istat. 2021a. *Impact of the Covid-19 epidemic on total mortality of the resident population*, March 5. https://www.istat.it.

Istat. 2021b. *Annual report 2021: The state of the nation*. https://www.istat.it.

Istat. 2022. *Total deaths during the period January 1st-May 31st, years 2022, 2021, and 2020 and average years 2015–2019*. https://www.istat.it.

Jiang, Nan, M. Alfred Wu, and W. Edmund Cheng. 2022. Social trust and stress symptoms among older adults during the Covid-19 pandemic: Evidence from Asia. *BMC Geriatrics*, April 15: 330. https://bmcgeriatr.biomedcentral.com.

JHU. 2019. *Inaugural global health security index finds significant gaps in preparedness for epidemics and pandemics*. Johns Hopkins Bloomberg School of Public Health, Oct 24. https://www.jhsph.edu/news/news-releases.

JHU. 2020. *Covid-19 and the long road to herd immunity*, April 30, https://hub.jhu.edu.

Kayano, Ryoma et al. 2019. *WHO Thematic Platform for Health Emergency and Disaster Risk Management Research Network (TPRN): Report of the Kobe expert meeting*. https://www.mdpi.com.

Kwok, Kin On, et al. 2020. Community responses during early phase of Covid-19 epidemic, Hong Kong. *Emerging Infectious Disease* 26 (7): 1575–1579.

Light, Ben. 2013. Digitally mediated social networking practices: A focus on connectedness and disconnectedness. In: *International Conference on Information Technology Interfaces*. https://ieeexplore.ieee.org.

Lobinska, Gabriela, et al. 2022. Evolution of resistance to Covid-19 vaccination with dynamic social distancing. *Nature Human Behavior* 6: 193–206.

Macmahon, Alle. 2020. Coronavirus: UK government's 'herd immunity' plan sparks fear and fury. *New Zealand Herald*, March 17. https://www.nzherald.co.nz.

Marvel, W., et al. 2020. The Covid-19 Pandemic Vulnerability Index (PVI) Dashboard: Monitoring county-level vulnerability using visualization, statistical modeling and machine learning. medRxiv [Preprint]. https://doi.org/10.1101/2020.08.10.20169649, update in: *Environmental Health Perspective* 129 (1): 17701 (2021 Jan).

Mazzola, Paolo, et al. 2016. Aging in Italy: The need for new welfare strategies in an old country. *The Gerontologist* 56 (3): 383–390.

Megna, Rosario. 2020. The first month of the epidemic caused by Covid-19 in Italy: Current status and real-time outbreak development forecast. *Global Health Research and Policy* 5: 43. https://doi.org/10.1186/s41256-020-00170-3.

Morgan, Craig, Tom Burns, Ray Fitzpatrick, Vanessa Pinfold, and Stefan Priebe. 2007. Social exclusion and mental health conceptual and methodological review. *The British Journal of Psychiatry* 191 (6): 477–483.

NYT, *New York Times*. 2020. Doubts on Wuhan death numbers, April 5. https://cn.nytimes.com.

Odone, Anna, Davide Delmonte, Thea Scognamiglio, and Carlo Signorelli. 2020. Covid-19 deaths in Lombardy, Italy: Data in context, *Lancet Public Health*, April 24. https://doi.org/10.1016/S2468-2667(20)30099-2.

Ortenzi, Flaminia, Emiliano Albanese, and Marta Fadda. 2020. A transdisciplinary analysis of Covid-19 in Italy: The most affected country in Europe. *International Journal of Environmental Research and Public Health* 17 (24): 9488. https://doi.org/10.3390/ijerph17249488.

Osborne, Geraint. 2020. *We can't stress the importance of social connection enough*. University of Alberta, May. https://www.ualberta.ca.

Pan, An, et al. 2020. Association of public health interventions with the epidemiology of the Covid-19 outbreak in Wuhan, China. *JAMA* 323 (19): 1915–1923.

Prante, L. Franz, Alexandro Bramucci, and Achim Truger. 2020. Decades of tight fiscal policy have left the health care system in Italy ill-prepared to fight the Covid-19 outbreak. *Inter Economics* 55 (3). https://doi.org/10.1007/s10272-020-0886-0.

qq.com. 2020. *An older person refused to return home after being discharged from a case of Wuhan trauma, Explained the Shanghai Psychological Response Team*. https://new.qq.com/rain/a/20200302A0OOCG00.

Reuters. 2020. *Why has Italy suffered so badly during the pandemic?* December 7. https://www.weforum.org/agenda.

Robb, E. Catharine, et al. 2020. Associations of social isolation with anxiety and depression during the early Covid-19 pandemic: A survey of older adults in London, UK. *Frontier Psychiatry* 11: 591120. https://doi.org/10.3389/fpsyt.2020.591120.

Santini, I. Ziggi, et al. 2020. Social disconnectedness, perceived isolation and symptoms of depression and anxiety among older Americans (NSHAP): A longitudinal mediation analysis. *Lancet Public Health* 5 (1): e62–e70.

Santini, I. Ziggi, et al. 2021. Social disconnectedness, loneliness, and mental health among adolescents in Danish high schools: A nationwide cross-sectional study. *Frontiers in Behavioral Neuroscience* 15: 632906. https://doi.org/10.3389/fnbeh.2021.632906.

Saraceno, Chiara, David Benassi, and Enrica Morlicchio. 2021. *Poverty in Italy, A regime approach*. Cambridge University Press, March 4, https://www.cambridge.org.

Schmidt-Sane, Megan, Leslie Jones, and Olivia Tulloch. 2020. *Key considerations: Emerging evidence on shielding vulnerable groups during Covid-19*. Social Science in Humanitarian Action Platform. https://www.preventionweb.net.

Schultze, Anna, et al. 2022. Mortality among care home residents in England during the first and second waves of the Covid-19 pandemic: An observational study of 4.3 million adults over the age of 65. *The Lancet Regional Health—Europe* 14: 100295. https://doi.org/10.1016/j.lanepe.2021.100295.

Sher, Leo. 2020. The impact of the Covid-19 pandemic on suicide rates. *QJM* 113 (10): 707–712.

Siu, Yuen Man, Yuan Cao, and H.K. David Shum. 2022. Perceptions of and hesitancy toward Covid-19 vaccination in older Chinese adults in Hong Kong: A qualitative study. *BMC Geriatrics*. https://doi.org/10.1186/s12877-022-03000-y

Sputnik. 2020. Swedish Model: The ruined economy will cause more deaths than Coronavirus, May 7. https://www.sott.net.

Statista. 2022a. *Covid-19 Coronavirus facts and figures*, Sep 2. https://www.statista.com.

Statista. 2022b. *Average living space of public rental housing tenants in Hong Kong from 2007 to 2021*. https://www.statista.com.

SWD, Social Welfare Department, HKSAR. 2022. *Social Security Allowance (SSA) Scheme*, September 5, https://www.swd.gov.hk.

Tognotti, Eugenia. 2013. Lessons from the history of quarantine: From plague to influenza A. *Emergency Infectious Diseases* 19 (2): 254–259.

Torres, L. Juliana, et al. 2022. Loneliness and social disconnectedness in the time of pandemic period among Brazilians: Evidence from the ELSI Covid-19 initiative. *Aging & Mental Health* 26 (5): 898–904.

Trust for London. 2022. *The age distribution of the population*. https://www.trustforlondon.org.uk.

UN, United Nations. 2020. *United Nations comprehensive response to Covid-19: Saving lives, protecting societies, recovering better*. https://www.un.org.

UNH, United Nations Habitat. 2020. *UN-Habitat Covid-19 response plan*, April. https://unhabitat.org.

United Nations Sustainable Development Group. 2020. The impact of Covid-19 on older persons. Policy brief. https://unsdg.un.org.

UM, University of Milan. 2020. *Swab from Milan boy, 4, tests positive to Coronavirus weeks before Wuhan outbreak*, December 3. https://www.news.com.au.

UO, University of Oxford. 2020. *Covid-19 government response tracker*. https://www.bsg.ox.ac.uk/research/research-projects/covid-19-government-response-tracker.

Vetter, David. 2019. How Hong Kong's public housing system works: Costs, waiting times and sales. *South China Morning Post*, Jan 19. https://www.scmp.com.

Wand, P.F. Anne, Biao-Liang Zhong, F. K. Helen Chiu, Brian Draper, and Diego De Leo. 2020. Covid-19: The implications for suicide in older adults. *International Psychogeriatric* 32 (10): 1225–1230.

WHO. 2019. *Health emergency and disaster risk framework*, Section 7.1, p. 15. https://apps.who.int.

WHO. 2022a. *Covid-19 dashboard. Overview*. https://Covid19.who.int.

WHO. 2022b. *Covid-19 cases and deaths with age and gender reported*. https://app.powerbi.com.

WHO. 2022c. *Covid-19 explorer*. https://apps.who.int/iris/bitstream/handle/10665/331773/WHO-2019-nCoV Adjusting_PH_measures-2020.1-eng.pdf

WHO. 2020. *Considerations in adjusting public health and social measures in the context of Covid-19 interim guidance.* Available at: https://apps.who.int/iris/bitstream/handle/1066.

WID, World in Data. 2022. *Hong Kong Coronavirus pandemic profile*, Sep 4. https://ourworldindata.org.

Worldometers. 2020. *Covid-19, Coronavirus pandemic.* https://www.worldometers.info.

Worldometers. 2022. *Coronavirus.* https://www.worldometers.info.

Worldmeters. 2023. *Population of Italy major cities. Extracted on 2023-06-01.* https://www.worldometers.info/world-population/italy-population/.

Wright, Nicola, and Theodore Stickley. 2013. Concepts of social inclusion, exclusion and mental health: A review of the international literature. *Journal of Psychiatric Mental Health Nursing* 20 (1): 71–81.

XH, *Xinhuanet.com.* 2020. Amendments to official Covid-19 deaths data in Wuhan, April 17. http://www.xinhuanet.com.

Yan, Bo, Xiao Min Zhang, Long Wu, Heng Zhu, and Bin Chen. 2020. Why do countries respond differently to Covid-19? A comparative study of Sweden, China, France and Japan. *The American Review of Public Administration* 50 (6–7). https://doi.org/10.1177/0275074020942445.

Yang, Juan, Xinhua Chen, Xiaowei Deng, Zhiyuan Chen, Hui Gong, Han Yan, Qianhui Wu et al. (2020). Disease burden and clinical severity of the first pandemic wave of Covid-19 in Wuhan, China. *Nature Communications* 11 (1): 5411. https://doi.org/10.1038/s41467-020-19238-2.

Chapter 7
Comparing Social Policy Responses Between Separate Crises: Taking the Case of Indonesia

Tauchid Komara Yuda

Abstract This article draws on an institutional approach to compare social policy responses and changes between the Asian Financial Crisis and the current Covid-19 Pandemic crisis in Indonesia. The two distinct crises led to distinct policy changes. First, during the Asian Financial Crisis, the response was to change two layers of social policy: social protection and health insurance due to emergency and uncertain situations. At the same time, the welfare institution, either state or informal network, to mitigate the crisis was inadequate. This social protection institutionalization was not conditioned as social rights and was pursued primarily due to clientelistic motives of politicians during competitive elections. Second, in contrast, during the Covid-19 crisis, the drastic change can be found only in labor market policies, which were restructured towards more flexible settings, driven by political interests embedded within a network of patronage that remains intact among oligarchs. Meanwhile, a "non-insider" had no real influence on policymaking. This illustrative case underscores the failure of democratization in empowering cross-class coalitions to promote a more protective welfare system against the influence of oligarchic power. Overall, the case of Indonesia offers an example of a welfare regime model firmly rooted in clientelism and moderately successful in the development of social welfare policies and programs.

Keywords Asian Financial Crisis · Covid-19 Pandemic · Policy responses · Social policy · Political clientelism

The move to pursue uniform and equal development initiatives in Indonesia has been confused with the Covid-19 Pandemic. After the first lockdown was imposed in April 2020, the economic sector suffered about a 5.3% reduction in GDP, with 1.77 million workers of all income levels being laid off and furloughed (Sparrow et al. 2020). The rapid economic downturns resulted in a slew of interconnected social problems, ranging from rising poverty rates to increasing economic disparities.

T. K. Yuda (✉)
Department of Social Development and Welfare, Universitas Gadjah Mada, Yogyakarta, Indonesia
e-mail: tauchidkomarayuda@ugm.ac.id

C. Aspalter (ed.), *Covid-19 Pandemic*,
https://doi.org/10.1007/978-981-99-2497-4_7

Under these circumstances, the government was pushed to maintain, extend, and introduce welfare benefits at the required levels to strike a fine balance between purchasing power parity and economic productivity. The major social policies include extended coverage of social assistance, wage subsidies, active labor market policy, and contribution exemption of health insurance for thirty million informal workers (Yuda et al. 2021a).

Looking at the economic shocks of 1998, which represents the first period of major social policy reforms in the country, the government has offered targeted welfare programs to legitimize the new democratic regime, along with a Structural Adjustment Program with the aim of recovering the national economic condition. (Aspinall 2014; London 2018; Murphy 2019; Rosser et al. 2016; Yuda 2019, 2021a). In responding to the crisis, the argument for change tends to prevail over the argument for continuity. The social transfer program, for example, has been rapidly expanding, from four temporary programs in 1998 to about fifty programs currently operating under all ministries (Kwon and Kim 2015) and reaching over ten low-income families (Yuda et al. 2021a).

Additionally, the multifaced effects of the crisis brought the government to the midst of a social insurance reform (Aspalter et al. 2017). Central to the reform agenda was reorganizing fragmented and segmented insurances into the National Social Security Administrative Body's (BPJS) control, which has been providing coverage to an increasingly large population group since 2014. The BPJS was then divided into two main programs, one for health (BPJS-Kesehatan) and one for employment-related insurance (BP-Jamsostek), with other features following suit soon after (Rosser et al. 2016). Despite this, social insurance schemes remain truncated due to the persistence of large subsistence economies (London 2018).

It is imperative to note that understanding social policy development in Indonesia also requires a deep comprehension of the transnational dimension of policy diffusion, which is essential for defining the reform outcome (Kaasch et al. 2019; Mok et al. 2021). The explanation is crucial because international bilateral donors, international financial institutions, multilateral agencies, non-governmental organizations (NGOs), and influential nation-states played an essential role in the early period of the reform. Although, the final adoption decision was driven more by the domestic elite interests (Aspalter 2021; Böger and Leisering 2020; Lavers and Hickey 2016, 2021). Nonetheless, transnational social policies would provide compelling case examples on the interplay of international organizations and domestic policy actors within an increasingly global context (Kuhlmann and Nullmeier 2021; Schmitt 2020).

However, the causal mechanism behind the past 'drastic' welfare reform cannot fully explain the social policy development in the current crisis. This is a crisis like no other, and Indonesia is not immune. The containment measures to curb the virus transmission have been increasingly devastating for millions of individuals living under restriction periods with little access to income. Particularly hard hit are labor-intensive industries and retail trade, which absorb a large scale of informal workers and serve as major driving components of the national economy (Sparrow et al. 2020). In previous crises, efforts to improve the national economy could be undertaken by empowering the informal sector through a regional-based community empowerment program promoting local industries (Kwon and Kim 2015). The current crisis is quite challenging because the efforts to revive the informal sector—most of which is concentrated in working areas, requiring intensive and face-to-face contact—must be operated under restriction.

Compared to the Asian Financial Crisis, introducing a new approach that leads to path-departing policy changes is unlikely, but it increases the likelihood of alternatives to the existing institutional settings becoming widely adopted (Cox 2004; O'Connor and Pierson 1995; Varjonen 2020). This phenomenon is "associated with the concept of path dependence and the idea that, once policies have created large constituencies and other institutional anchors, path-departing change becomes rare" (Béland et al. 2021: 251). However, here and in other emerging economies whose social policies are still relatively new (institutionalized in the last two decades), social policy responses pursued are not fully path-dependent social policy development. Instead, there is a fusion of extensions of existing programs and reinvention, making the Indonesian case an interesting case to study.

By drawing on two comparative analyses of the crisis between the past rounds of economic crunches and the current pandemic crisis, this analysis inevitably focuses on the very different paths to welfare regime change of the two periods. The first succeeded in embracing democratization sufficiently to respond to wider socio-political forces expanding the state-sponsored welfare policies, whilst social policy responses during the current pandemic seem to be the result of a critical juncture created from the interplay of institutional legacies and threat-rigidity logic. The threat-rigidity logic means that "during moments of emergency and uncertainty, humans tend to stick to what they know best" (Starke, cited in Moreira and Hick 2021: 262). Given that the change is not driven by the tension of macro-level political and economic changes, the explanation of the social policy responses to the Covid-19 crisis can be argued as a quasi-path dependent driven reform. This implies that policy decisions are dependent on the combination of "previous experiences" made in the past and situational emergencies.

In a broader discussion, the "previous experiences" here must encompass the established social policy, as well as the multiple political settings shaping the policy. Indonesia lacks a comprehensive organized labor movement, has strong business influence in politics, and has a political party system that does not favor parties with strongly egalitarian or redistributive ideologies. Due to this reason, the Indonesian social policies during pandemic crises are developed based on market growth. The generous social support for the local government is an exception to the general trend. There is, for example, the Jakarta district, but the social assistance package supplied is inadequate and may not last. In general, Indonesia is a typical "universalist" developmental welfare regime at the national level (Yuda and Kühner 2022). Understanding past drivers of social policy responses as a loop to look at analyzing pandemic crises will provide a broad term of reference to understanding "the perceived and real 'perimeter' of present policy choices and offer effective policy advice to today's decision-makers" (Yang and Kühner 2020).

Overall, the discussion on Indonesia provides a model of a Southeast Asian country that has been relatively successful in developing a wide range of social welfare policies and programs anchored in a rudimentary democracy system and very much grounded in clientelistic governance.

The Paths to Change

This article draws on an institutional approach to compare social policy responses and changes in two periods of crisis (1998 and the Covid-19 Pandemic) in Indonesia. Much of the scholarship on this subject focuses on advanced democratic and capitalist countries (mainly Europe) and argues that a radical and abrupt social policy change is unlikely to occur (Cox 2004; O'Connor and Pierson 1995). This argument is often associated with the path-dependence thesis, which suggests that some of the established social policy programs, for generosity and particular value embedded reasons, can prevail in the long run as they have created "large constituencies and other institutional anchors" (Béland et al. 2021: 251). This means that attempts to redesign institutions would always be constrained in what we can conceive with these embedded political interests and sociological constraints (Murphy 2010; Varjonen 2020). Pierson (1994) calls such constraints as 'lock-in effects.'

Such a premise is relevant to the idea of stickiness (Cox 2004), which suggests that in a democratic society, social policy is stable over time. The stickiness of social policy, as exemplified in the plethora of institutional studies citing social-democratic welfare state regimes, arises because cross-class coalitions supporting the ideas of social solidarity have done much to promote their interest through their political channels in parliaments. They also "vehemently resist any change that could weaken the institutional structure" (Ozkan 2015: 127).

As with *The Three Worlds of Welfare Capitalism*, literature that assumes the welfare state as an inherently frozen landscape has been challenged by another stream of thought which perceives social policy institutions as much less stable (Hacker 2002; Mahoney 2017; Mahoney and Thelen 2009). Causal accumulation, such as time, historical sequences, and regularities of change continually—which all are called endogenous factors—can drive gradual changes (Starke 2006). These gradual changes can be further classified into three modes: "conversion (revising the goals of a policy without formally replacing it), layering (adding new elements to existing policy legacies without immediately displacing them) and policy drift (not adapting existing programmes to a new context that alters their impact and meaning)" (Béland and Powell 2016: 736).

Abrupt changes leading to institutional transformation may happen when the existing arrangement meets exogenous pressure (for example, an economic crisis). Institutional transformation reflects what Mahoney and Thelen (2009) call the 'displacement mode,' which means removing the existing institutions by introducing new ones. Yet, as Varjonen (2020: 2) suggested, "exogenous factors became significant only after endogenous developments had begun a cumulative process of divergence from the old path," as well as very depending on its pressure. In the context of the Covid-19 crisis, the strong pressure from economic contraction does not necessarily produce drastic changes, but there is the layering mode, which means that self-reinforcing properties of the previous institutions (developed world) or threat-rigidity logic (developing countries) make drastic reform unlikely. Threat-rigidity refers to the tendency for policymakers to pay attention to what they know best when faced with emergencies and uncertainty (Moreira and Hick 2021).

Much work is still needed to explain social policy changes in the Global South, which shows a different version of the political-economy structures of the countries found in the West. For instance, there has been the rise of sustained conservative party democracy, but it has faced weak opposition, whilst the social policies are conditioned under a clientelistic mode of governance (Hadiz 2003; London 2018; Rosser et al. 2016). A government that is relatively isolated from interest groups can bring possible changes to the social policy design at any time in tune with the political dynamics.

Studies on the welfare regime changes in the developing world were extensively explored after two publications by Barrientos and Hulme (2009) and Mares and Carnes (2009), which provided important clues for firmly arguing welfare regimes' institutional elasticity (Dorlach 2020; Lavers and Hickey 2021). They argued that welfare institutions in developing countries might change drastically as a result of economic liberalization, global financial crisis, democratization, and intensified international organization activities at the domestic level. The changes can be proven by the significant reforms that most Global South countries have experienced in recent years, with the nature, extent, and timing varying across countries.

In line with the said argument, Indonesian social policy responses leading to re-designing the welfare system post-Asian Financial Crisis were possible because previous social provision had only isolated small constituencies such as civil servants, military personnel, and employees of large firms through Civil Servant's Social Insurance (ASKES), Indonesian Armed Forces Social Insurance (ASABRI), and Employees Social Insurance (ASTEK/JAMSOSTEK). Such a vacuum of generous and universal social policies provided more room for policy restructuring when the crisis came, while democratization gave way to the institutionalization of the provisional social safety nets to establish welfare state institutions in a range of directions. Despite the little change occurring beyond the bounds of their productivist institutions, such change does not necessarily lead to effective policies, making it fail in promoting social citizenship. Pervasive clientelistic motives of the surviving-conservative elites of past authoritarian governments have been the cause of policy ineffectiveness.

The case of Indonesia presented here is quite contrary to Pierson's argumentation citing European welfare states, in which previous 'generous' social policies have created a shared attachment among cross-class coalitions (Piesron 2004). Under such social constraints, "change agents do not directly challenge or attack the pre-existing institution; instead, they introduce a new institution that undertakes a similar function as the pre-existing institution" (Ozkan 2015: 127). Previous studies examining policy responses during pandemics in East Asia relied on this premise (Soon et al. 2021), given those self-reinforcing properties of institutionalized policies. Despite being in the same region, here in Indonesia, the decision to make a response is more caused by the interplay of institutional legacies and threat-rigidity logic. The evidence to support this argumentation is provided in the subsequent section.

The Evolution of Indonesian Social Policy

Indonesian social policy followed a similar trajectory as the rest of the large East Asian countries. Pioneered in the final years of Sukarno's Guided Democracy and incubated further under the military-authoritarian regime of President Suharto, the Indonesian social policy design was implemented under the productivist regime framework (Holliday 2000). Such design was often referred to as the East Asian model (Aspalter 2006) or the developmental model (Kwon 2009) up to the early 2000s. This type is characterized by its application of targeted and limited services to the productive population (for example, formal workers in large companies, civil servants, and military personnel). These early forerunners of productivist welfare architects assumed that social policy should be limited only to those who can contribute to economic growth. Meanwhile, means-tested and low benefits provided to 'outsiders' were aimed at encouraging them to participate in the formal labor market (Holliday 2000).

The first precedents of formal social protection in Indonesia were mandatory pension savings for military personnel and civil servants, or TASPEN (1963), which were then added with mandatory contributions for health insurance (ASKES), including their families in 1968. By 1971, the social protection system was updated by providing the military with a separate pension fund through ASABRI. In the same period, social protection for private employees in large firms and state-owned companies, namely ASTEK, was introduced, which transformed into JAMSOSTEK in 1992. It provides old-age provident funds, health insurance, and defined-benefit pensions.

Given the limited scope of benefits, families and communities carried the heaviest burden of welfare provision. A notable example of community-based health care was community-health posts called '*posyandu*' that provide basic health services (for example, childcare, maternal care, elderly care, immunization, infant nutrition improvement, and family planning). Volunteers and medical professionals supported this initiative, which was to operate following the previously mentioned health-related programs (Berenschot et al. 2018).

It is worth noting that, during that period, many international insurance companies tried to expand their product to Indonesia, which was considered a growing insurance market in Asia. A clear example can be found in the health sector. As noted by Gough (2004: 175), "Indonesia permitted for-profit hospitals in 1988, extended this to foreign investment in large hospitals in 1994 and, in 2003, will permit unrestricted foreign investment in all health care."

The oil-crisis induced inflation in the 1990s brought the high economic growth to a standstill. Responding to this situation, ASKES expanded its benefits and coverage to non-productive parts of the population, especially to people with incomes below certain thresholds (Fossati 2017). They were granted additional broad services through the Public Health Maintenance scheme (*Jaminan Pemeliharaan Kesehatan Masyarakat*—JPKM). While the benefits continued to expand, the government transformed ASKES into new ASKES in 1992, which was reorganized in 2014 into a new label called BPJS-Kesehatan. The latter is a public institution responsible for running the Universal Health Care System (*Jaminan Kesehatan Nasional*—JKN). During the same time, the coverage of JAMSOSTEK was expanded to workers and their families. However, workers in the informal sector were not covered by the system. Thus, their families did not have access to the required levels of protection.

Taken collectively, such expansion did not cause the welfare regime to shift beyond the bounds of the productivism legacies continuum until the Asian Financial Crisis in 1998. The crisis halted the improvements in social development and poverty reduction as the GDP drastically dropped to the lowest level since 1961 (Fig. 7.1), wages eroded, unemployment rose (from approximately 4.5 million in 1996 to 10.9 million in 1998), inflation increased, and formal sector wages fell drastically by 34%, resulting in a massive shift of the job sector to informal and even agricultural sectors. The economic downturn hardship strained the authoritarian Suharto regime, which lost its legitimacy and control for the first time in 32 years. In May 1998, Suharto stepped down amid widespread riots.

After the fall of Suharto, the country's economic system was reformed in tune with the neoliberal agenda, and a Social Safety Net program (*Jaring Pengaman Sosial*-JPS) was introduced to protect low-income households during the economic transition period. JPS consisted of (i) subsidized rice for the poor (OPK), (ii) a health card entitling the poor to free services (JPSBK), (iii) scholarships for children from low-income families (JPS-BO), (iv) block grants and the extension of micro-scale

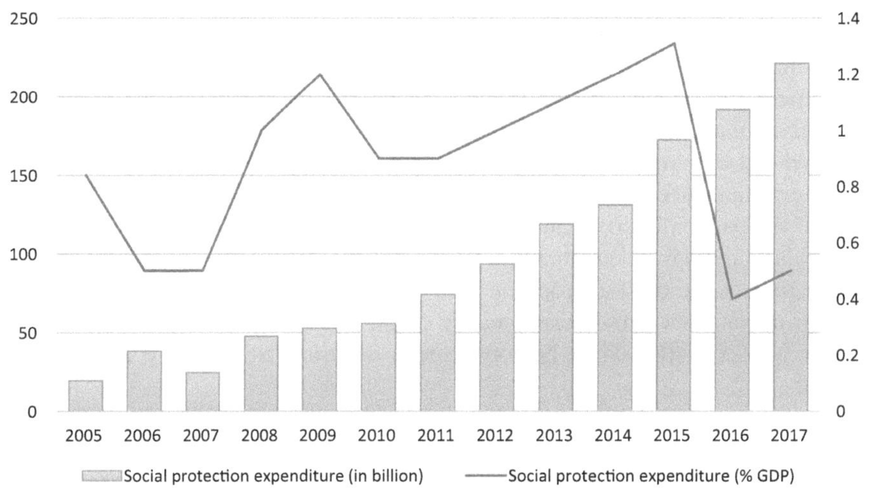

Fig. 7.1 GDP per capita growth (annual %). *Source* World Bank (2019)

credit for the informal sector, and (v) a work creation program (Padat Karya). JPS was originally meant to be temporary, given that the existing social protection system was unable to provide the poor and informal sector with substantial protection (Kwon and Kim 2015). However, the safety nets (except Padat Karya) were instead institutionalized by President Susilo Bambang Yudhoyono (2004–2014) and continued by his successor, Jokowi (2014-present). The social safety nets, as well as their new names, are as follows: (i) Raskin (2002)/food electronic voucher (2017), (ii) Askeskin (2005)/Jamkesmas (2007), (iii) Bantuan Operasional Sekolah (BOS) (2004), and (iv) PNPM Mandiri (2006)/BSPS/Kotaku (2014), coupled by some other new programs. The unconditional cash transfer (Bantuan Langsung Tunai-BLT) in 2005 and the conditional cash transfer or Prosperous Family Program (Program Keluarga Harapan-PKH) in 2007, both of which were introduced to mitigate the effects of rising oil prices, got the highest budget allocations.

Another important leap was the public insurance reform, which attempted to expand services with a more universalistic feature, with the poor families being exempted from paying the contribution. The reform was carried out by merging four separate social insurance (JAMSOSTEK, TASPEN, ASABRI, and ASKES) into one single administrative body, BPJS. BPJS was then divided into two areas: national health insurance (BPJS-Kesehatan) and employment-related insurance (BPJS-Ketenagakerjaan) (see Table 7.1). Despite this, universal coverage was almost successfully achieved in health care, while employment insurance coverage was still limited to formal workers. Although Law No. 40/2004 on National Social Security (NSS), which mandated social insurance integration, was passed in 2004, it was stalled for more than a decade due to political constraints (further explanation is provided in the next section), making low-income families who were not under the poverty line unprotected till 2014.

After 2014, the development of social policy shows a shift in the paradigm of the welfare approach, which fits the quasi-inclusive perspective. The term 'quasi-inclusive' means that the expansion of social policy has not fully reached the unemployed and informal workers. BPJS-Kesehatan is the only universal program that covers the entire population. Up to 2020, it has reached 83.4% of the total population, given that it provides a voluntary insurance program that offers services to registered self-employed individuals.

This explains the evolving institution. Drawing implications from this during the shock of the pandemic crisis, there is little time for the government to adjust their policy to fit the unpreceded situation. Extension in features and coverage with little modifications is the most appropriate path forward. In this sense, informal workers and their dependents remain excluded by social protection even if, in principle, as stated in Law No. 40/2004 on National Social Security (NSS), everyone should be included.

Table 7.1 Integration and restructurization plan of the prior segmented social insurance system under NSSS

Administering body prior to BPJS	Target	Sector	Current administering body
TASPEN	Civil Servants	Life	BPJS-Ketenagakerjaan (Employment-related Insurance)
		Work Accidents	
		Old Age Pension	
ASABRI	Military and Police	Life	
		Work Accidents	
		Old Age Pension	
JAMSOSTEK	Private Formal Sector Employees	Life	
		Work Accidents	
		Old Age Pension	
		Health	BPJS-Kesehatan (National Health Insurance)
ASKES	Civil Servants	Health	
JAMKESMAS/ASKESKIN	Near poor and poor	Health	

Sources Modified from Van-Diermen (2018) and Yuda (2019)

Shaping Policy Responses: Comparative Cases from Two Crises

The Asian Financial Crisis

A crisis, as debated by institutionalist scholars, refers to a critical juncture that opens the windows of opportunity for the country to macro system changes. As documented in many studies (Aspinall 2014; Fossati 2017; Hadiz 2013; Mackie 2010), right after Suharto stepped down, pressures for greater democratization began to mount, but they did not automatically make civil society and opposition parties gain the ground. This explanation rests on the democratic consolidation thesis, which argues that even though authoritarianism was overthrown in 1998, many of the core ideas and institutions President Suharto had introduced continued. The cross-class coalition supporting the ideas of social redistribution was underdeveloped and subordinated during this time. The following political climate "instead offered a majority of the political actors and bureaucrats previously involved in policymaking lucrative opportunities for reclaiming power" (Yuda 2021b: 2) through democratic competition. It was in the context of these changes that the transformation of the Indonesian welfare system was carried out. It achieved so by pushing the productivist welfare regime to take unprecedented steps ahead in providing social protection to more people.

The policy responses leading to welfare reform were divided into two layers of social protection, namely social assistance and social insurance. The first began under the transitional government of BJ Habibie (affiliated with the Golkar, a political machine of Suharto's regime) that took office in 1998. The Social Safety Net package (JPS-Jaring Pengaman Sosial), consisting of key five targeted social protection schemes (OPK, JPS-BK, JPS-BO and Padat Karya) for the poor, was introduced as an emergency relief scheme. This program was funded by the World Bank's loan offering scheme of US$600 million and supported by the ADB in providing technical assistance to enhance the effectiveness of program targeting. A study by Kwon and Kim (2015: 431) found that "despite assistance from international organizations, the targeting system for the program on social safety nets was evaluated as sub-standard." The situation was compounded by the mis-targeted and uneven distribution of JPS due to the unavailability of poor household datasets. The distribution relied only on the family planning program data, which were not yet updated.

In addition to what had been viewed as an economic and political stabilizer, JPS was considered a political machine for politicians to reach out to the poor voter. Being eminently political, JPS was permanently institutionalized with detailed scopes and features, as displayed in Fig. 7.2.

In further discussion, the expansion of the JPS and its redesign into its present form in 2004–2005 (see Fig. 7.2) has been closely linked to the upward spiral in fuel prices that directly led to public disorder in 2005. Equally important, such attempts at institutional realignment were followed by the national-scale census of poor households (July–September 2005) for the first time, which resulted in a 'PSE05 database.' This dataset was used as a reference to distribute existing social benefits, including additional schemes, namely unconditional cash transfers (*Bantuan Langsung Tunai*,

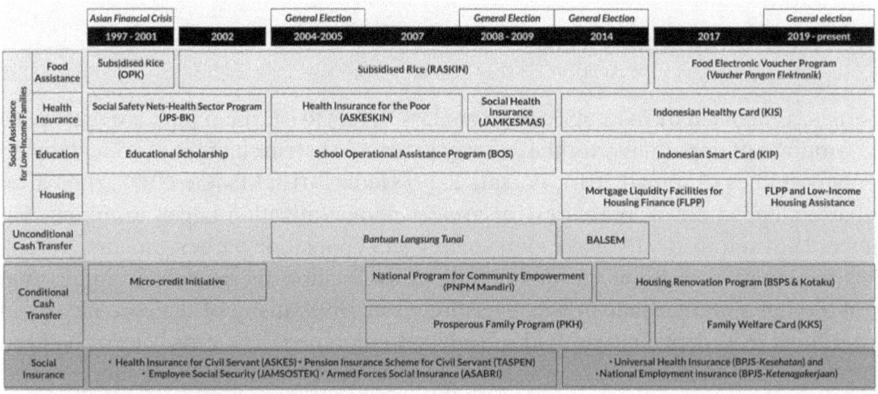

Fig. 7.2 The institutionalization process of targeted social protection in Indonesia post-Asian financial crisis. *Source* Modified from Yuda (2021a)

BLT), for that period, at the level of detail required. The BLT benefits were monthly cash transfers amounting to US$10.50, which targeted 15.5 million poor households all over the nation.

While BLT has been institutionalized, another feature of the cash transfer program that put forward the conditionality principle was introduced in 2007, namely the Program Keluarga Harapan (PKH). The original PKH was introduced as a poverty alleviation instrument in response to the crisis, but consultation on the feasibility of PKH was just undertaken around 2006 with the ADB and World Bank after learning that conditional cash transfers (CCTs) were succeeding in reducing poverty in Latin America. ADB and World Bank were the key external partners supporting PKH implementation in terms of technical assistance and financial support.

The time constraint of the PSE05 survey, coupled with a different understanding of poverty between community, local authorities, and the national government, led to continuous errors in social protection targeting (Alatas et al. 2016). Social conflicts, in turn, were unavoidable (Bazzi et al. 2015). To prevent the continued social conflicts, the government decided to update the beneficiary lists through the second wave of a national poor household survey in 2008–2009, which resulted in the PPL08 database. Nonetheless, the problem of mistargeting was reported again. As a policy response, in 2010, the PPL08 was upgraded and integrated into the Unified Targeting System (Alatas et al. 2016) and further upgraded in 2011 into the PPLS database. This new database system was managed by the National Team for the Acceleration of Poverty Reduction (*Tim Nasional Percepatan Penanggulangan Kemiskinan*, TNP2K) and used as the reference for distributing social protection benefits.

Consistent with the literature on this subject, democratization has intensively nurtured electoral competition, which, at certain moments (for example, around election season), has caused rising social protection expenditure. The illustration can be seen in Fig. 7.3, suggesting that social protection expenditure per GDP significantly increased ahead of the 2009 and 2014 elections. This process is outlined by the recent work of Lavers and Hickey (2021), who argued that as the political-economic system was restructured, traditional institutions lost their relevance in social risk internalization, enabling social protection to be expanded. Moreover, democracy enables the ruling political regime to define to whom the social benefits are targeted.

The idea of restructuring the second layer of social policy, namely social insurance, also began to consolidate in 1999 under the BJ Habibie Administration. Supported by the International Labor Organization (ILO), a national steering committee founded by the Ministry of Manpower and Transmigration (*Kementerian Tenaga Kerja dan Transmigrasi*, Kemenakertrans) explored the options for reforming JAMSOSTEK through the mega shift project, 'Restructuring of the Social Security System' (Kwon and Kim 2015). This project, at its core, aimed at initiating an inclusive social insurance system reaching more economic sectors.

Social unrest and the continued severity of the 1998 crisis provided a 'critical juncture' for President Abdurahman Wahid (1999–2001) to follow up the aftermentioned mega shift project, which was then continued by his successor, President Megawati Sukarnoputri (2001–2004) right after Wahid's ouster (Aspinall 2014). Discussed with labor unions, business representatives, and various international organizations (ADB,

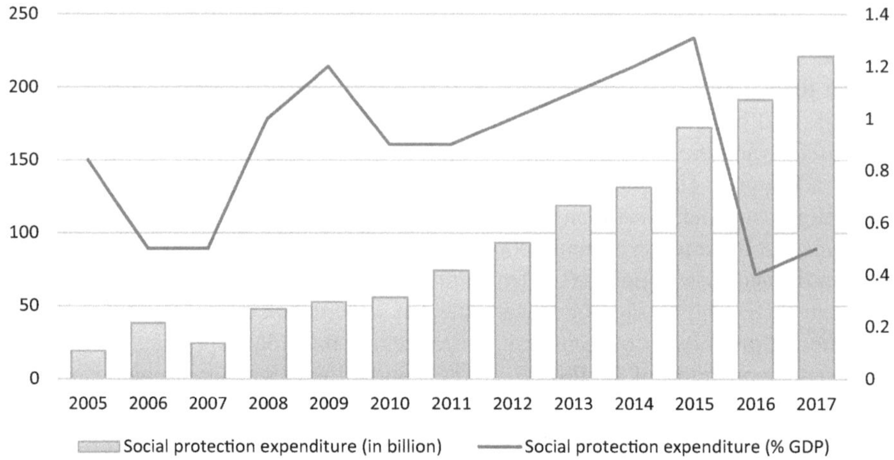

Fig. 7.3 Public social protection expenditure. *Sources* ADB (2019), ILO (2017) and Widjaja (2012)

GIZ, WB, WHO and EU), the ambitious plan to restructure the fragmented social insurance into one single administrative body covering the entire population ended up with the issuance of Law No. 40/2004 on National Social Security (NSS) (Kwon and Kim 2015). This law mandates the government to merge separate social insurance and establish BPJS to run the new integrated system (see Fig. 7.2 above). A greater initiative by Megawati finalized the draft national social security system to reflect the intentions of her party, the Indonesian Democratic Party of Struggle (PDI-P), to win the first democratic presidential election in Indonesian history in 2004 (Fossati 2017). Unfortunately, considerable efforts to attract the heart of informal and poor families ended with no benefit, as voters elected former army general Yudhoyono from the Democratic Party. Apart from political motives, the process of this social insurance restructuring reflects similar experiences in other Global South countries, as does the influential role played by international development agencies working on social protection (Schmitt 2020).

From this, it can be argued that the welfare reform, especially in the first phase, was not necessarily a democratization effect; instead, it was instrumental. It served as an emergency social strategy and 'sedative' when the government-run Structural Adjustment Program was used to restore the slumping economic condition. Tied to this, social policy literature extended the standard explanatory model of social policy by giving particular attention to the importance of international actors' influences in social policymaking despite the role of domestic elites (both national and local) who benefited from the reform, especially when it came to institutionalization (Holden 2015; Kaasch et al. 2019; Seekings 2019).

There have been many studies highlighting the institutional context in which strategic interactions of external and domestic actors take place in social policy-making. For example, Brooks (2015), Sugiyama (2011) and Schmitt (2020) find the positive effect of their presence in social security legislation against inclusive coverage agendas. Despite this, "recent welfare state expansion in the Global South has been unique in its reliance on social assistance (rather than social insurance) on the path towards universalism" (Dorlach 2020: 3).

The recent work by Yuda (2021b) further explains that the political process behind this expansion scenario emphasizing social assistance is linked to the political motives of domestic elites to integrate more economically marginalised groups as their political constituencies. This indicates that social policy models driven and promoted by international actors are not simply translated into domestic policies but have been fine-tuned to political interest rather than related directly to the social-economic context. In other words, international organizations have to find ways of negotiating their agendas in a context where often the more powerful political interest of domestic actors has been present together with heightened electoral competition. We take a brief detour through some cases of social policy dynamics, which offer good convictions to elucidate the external and domestic actors' relationships in shaping policy responses which gave way to a more long-term trajectory of welfare state development.

Although the NSSS law was passed, the administration of Susilo Bambang Yudhoyono (2004–2014), a new president democratically elected for the first time since the country's independence in 1945, delayed implementing the law. It resulted in an additional ten years of a universal social policy vacuum. Instead, the national government, supported by the local government, renewed the World Bank-sponsored social safety nets (Fig. 7.3). It is indicative of the importance of residual-like social protection as means to consolidate popular support during the periods of democratization and economic recovery. Successful implementation of the NSSS law found its momentum ahead of the 2014 presidential election.

Several studies (Aspinall 2014; Murphy 2019; Yuda 2019) point out the new political dimension of JPS institutionalization and underline why SJSN did not immediately gain political importance under the Yudhoyono Administration. The institutionalization of social assistance, however, was seen to be more lucrative to Yudhoyono's political standing, and the follow-up of Megawati's claimed legacy (the SJSN law) would be especially vulnerable to developments that make it hard for President Yudhoyono to continue to deliver patronage benefits. In the months before the general election of 2009, the public was surprised by the degree of Megawati's support for Yudhoyono's non-contributory programs. This raised questions, given that Megawati and her Indonesian Democratic Party of Struggle (PDI-P) were the most vocal voice against non-contributory social programs whilst urging support toward the immediate implementation of the NSSS law. This attitude arose predictably because Megawati would not have benefited politically in the upcoming election of 2009 if she kept in its undertaking. Unfortunately, an effort to increase her political image favoring poor groups did nothing, given that Yudhoyono won the election again.

A further impetus came in the form of mass pressure in 2010, when the Social Security Action Committee (KAJS, Komite Aksi Jaringan Sosial) comprised of 67 civil society, student, and labor organizations joined forces with sympathetic members of parliament to stage a demonstration on the grounds of parliament, urging legislators to implement NSSS. The pressure resulted in a successful decision in

2011, when the Law on Social Security Providers (BPJS) was approved (Joedadibrata 2012; Torheim 2013). The public was optimistic about the new law's quick adoption. However, the plan was re-stalled until 2014. Also apparent in that process was Yudhoyono and his Democratic Party's strategy to win the hearts of many people in the 2014 election, as Megawati did during her administration. Unfortunately, the Democratic Party lost the election, and President Jokowi, a controversial and populist leader from the PDI-P, was elected.

Under the Jokowi government, Susilo's legacy was redesigned and complemented with new features, such as unemployment benefits installed under BPJS-Ketenagakerjaan. Although he made no overall substantial difference (see Fig. 7.3), social provision was successfully expanded to broader swathes of the population.

In summary, there are two key features that can be highlighted in the first wave of social policy responses. First was the increase of the centrality of the social insurance system for welfare provision. The second feature was the rapid growth of social assistance for families with incomes below certain thresholds. The initiation of the welfare beneficiary database and its improvement, that has been deployed during the past two decades, could also be acknowledged as another essential feature of the welfare regime change in this country.

Overall, social policies originated in a condensed period during the Asian economic crisis and the mid-2000s but have since become a vital layer providing safety nets amidst the current pandemic crisis. The episode of continuity and change in Indonesian social policy during the pandemic, including institutional factors which have shaped the Indonesian response, will be discussed in the next section.

The Covid-19 Crisis

The outbreak of the Covid-19 Pandemic has brought about devasting public health and economic crisis. Indonesia, the world's fourth most populous nation, has been one of the most severely impacted nations in almost every sector.

Criticism of the Indonesian government in their response to outbreaks, particularly from epidemiologists and other public health experts, surged when the virus first began to spread across East Asia in January and February 2020. They highlighted Terawan, the former Health Minister, for his outlandish claims stating that Indonesia would be immune to infections due to its good diets and faith. His attitude of denial was also reflected in his response to a study by researchers at Harvard University's T.H. Chan School of Public Health, which predicted that the virus would spread all over the nation by the end of February. He insulted the report and challenged the researchers to prove and present their study (Fealy 2020; Olivia et al. 2020; Sparrow et al. 2020).

The government's attitude of denying the potential transmission of the virus did not stop there. Around February, unscientific and controversial speculation of other public officials was re-thrown. They said the tropical climate and the population's ethnic characteristics offered sufficient protection from the virus.

Attitudes discrediting the virus reached a peak when President Jokowi offered travel discounts of up to 30% to foreign tourists in February 2020. About US$8 million was allocated to tourism promotion (Fealy 2020). This policy contradicted those of the neighboring countries, which were preparing for social restrictions.

Confidently showing zero cases of transmission, the government convinced the public that Indonesia was a safe tourism and investment destination. WHO doubted the claim and issued a stern warning to the government, urging the officials to adopt more serious measures to withstand the great potential for virus' transmission across the region.

On March 2, the first two cases of Covid-19 in Jakarta were confirmed (registered). However, instead of avoiding the panic, Jokowi withheld the information regarding virus transmission by not declaring a public health emergency. As the transmission grew worse, especially in the Greater Jakarta region, which suddenly became the epicenter of the outbreak, the government finally faced pressure to forgo its plan to give a permit to foreign tourists to enter the country. However, due to escalating tensions between national and regional authorities seeking adequate steps to cut infection cases, social restrictions, a WHO-recommended mitigation tool, were stalled in their implementation.

Jakarta's Governor Anies Baswedan pioneered social restriction measures for the first time in Indonesia through the Large-Scale Social Distancing (PSBB) program. He intended to apply PPSSB earlier, but he did not receive approval from the Health Ministry, so PSSB was implemented on March 20, 2020. With the informal economy reaching a significant portion (55.7%), PSBB led to many people losing their livelihoods. Ad-hoc social protection packages were then rolled out, including unconditional cash transfers (BST), food subsidies, and educational assistance (KJP for elementary school students up to high school levels and KJMU for higher education students), targeting 2.4 million households. After Greater Jakarta, other regions such as West Java, Gorontalo, and West Sumatra followed suit.

Despite gaining approval, measures taken by Anies and other local governments received heated criticism from Jokowi and his supporters, who did not fully agree with the lockdown implementation. A notable reason for this opposition was the sizable economic contribution of the regions, especially Jakarta, to the national economy. Realizing that the virus had reached all regions of the country, on April 3, 2021, the president finally released the regulation to pave the way for large-scale social restrictions (PSBB), which was equivalent to a partial lockdown. This delayed response hindered the initiation of the necessary measures to curb the virus transmission.

It was not hard to assume why Jokowi was opposed to a lockdown. His background as a businessman and his presidential career, which was supported by a circle of oligarchs, extensively influenced his decision making that would have prioritized market interest. What was even more surprising was that the composition of the National Economic Recovery and Covid-19 Response Team, established in July, was dominated by businesspersons over public health experts. This reflects a re-enabled developmentalism-related logic configuration.

Overall, Indonesia's prospects of containing the virus were substantially weakened due to late responses and a lack of stringent containment measures, which were

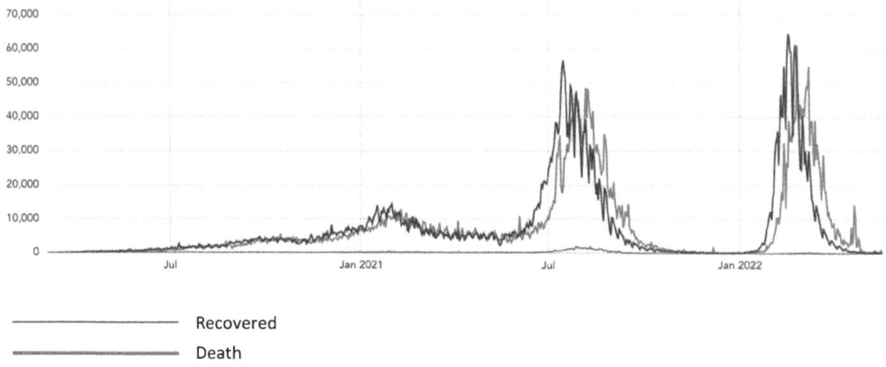

Fig. 7.4 Number of new registered Covid-19 cases per day in Indonesia (April 2020–May 2022). *Source* Satgas Covid-19 Republik Indonesia (2021)

aggravated by a shortage of supporting medical equipment during the first several months of the pandemic. Figure 7.4 shows a large rise in verified Covid-19 cases, demonstrating the virus' uncontrolled transmission and high fatality rate compared to other Southeast Asian countries.

With the implementation of the first lockdown in April 2020, Indonesia's economy suffered a 5.3% reduction in GDP, with 1.67 million workers of all income levels being laid off and furloughed. The rapid economic downturns generated intersecting social problems which compounded each other, ranging from the increased poverty rate (0.56%), increased economic inequality (0.001%) and increased criminality rate (19.72%), as compared with September 2019. Moreover, household consumption, which contributes to more than half of the national GDP, fell by 3.6% year-on-year in the fourth quarter, falling from 4.1% in the previous quarter. Under these circumstances, the remaining option was to raise large government deficits to escalate more social protection spending and maintain the purchasing power parity of Indonesia at the required levels.

Beginning with the issuance of the Law of the Republic of Indonesia No. 1 of 2020, the national financial allocation was prioritized for public healthcare, economic recovery, and social protection under the regulation. The national budget deficit limit was also stipulated, enabling the deficit to exceed 3% of GDP in the period of handling the transmission and its effect cause. However, in 2022, the budget deficit was allowed at a maximum of 3% of GDP.

With the financial boost received amounting to US$27.43 billion in the first period of the outbreak, US$7.44 billion was allocated to the Social Safety Net (SSN), while US$4.85 million was allocated for public health support. Other budgets were allocated to enable the quick recovery of the industrial sector (US$4.74 million) and the overall national economic performance (US$10.15 million).

It is worth noting here that the basic similarity of experiences in past crises reflected the role of international organizations as one of the drivers of social policy expansion. During the pandemic, the international organizations came back to experiment with, or support, new forms of social provision in various ways. The World Bank, for example, provided a loan totaling US$400 million to extend the PKH coverage from 6 to 10 million households. The fund was also used to update Indonesia's Social Registry (DTKS), which was used as a reference for social protection targeting. ADB also granted US$2.03 billion to the Indonesian government—one of its key allocation targets was the vaccine initiative, offering rapid support to counter the severe health impacts. In addition to financial support, technical assistance was also given, such as by ADB. In collaboration with the Indonesian Employers' Association (Apindo) and trade union confederations, ADB provided huge scale training to labor inspectors, professionals and other representatives of workers to promote increased health and hygiene culture at workplaces as part of supporting the economic recovery.

Another case has been the effort of the Australian Government to support WHO in providing technical support to the Indonesian Government through the Ministry of Health for strengthening information systems and surveillance, laboratory capacity building, and infection prevention and control. Recently, the assistance has been directed towards the vaccination initiative, coupled with the deployment of health experts to locations not yet reached by WHO or other international organizations.

Despite intensified external assistance, among middle-income countries in the Southeast Asia region, Indonesia (see Table 7.2) has the second-lowest spending rates for tackling the pandemic in the first year but rose to a little below Malaysia in the second year. The convergence largely occurred as Malaysia's spending significantly dropped from 10% in 2020 to 5.3% in 2021. Meanwhile, the Philippines made the least changes in their spending, which did not exceed 3%. Thailand is the only country that has consistently managed to maintain above-average spending levels to mitigate the pandemic.

Reflecting on the welfare regime changes during a pandemic, when it comes to a crisis, scholars often stick to the cognitive framework based on the long-term reproduction of an established welfare institutional pattern (Soon et al. 2021). In the following discussion, for example, the creation of a new feature tailored to a pandemic

Table 7.2 Summary of fiscal measures in response to the Covid-19 pandemic

Country	Additional spending or foregone revenues (% GDP)					
	Total		Health sector		Non-health sector	
	2020	2021	2020	2021	2020	2021
Indonesia	2.4	4.5	0.5	1.8	2.0	2.7
Thailand	8.2	11.4	N/A	N/A	N/A	N/A
Malaysia	10.00	5.3	N/A	0.3	N/A	5.0
Philippines	2.2	2.7	0.3	0.4	1.9	2.3
Average	5.7	5.97				

Source IMF (2021)

crisis was developed from established social policies (see Table 7.3). The exceptions have been Kartu Prakerja, Temporary Wage Subsidies, and other temporarily social assistances (internet quota subsidies and six-month tax exemption**). Kartu Prakerja was labelled as the Active Labor Market Policy (ALMP) and was operated by providing cash transfers amounting to US$67.60 per month. This scheme was also coupled with vocational training run by the Ministry of Labor in collaboration with designated private job training agencies. Meanwhile, the Temporary Wage Subsidy was operated by granting US$42.07 for four months to qualified formal workers, referring to those who were previously registered in the BPJS-Ketenagakerjaan scheme.

In analyzing the policy responses, it is essential not to rely on policies made as references in this study alone. The importance of oligarch forms of power could give an initial clue about the choices in relation to policies made by rulers in the context of labor market liberalization. The recent Indonesian experience on the issuance of Omnibus Law on October 5, 2020, provides sufficient empirical evidence to support this argument.

No one thought that the introduction of Kartu Prakerja was part of the Jokowi regime's plan to promote labor market deregulation. Instead of expanding the labor market during and after the epidemic, this bill contains too much labor-related relaxation as a means of attracting investment. The bill's major focus is on loosening the rigorous hiring and firing laws, including severance pay, which were thought to deter prospective investors from investing in Indonesia. As a result, Prakerja might be viewed as a 'sweetener' to the harsh reality that domestic employees, particularly in the informal sector, would confront in the near future while competing with international labor. Observers also pointed out that only businessmen and a limited group of elites were engaged in the bill's formulation, which was kept secret from the public until its legalization. Surprisingly, attempts at public opinion manipulation were also made by paying roughly US$101 to some influencers and buzzers. They were required to use the hashtag #IndonesiaNeedsJobs on social media to indicate their support for the new bill.

Overall, this controversial labor market restructuration illustrates the welfare state regression, which was intentionally hidden behind a veil of social safety nets extension in the name of salvaging the key parts of the national economy.

This is all the more troubling because Jokowi's close relations with the oligarchic alliance power during his presidency have contributed to a relatively disappointing performance in managing health policies. A recent example is the dominance of the oligarchic alliance power over the Polymerase Chain Reaction (PCR) test policy for aircraft passengers or others. Tied to this, many numerous sources reporting some large firms controlling the supply chains of the PCR service were closely affiliated with or owned by high-ranking officials and politicians in Indonesia. This 'profit-making' motivation of elites has hampered any measure to reduce the unreasonable and high PCR test price, especially in the first period of the outbreak, where the price amounted to US$175.42. It was then reduced to US$63.15 in October 2020 and continued to be brought down to around US$21.5 after receiving widespread

Table 7.3 Outline of social protection measures during Covid-19 by component

Social assistance	Health	Education	Active labor market	Pension	Unemployment
• BPNT (food subsidies) • Program Kaluga Harapan/Kartu Keluarga Sejahtera (conditional cash transfer) • Bantuan langsung Tunai (unconditional cash transfer) • National Program for Community Empowerment	• JKN (national health insurance; compulsory for the formal sector, voluntary for others) • JKN-sponsored Program for the poor	• Indonesian Smart Card (Scholar-ship for the poor) • Free primary and junior secondary education	• Program BLK (job Training Programs)	• BPJS-Ketenaga-kerjaan Program	• Jaminan Kehilangan Pekerjaan (unemployment benefits)

Source Author compilation

criticism. On the other hand, reports linking PCR regulation to elite entrenched interests emerged piecemeal.

One question remains unanswered: does the Indonesian welfare regime's approach to social policy remain to be a developmental-centered approach? The introduction of Kartu Pra-Kerja implies that Indonesia has been adopting developmental ideas in governing welfare, and its other new extended programs are not meant to be generous. The overall program, though making a clear improvement in social spending, is certainly not any kind of social policy system on Welfare state regime lines. However, it has become a widespread concern among scholars that once particular policy areas are examined further, the general character of the welfare regime tends to break down. The welfare regime analysis is most useful when it helps us understand how a country organizes its welfare system and grants social provision to citizens. In the case of Indonesia, the pandemic has led the welfare system to serve more instrumental purposes—facilitating labor market engineering for attracting foreign and domestic investment and protecting purchasing power parity of households. In this sense, this paper regards Indonesia as a protective-developmental welfare regime.

Despite the political controversy working behind the response, it can be summarized that the welfare institutional change displayed during the welfare regime during the crisis obviously reflects policymaking that relies on the combined logic of institutional legacies and threat-rigidity logic. The new introduction may only happen when the existing welfare arrangement has been inadequate to respond to the emerged social risk.

Lessons Learned

This comparative analysis of the two crises of different periods in Indonesia suggests two distinct pathways to the policy response. During the Asian Financial Crisis, the response was to change to two layers of social policy—social protection and social insurance. The former was made possible by the emergence of urgent and uncertain situations when the welfare institution, whether state or informal network, to mitigate the crisis was inadequate. This period of social protection lasted, but it was not conditioned as a set of social rights with any prospect of permanence. Progress toward institutionalization was eventually made, but mostly as a result of a tug-of-war between politicians' clientelistic interests and extremely contested elections.

The subsequent leap of the reform was on social insurance due to the political structure of the regime, which was largely detached from the interested group (Hadiz 2003), social insurance reform could not be presented as a response to the demand of the cross-class coalition of the leftist movement for welfare, even in terms of democratization. Additionally, the case presented here also produced the belief that social policy reforms were effectively made only after "endogenous developments had begun a cumulative process of divergence from the old path" (Varjonen 2020: 2). As previously stated, Indonesia began to modify its social policies in the 1970s. In the early 1990s, similar programs were expanded to include larger portions of the productive population. The government restructured social insurance in 2004 to make it available to all sectors for the first time. This has largely slipped the attention of many institutional accounts in the developing world.

During the pandemic crisis, the social policy responses have implemented only minor adjustments to the broader welfare system. The explanation of this may rest on two arguments. First is the threat-rigidity logic, which means that governments are unlikely to experiment with new approaches that may bring unknown risks. They stick to their cognitive frame of reference, shaped by legacies (Soon et al. 2021). The second argument is the path-dependence logic, given that social policy and the political interest of predatory elites have become 'interwoven' and mutually interdependent institutions, especially in the context of social protection, which is essential for the patron-client relationship's survival. Attention to the latter will advance our understanding of path-dependence theories that are attached to patron-client motives instead of social rights defense, as theorized by many scholars. This issue is left fuzzy in many institutional works which are largely centered on the European welfare states.

The drastic change is only found in the labor-market policy that was restructured into more flexible settings. Significantly, as explained above, the restructuring, preceded by the introduction of Kartu Prakerja (Active Labor Market Policy), reflects the continuing salience of the interests that had been embedded in the established network of patronage that remains intact among policy actors and their association with oligarchs. The 'outsider' had no real capacity to influence policymaking. The situation exemplifies institutional stagnation resulting from historical failure of democratization to effectively empower cross-class coalition to promote more protective welfare system against the influence of oligarch power.

Despite the different pathways, transnational dimensions are very much attached to social policy development in Indonesia during periods of crisis. This indicates the importance of understanding the impact of external factors on national policy making. Tied to this, Shriwise (2020: 30) noted that "[international organizations] may act independently in line with their own interests or as instruments of powerful nation-states, and they may also act in line with broader institutional norms and practices over time." Notable examples of the first argument are the World Bank and IMF. Their activities in this country intensified during the crisis as the importance of Indonesia as a growing market for products expansion of the developed world. By helping the country extend social transfers to low-income families, this solution expectedly maintains the households' purchasing power parity, which is essential for investment and market expansion.

Taking a different route from financial agencies, UN-sponsored international organizations such as WHO, ILO, UNDP and other bilateral and multilateral organizations urged the government to support more comprehensive approaches to social policy to advance the social rights of individuals. As demonstrated in the examined Asian Financial Crisis case, where interest and ideas on how best to restructure social protection targeting larger sectors of the population were negotiated between international organizations and domestic actors, these organizations were concerned with the universal health and employment-related protection. However, the more common case is that international organizations' recommendations are often not perfectly institutionalized unless their prescription is in line with the political actors of interest. The case of labor market restructuring could be a recent illustration of how decommodification measures suggested by ILO have been deflected by predatory elite interest, hidden behind a veil of economic recovery policy.

Overall, what matters the most in explaining the potential causes favoring and precluding welfare institutional change in Indonesia—including variations in policy outcomes that are formed out of the two crises—is not an attachment to path dependence or the self-reinforcing mechanisms that have been negotiated between state and consolidated cross-class coalition. Instead, it is the oligarchic power and its extension to ruling political parties that need to be examined more thoroughly to explain the path of the welfare changes and policies in the country. In addition, the emergence of the pandemic has paved the way for an entrenched system of oligarchic power whereby the oligarchs attempted to reorganize their domination.

References

ADB, Asian Development Bank. 2019. *Social protection expenditure in Asia and the Pacific*. https://data.adb.org

Alatas, V., A. Banerjee, R. Hanna, B. A. Olken, R. Purnamasari, and M. Waipoi. 2016. Self-targeting: Evidence from a field experiment in Indonesia. *Journal of Political Economy* 124(2), https://doi.org/10.1086/685299.

Aspalter, C. 2006. The East Asian welfare model. *International Journal of Social Welfare* 15 (4): 290–301.

Aspalter, C., ed. 2021. *Financing welfare state systems in Asia*. Oxon: Routledge.

Aspalter, C., K. Teguh-Pribadi, and R. Gauld. (eds.). 2017. *Health care systems in developing countries in Asia*. Oxon: Routledge.

Aspinall, E. 2014. Health care and democratization in Indonesia. *Democratization* 21(5). https://doi.org/10.1080/13510347.2013.873791.

Barrientos, A., and D. Hulme. 2009. Social protection for the poor and poorest in developing countries: Reflections on a quiet revolution. *Oxford Development Studies* 37 (4): 439–456.

Bazzi, S., S. Sumarto, and A. Suryahadi. 2015. It's all in the timing: Cash transfers and consumption smoothing in a developing country. *Journal of Economic Behavior and Organization*. https://doi.org/10.1016/j.jebo.2015.08.010.

Béland, D., B. Cantillon, R. Hick, and Moreira, A. 2021. Social policy in the face of a global pandemic: Policy responses to the Covid-19 crisis. *Social Policy and Administration* 55(2). https://doi.org/10.1111/spol.12718.

Béland, D., and M. Powell. 2016. Continuity and change in social policy. *Social Policy & Administration* 50 (2): 129–147.

Berenschot, W., R. Hanani, and P. Sambodho. 2018. Brokers and citizenship: Access to health care in Indonesia. *Citizenship Studies* 22 (2): 129–144.

Böger, T., and L. Leisering. 2020. A new pathway to universalism? Explaining the spread of 'social' pensions in the Global South, 1967–2011. *Journal of International Relations and Development* 23 (2): 308–338.

Brooks, S. M. 2015. Social protection for the poorest: The adoption of antipoverty cash transfer programs in the Global South. *Politics and Society* 43(4). https://doi.org/10.1177/0032329215602894.

Cox, R. H. 2004. The path-dependency of an idea: Why Scandinavian welfare states remain distinct. *Social Policy and Administration* 38(2). https://doi.org/10.1111/j.1467-9515.2004.00386.x.

Van Diermen, M. 2018. Welfare in transition: The political economy of social protection reform in Indonesia. *Thesis*, The University of Adelaide. https://digital.library.adelaide.edu.au.
Dorlach, T. 2020. The causes of welfare state expansion in democratic middle-income countries: A literature review. *Social Policy and Administration*. https://doi.org/10.1111/spol.12658.
Fealy, G. 2020. Jokowi in the Covid-19 era: Repressive pluralism, dynasticism and the overbearing state. *Bulletin of Indonesian Economic Studies* 56(3). https://doi.org/10.1080/00074918.2020.1846482.
Fossati, D. 2017. From periphery to centre: Local government and the emergence of universal healthcare in Indonesia. *Contemporary Southeast Asia* 39(1). https://doi.org/10.1355/cs39-1f.
Gough, I. 2004. Welfare regimes in development contexts: A global and regional analysis. In: *Insecurity and welfare regimes in Asia, Africa and Latin America*, eds. I. Gough and G. Wood. Cambridge: Cambridge University Press.
Hacker, J.S. 2002. *The divided welfare state*. Cambridge: Cambridge University Press. https://doi.org/10.1017/cbo9780511817298.
Hadiz, V. R. 2003. Reorganizing political power in Indonesia: A reconsideration of so-called "democratic transitions". *Pacific Review* 16(4). https://doi.org/10.1080/0951274032000132272.
Hadiz, V. R. 2013. The rise of capital and the necessity of political economy. *Journal of Contemporary Asia* 43(2). https://doi.org/10.1080/00472336.2012.757433.
Holden, C. 2015. Global social policy in the making: The foundations of the social protection floor, by Bob Deacon, Bristol: Policy Press. *Social Policy and Administration* 49 (3): 412–413.
Holliday, I. 2000. Productivist welfare capitalism: Social policy in East Asia. *Political Studies* 48 (4): 706–723.
ILO. 2017. *World social protection report data*. http://www.social-protection.org.
IMF. 2021. *Database of fiscal policy responses to Covid-19*. https://www.imf.org.
Joedadibrata, D. 2012. A study of the shift towards universal social policy in Indonesia. *Master thesis*, International Institute of Social Studies, Rotterdam, https://thesis.eur.nl/pub/13046.
Kaasch, A., M. Koch, and K. Martens. 2019. Exploring theoretical approaches to global social policy research: Learning from international relations and inter-organisational theory. *Global Social Policy* 19(1–2). https://doi.org/10.1177/1468018119845570.
Yuda, T.K., and S. Kühner. 2022. Bringing Indonesia into the global welfare regime debate: A literature review and future research agenda. *Asian Social Work and Policy Review*. https://doi.org/10.1111/aswp.12275.
Kuhlmann, J., and F. Nullmeier. 2021. A mechanism-based approach to the comparison of national pension systems in Vietnam and Sri Lanka. *Social Policy and Administration*. https://doi.org/10.1111/spol.12691.
Kwon, H.J. 2009. The reform of the developmental welfare state in East Asia. *International Journal of Social Welfare* 18 (1): 512–521.
Kwon, H.J., and W.R. Kim. 2015. The evolution of cash transfers in Indonesia: Policy transfer and national adaptation. *Asia and the Pacific Policy Studies* 2 (2): 425–440.
Lavers, T., and S. Hickey. 2016. Conceptualising the politics of social protection expansion in low-income countries: The intersection of transnational ideas and domestic politics. *International Journal of Social Welfare* 25(4). https://doi.org/10.1111/ijsw.12210.
Lavers, T., and S. Hickey. 2021. Alternative routes to the institutionalisation of social transfers in Sub-Saharan Africa: Political survival strategies and transnational policy coalitions. *World Development*. https://doi.org/10.1016/j.worlddev.2021.105549.
London, J. D. 2018. *Welfare and inequality in marketizing East Asia*. https://doi.org/10.1057/978-1-137-54106-2.
Mackie, J. 2010. Patrimonialism: The new order and beyond. In: *Soeharto's new order and its legacy: Essays in honour of Harold Crouch*, eds. E. Aspinall and G. Fealy. https://doi.org/10.22459/snol.08.2010.06.
Mahoney, J., and K. Thelen. 2009. Explaining institutional change: Ambiguity, agency, and power. In: *Explaining institutional change: Ambiguity, agency, and power*, ed. J. Mahoney and K. Thelen. https://doi.org/10.1017/CBO9780511806414.

Mahoney, J. 2017. Shift happens: The historical institutionalism of Kathleen Thelen. *PS - Political Science and Politics* 50(4). https://doi.org/10.1017/S1049096517001494.
Mares, I., and M. E. Carnes. 2009. Social policy in developing countries. *Annual Review of Political Science* 12. https://doi.org/10.1146/annurev.polisci.12.071207.093504
Mok, K. H., Ku, Y.-W., Yuda, T. K. 2021. Managing the Covid-19 pandemic crisis and changing welfare regimes. *Journal of Asian Public Policy* 14(1). https://doi.org/10.1080/17516234.2020.1861722.
Moreira, A., and R. Hick. 2021. Covid-19, the Great Recession and social policy: Is this time different? *Social Policy and Administration* 55(2). https://doi.org/10.1111/spol.12679.
Murphy, J. 2010. Path dependence and the stagnation of Australian social policy between the wars. *Journal of Policy History* 22(4). https://doi.org/10.1017/S0898030610000229.
Murphy, J. (2019). The historical development of Indonesian social security. *Asian Journal of Social Science* 47(2). https://doi.org/10.1163/15685314-04702005.
O'Connor, J., and P. Pierson. 1995. Dismantling the welfare state? Reagan, Thatcher, and the politics of retrenchment. *Contemporary Sociology* 24(5). https://doi.org/10.2307/2077364.
Olivia, S., J. Gibson, and R. Nasrudin. 2020. Indonesia in the time of Covid-19. *Bulletin of Indonesian Economic Studies* 56(2). https://doi.org/10.1080/00074918.2020.1798581.
Ozkan, R.O. 2015. Welfare regime change—or lack of change—in unemployment compensation. *International Journal of Social Welfare* 25 (2): 126–135.
Pierson, P. 1994. *Dismantling the welfare state?: Reagan, Thatcher and the politics of retrenchment*, New York: Cambridge University Press.
Pierson, P. 2004. Positive feedback and path dependence. In: *Politics in time: History, institutions, and social analysis*, ed. P. Pierson. Princeton: Princeton University Press.
Rosser, A., M. Van Diermen, and J.-H.Choi. 2016. Beyond predatory productivism?: The political economy of welfare capitalism in post-new order Indonesia. *Asia Review* 5(2). https://doi.org/10.24987/snuacar.2016.02.5.2.157.
Satgas Covid-19 Republik Indonesia. 2021. *Peta sebaran Covid-19.* https://Covid19.go.id.
Schmitt, C. 2020. From colonialism to international aid. In: *From colonialism to international aid: External actors and social protection in the Global South*, ed. C. Schmitt. Cham: Springer.
Seekings, J. 2019. The limits to 'global' social policy: The ILO, the social protection floor and the politics of welfare in East and Southern Africa. *Global Social Policy* 19(1–2). https://doi.org/10.1177/1468018119846418.
Shriwise, A. 2020. Advancing transnational approaches to social protection in the Global South. In: *From colonialism to international aid: External actors and social protection in the Global South*, ed. C. Schmitt. Cham: Springer.
Soon, S., C. C. Chou, and S. J. Shi. 2021. Withstanding the plague: Institutional resilience of the East Asian welfare state. *Social Policy and Administration* 55(2). https://doi.org/10.1111/spol.12713.
Sparrow, R., T. Dartanto, and R. Hartwig. 2020. Indonesia under the new normal: Challenges and the way ahead. *Bulletin of Indonesian Economic Studies* 56(3). https://doi.org/10.1080/00074918.2020.1854079.
Starke, P. 2006. The politics of welfare state retrenchment: A literature review. *Social Policy and Administration* 40 (1): 104–120.
Sugiyama, N. B. 2011. The diffusion of conditional cash transfer programs in the Americas. *Global Social Policy* 11(2–3). https://doi.org/10.1177/1468018111421295.
Torheim, R. 2013. Foundations of a welfare regime: The case of Indonesia. Thesis, University of Oslo. https://www.duo.uio.no/handle/10852/36942.
Varjonen, S. 2020. Institutional evolution and abrupt change: Reforming the administration of social assistance in Finland. *International Journal of Social Welfare* 29 (1): 62–70.
WB, World Bank. 2019. *GDP per capita growth.* https://data.worldbank.org.
Widjaja, M. 2012. Indonesia in search of a placement-support social protection. *ASEAN Economic Bulletin* 29 (3): 184–196.

Yang, N., and S. Kühner. 2020. Understanding social policy divergence in East Asia. *The Social Policy Blog*. https://socialpolicyblog.com/2020/05/11.

Yuda, T.K. 2021a. The complementary roles between clientelism and familism in social policy development. *Social Policy & Administration* 55 (3): 1370–1392.

Yuda, T.K. 2021b. The limits of healthcare reforms in Indonesia: Interrogating the Dutch Colonial legacies' influence within the logic and principles of welfare. *International Journal of Social Welfare* 31 (2): 236–247.

Yuda, T.K., and S. Kühner. 2022. Bringing Indonesia into the global welfare regime debate: A literature review and future research agenda. *Asian Social Work & Policy Review*. https://doi.org/10.1111/aswp.12275.

Yuda, T. K., and J. D. Nurhadi. 2021a. Examining emerging social policy during Covid-19 in Indonesia and the case for a community-based support system. *Asia Pacific Journal of Social Work and Development* 31(1–2). https://doi.org/10.1080/02185385.2020.1829499.

Yuda, T. K., P. P. Pratiyudha, and K. A. Kafaa. 2021b. Managing social policy in the emerging welfare regime of governance: What Indonesia can learn from South Korea's experience. *International Social Work*. https://doi.org/10.1177/00208728211011634.

Yuda, T. K. 2019. Welfare regime and the patrimonial state in contemporary Asia: Visiting Indonesian cases. *Journal of Asian Public Policy* 12(3). https://doi.org/10.1080/17516234.2018.1462685.

Part III
Country Case Study Chapters on the Pandemic Itself (With Additional Focal Points)

Chapter 8
The Pandemic in Mainland China: With Special Reference to Rising Relative Poverty

Tao Liu

Abstract Two important events in 2020 have affected the development trajectory and path of China's social policy: the first is that the Chinese government announced the eradication of absolute poverty; the second is the outbreak of Covid-19 and the subsequent stringent social control measures. This paper focuses upon the issue of relative poverty in China in the post-poverty era since 2020. Concretely, this research mainly highlights the relative poverty caused by the Covid-19, such as the rising unemployment rate and relative poverty caused by strict lockdown and shutdown measures. At the same time, this research studies how China's social insurance and social assistance cope with the rising relative poverty in the crisis period, and the implementation of some special economic, fiscal, and social policies also helps to alleviate the consequences of the relative poverty during the pandemic. Moreover, this paper also introduces the relative poverty independent of the Covid-19 Pandemic, that is, the problem of "*secondary poverty*" and expenditures-related poverty mentioned in the Chinese context. Some households fall into the poverty trap not because of low income, but because of the severe diseases and long-term care of family members, which need to be solved by the innovation of China's social policy system.

Keywords Covid-19 pandemic · China · Relative poverty · Lockdown · Policy response · Social policy

2020 is a year of special significance in the history of China's social policy: the Covid-19 Pandemic first broke out in Wuhan, China, which "dragged" the whole country into the crisis management and crisis response mode. China's welfare regime began to respond to the unpredictable social crisis and a large number of social risks based on the emergency. Surprisingly, the pandemic did not disrupt the development pace of the Chinese government. On the contrary, China's ruling elite group continued to promote the grand plan of eradicating poverty which has been proposed before the outbreak of the pandemic. In the same year, the Chinese government announced the

T. Liu (✉)
School of Public Affairs, Zhejiang University, Hangzhou, China
e-mail: taoliu1975@zju.edu.cn

C. Aspalter (ed.), *Covid-19 Pandemic*,
https://doi.org/10.1007/978-981-99-2497-4_8

elimination of poverty according to the original plan. So far, China has entered the post-poverty era. However, it should be noted that poverty here refers to absolute poverty. Relative poverty exists in any human society, and of course, it will continue to exist in China and even in the post-poverty era. The superposition of the two historic events constitutes an unusual year for China's social policy.

This chapter will specifically address the following two issues: first, how China's socioeconomic and welfare regime responds to the special emergency of the pandemic and uses institutionalized means to reduce the social risks within the crisis; second, how China's socioeconomic and welfare regime responds to the special phenomenon of relative poverty alongside the Covid-19 Pandemic. Considering that the pandemic, a social emergency crisis, is also an important reason for the rise of relative poverty, China's relative poverty since 2020 must include both conventional relative poverty and special forms of relative poverty induced by the pandemic and rigorous measures of containing the spread of corona virus. Considering the inseparable relationship between the pandemic and relative poverty, this chapter focuses on the analysis of relative poverty during the pandemic.

China's social policy response mechanism is also limited to the special field of coping with relative poverty alongside the pandemic, and less involved in medical insurance, public health and pandemic prevention and some other areas. The study shows that the pandemic is a special inducement to the rise of relative poverty. The rising unemployment rate caused by the pandemic, the closure of small and micro enterprises and the suspension of factories have exacerbated the situation of relative poverty. China's comprehensive social safety net plays an important social function to alleviate the rising relative poverty rate in the society, but it cannot completely eliminate the negative social consequences of the pandemic. The development of China's relative poverty still largely depends on when China can get out of the predicament of the pandemic.

Relative Poverty in the Modern Society: Notions and Concepts

Poverty can be divided into two main types: absolute poverty and relative poverty (Foster 1998; Madden 2000). The definition of absolute poverty is relatively clear and fixed. It mainly refers to the serious material shortage faced by residents and social groups, and the lack of the most basic material conditions for survival. Absolute poverty is often associated with hunger or famine in human societies. The material reserves and monetary reserves of people cannot meet the basic living conditions of mankind. According to the definition of the United Nations, absolute poverty is "a condition characterized by severe deprivation of basic human needs, including food, safe drinking water, sanitation facilities, health, shelter, education and information."[1] The measurement of absolute poverty is also relatively simple and transparent. For example, the World Bank defined the international absolute poverty line as US$1.90

per day in 2015 and established the global poverty standard in the form of monetary income.[2] Absolute poverty has a certain universality, objectivity, and commensurability. By using relatively simplified quantitative indicators, countries all over the world can compare the development status of absolute poverty. In general, the main problem faced by developed countries and high-income countries is not absolute poverty, but relative poverty. As a newly industrialized country that is very close to the high-income threshold, China, like most OECD countries, faces mainly the problem of relative poverty (Ravallion and Chen 2011; Moller et al. 2003).

Compared with absolute poverty, relative poverty is much more complex and contains more aspects. A country can claim to have largely eliminated absolute poverty within its sovereign borders, but it can never claim to have eliminated relative poverty completely. Relative poverty as such cannot be eliminated due to its "relativity." It can only be said that relative poverty has been alleviated and reduced, rather than the vanishing relative poverty. Relative poverty reflects the relative relationship between income groups in a society. Its core focus is the relationship between low-income groups and other social groups. It is precisely because relative poverty measures the intra-group difference in income and assets, so there is relative poverty in both poor and affluent countries. Relative poverty exists even in the wealthy Nordic Scandinavian welfare states (Gustafsson and Pedersen 2018).

The measurement indicators of relative poverty are relatively diversified, and unlike the measurement indicators of absolute poverty, relative poverty does not have a completely unified set of measurement indicators. The standard of relative poverty is largely influenced by some international organizations and supranational entities. For example, OECD usually takes 40–60% of median household income in its member states as the standard of relative poverty,[3] while the European Commission also takes 60% of the median household income as the threshold of relative poverty of EU Member States. Additionally, it is also suggested to use 40 and 50% of the median household income as reference indicators by the European Commission (Van Vliet and Wang 2015).

The report on global poverty released by the World Bank in 2018 sets different relative poverty thresholds according to different income levels of different countries in addition to the global absolute poverty bottom line. For example, the relative poverty line in low- and middle-income countries is US$3.2 per day, the relative poverty line in upper-middle-income countries is US$5.5 per day, and the relative poverty line in high-income countries is US$21.7 per day (WB 2018).

In addition to the above-mentioned "hard indicators" measuring relative poverty, relative poverty also reflects a complex living state that can be linked with different "soft indicators." Relative poverty also requires some qualitative and theory-based analytical description. For example, from a sociological perspective, relative poverty is often associated with social exclusion (Kabeer 2000; Notten and de Neubourg 2011; De Haan and Maxwell 2007; Halleröd and Larsson 2008), which means that people suffering from relative poverty cannot fully participate in economic, social, and cultural life. Relative poverty can be exacerbated by lack of equality of opportunity, such as lack of educational opportunities. Relative poverty may also be affected by important events in the individual life course. For example, a middle-income household may be greatly affected by the severe illness of family members and the resulting "out-of-pocket expenses" when their country lacks a comprehensive medical insurance system. A relatively prosperous agricultural-industrial area may be affected by extreme weather such as hail and floods, and its production may be greatly reduced. If a country does not establish a corresponding agricultural catastrophe insurance scheme, the entire disaster-affected area may temporarily fall into relative poverty. Relative poverty is strongly affected by various disasters, crises, natural and social risks, and therefore multiple factors may lead to the rise of relative poverty. The intervention of the state is also an important factor affecting relative poverty. If the state establishes a wide range of support and assistance systems and risk adjustment systems by intervening in the field of individual social life, then relative poverty may be alleviated. On the contrary, relative poverty may rise in case of the absence of public assistance and social protection, even in the affluent countries from the Global North (Kangas and Palme 2000).

Compared with the definition and measurement of absolute poverty, relative poverty displays its diversity. The synthesis of multi-dimensional indicators helps to measure the relative poverty of residents. In general, income is still the most important measure of relative poverty. The poverty threshold or social assistance threshold based on a certain percentage of the median household income, or the national average income is the common practice of most OECD countries. The World Bank determines the relative poverty standard for countries with different levels of development according to a lump-sum income, which is still a relatively rare practice. If relative poverty reflects not only a static state, but a dynamic momentum, then social factors in a broad sense, especially the institutional arrangements of social policy and public policy, are also relevant reasons alleviating relative poverty. For example, whether a country's medical security system is complete and sound, whether a country has a well-functioning old-age protection system, and whether a country has established a wide range of old-age service facilities, especially the long-term care insurance, and these multiple factors will inevitably affect the development of relative poverty.

The Rising Relative Poverty During the Covid-19 Pandemic and China's

Social Policy Responses

In January 2020, the corona virus broke out in Wuhan, the capital city of Hubei Province, China. The new pandemic spread rapidly to other cities in Hubei and other provinces and cities in China, and even evolved into a protracted global pandemic. Due to China's unique party-government integration model and strong national and social mobilization capability, China controlled the first wave of the pandemic within three months, while implementing the world's most stringent "dynamic zero Covid-19 strategy." Afterwards, the second and third waves of pandemic broke out in many places in China. China's epidemic center has shifted from Wuhan to Shijiazhuang, Changchun, Nanjing, and other places. At present, China's megacity Shanghai is suffering from the severe impact of a new wave of pandemic, and China's "dynamic zero Covid-19 strategy" is also undergoing a severe test.

The pandemic-related crisis has greatly impacted the normal social and economic order and caused great anxiety and panic in the public perception world. The stringently enforced social distance has also forced hundreds of millions of practitioners to leave the workplace temporarily, and their families have become temporary "shelters" and "office places," while employees who cannot complete their professional tasks through "home-office model" have become the "victims" of the pandemic. Faced with forced shutdowns and income disruptions, a large number of temporary workers and flexible employees have become losers in the crisis, and their livelihood has become a huge social problem.

The "zero Covid-19 strategy" strictly implemented by various local governments in China and the accompanying curfew and lockdown have also greatly deteriorated people's living conditions, and a large number of service industries such as the catering and the film and entertainment industry have been nearly devastated. With the emergence of the second wave, the third wave and even the fourth wave of the pandemic, the lockdown plan originally thought to be temporary and short-term has now shown a long-term trend, and the living conditions of specific groups and industries have been affected by the pandemic for a long time. In recent human history, the wave of unemployment caused by the Covid-19 Pandemic can even be compared to the Great Depression of the 1920s and 1930s (Selgin 2021). To sum up, the pandemic is not only an epidemiological crisis, but also a social crisis. The social consequence of the pandemic is the rise of relative poverty.

Next, this paper will analyze the rise of relative poverty during the Covid-19 crisis from different levels.

An Overview of China's Relative Poverty Development During the Covid-19 Pandemic

Since China does not set a poverty line or a relative poverty line, neither at the national level nor at the local level, there is such a standard line, so it is impossible to describe China's relative poverty through a unified scale. However, China established the urban Minimum Living Standard Scheme (MLSS, in Chinese "Dibao") in 1999 covering the urban households and residents whose income falls below the minimum acceptable standard of living according to local conditions, and since then this system has also been extended to rural areas in 2007 (Liu and Sun 2016; Leisering et al. 2017), so China has formed a dual basic income security system, which is equivalent to the social assistance in OECD countries (Leisering et al. 2006). In addition to the urban and rural minimum living security system, China's social assistance also includes the assistance for extremely poor households—the so called "tekunhu." Literally, "tekunhu" refers to those households who face special difficulties in life. Their living standards are not only lower than the Dibao-line, but also close to the bottom line of physical survival. Moreover, China also has a separate temporary assistance scheme, that is, relief for people who are not registered in the city, this system mainly covers the basic living needs of floating population from other cities or villages. The comprehensive application of these composite indicators can well reflect the development state and dynamic of China's relative poverty. Methodologically, this paper mainly selects the data of the MLSS, the Assistance for the Extremely Poor (AEP) and the Temporary Assistance (TA) in the years before and during the pandemic to describe the change of China's relative poverty. When accessible, some social assistance programs also include the data of 2021, and most social assistance programs only have the data of 2020, because the social assistance data of 2021 has not been fully released so far.

Based on the author's synthesis of data released by the Ministry of Civil Affairs (MOC) and government statistical bulletin over the past years, this study shows the development of China's Minimum Living Standard Scheme (MLSS) before and after the pandemic. Figure 8.1 shows that before the pandemic, the number of households receiving MLSS in both urban and rural areas in China continued to decline. From 2019 to 2020, the number of households receiving MLSS in urban areas dropped slightly from 5.25 million to 4.89 million, while the number of households receiving MLSS in rural areas increased from 18.92 million to 19.85 million in the same period. The development in rural areas shows that the relative poverty in rural areas has risen again in the first year after the outbreak of the Covid-19 Pandemic.

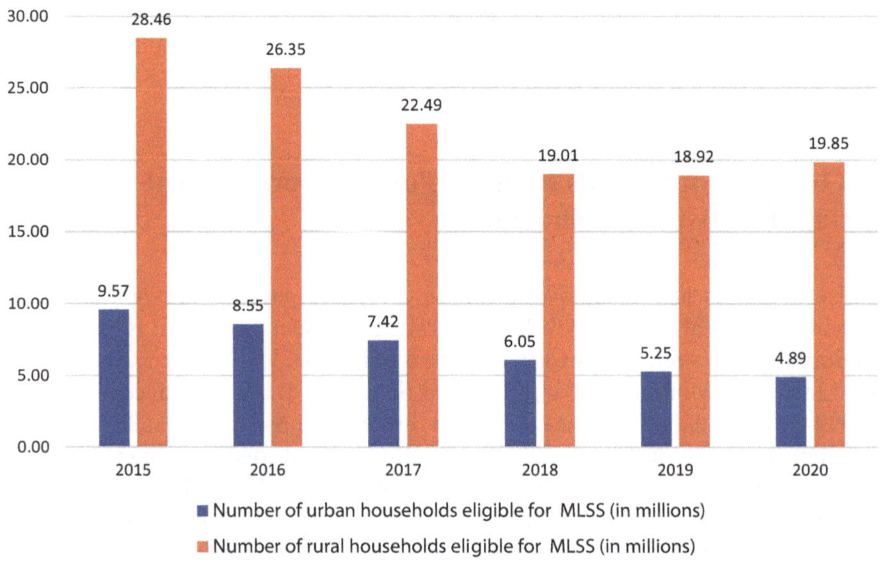

Fig. 8.1 Changes in the number of households receiving MLSS (Dibao) in urban and rural China from 2015 to 2020. *Source* Author's own compilation[4]

However, if the data are extended to March 2022, the impact of the pandemic on China's relative poverty will be more obvious. Figure 8.2 shows the changes in the number of people receiving MLSS in China from 2015 to March 2022. According to the data of the MOC, the number of people receiving MLSS in both urban and rural areas continued to decline before the pandemic, and then there was a "reversal of development." In 2020, the number of people receiving MLSS in cities was 8.05 million, and in 2021 it was 7.38 million, while the latest data showed that the number of people receiving MLSS rose again to 7.94 million. In 2020, the number of people receiving MLSS in rural areas was 36.21 million, 34.74 million in 2021, and 35.97 million in 2022. If the number of people receiving MLSS is used as the relative poverty standard, the relative poverty in both urban and rural areas has increased from 2021 to 2022, which shows the impact of the pandemic on the relative poverty in urban and rural areas.

In addition to MLSS-schemes, the Assistance for the Extreme Poor (AEP, tekun) in rural China is an important yardstick reflecting the relative poverty in rural areas, which measures the poor who are close to the physical bottom line of survival. The trendline in Fig. 8.3 shows that from 2015 to 2019, the number of rural residents receiving AEP decreased from 5.17 to 4.39 million, and the data rose inversely to 4.46 million in 2020, which shows clearly that the number of rural residents facing special poverty in the pandemic has increased. Figure 8.4 shows that the number of residents receiving AEP in the urban areas has continued to increase from about 254,000 in 2017 to 312,000 in 2020, both before and after the pandemic.

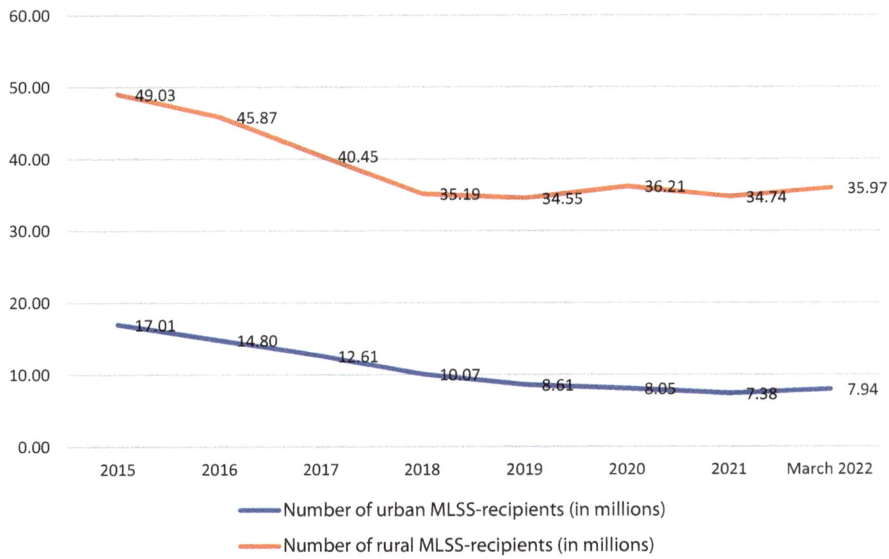

Fig. 8.2 Changes in the number of people receiving MLSS (Dibao) in urban and rural China from 2015 to March 2022. *Source* Author's own compilation

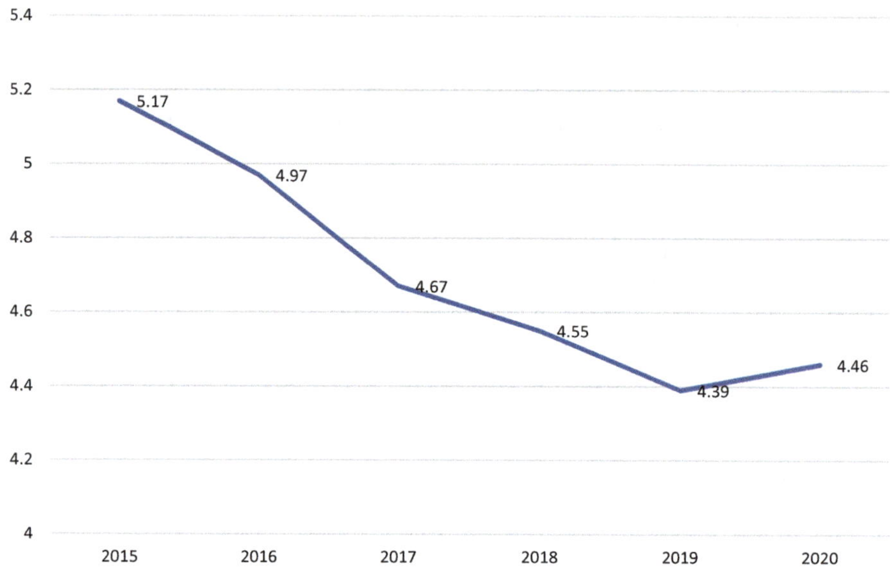

Fig. 8.3 Number of rural residents of receiving assistance for the extremely poor (AEP, Tekun) from 2015 to 2020 (in millions). *Source* Author's own compilation

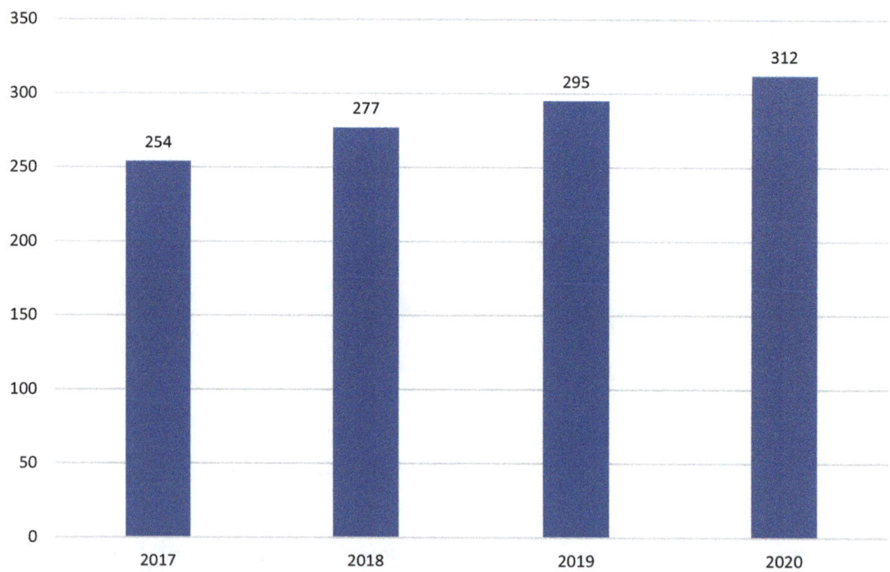

Fig. 8.4 Number of urban residents of receiving assistance for the extremely poor (AEP, Tekun) from 2017 to 2020 (in thousands). *Source* Author's own compilation

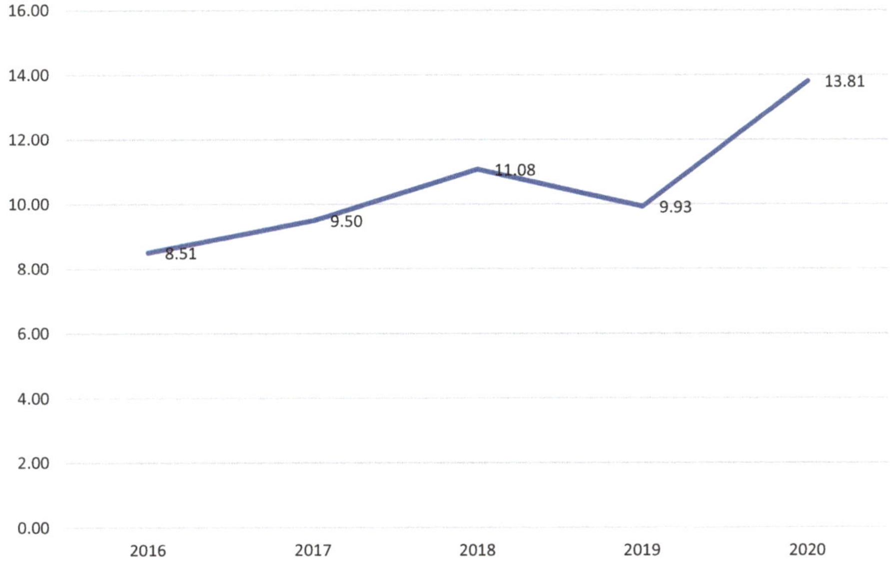

Fig. 8.5 Number of the Chinese residents of receiving temporary assistance (TA) from 2016 to 2020 (in millions). *Source* Author's own compilation

If the MLSS system better reflects mid- to long-term poverty or persistent "chronic poverty," then Temporary Assistance (TA) can better reflect short-term poverty or how sudden social crises (such as economic and pandemic crises) created new poverty. Figure 8.5 shows that the number of the recipients of TA dropped from 11.08 million in 2018 to 9.93 million in 2019 but rose to 13.81 million a year after the outbreak of the Covid-19 Pandemic. The surge in TA-recipients shows that the Covid-19 has directly caused the rise of relative poverty in China.

The Impact of the Covid-19 Pandemic on the Job Market and People's Livelihood: The Phenomenon of "Poverty Caused by the Pandemic" (in Chinese: Inyi Zhipin)

In the more than two years since the outbreak of the pandemic, and with the continuous shift of the "epicenter" of the pandemic, various parts of China have been affected by the pandemic in different time periods. In terms of the impact of the pandemic on the labor market and unemployment, the problems faced by urban and rural areas are also different, so the development of relative poverty also shows different trajectories.

In the Urban Spaces

In the urban spaces, due to strict quarantine measures and even periodic measures of city-wide lockdown in various mega cities like Beijing, Nanjing and Shanghai, economic and commercial activities seemed to have "hit the pause button" under the instantaneous impact at different times. For factories and companies, strictly enforced quarantine and social distancing policies mean shutdowns of production and work. Some large or medium-sized state-owned enterprises are still able to implement the continued remuneration or provide income compensation for their employees during the crisis, while small and micro enterprises and private enterprises are often unable to pay workers and provide income-replacement compensation. In addition, due to the termination of commercial activities and bank credit activities, the liquidity of the financial market has been greatly tightened, which means that many troubled small and micro enterprises cannot obtain loans from the financial market, and many small enterprises are facing survival crisis or even forced to declare bankruptcy. The economic depression also directly leads to the increase of urban unemployment and the emergence of new urban poverty. However, the impact of the Covid-19 Pandemic in various occupational fields is also significantly different. Some fields, such as government departments and public institutions, are less affected, while manufacturing and service industries have been hit harder. Some specific service industries, such as catering and entertainment industries, tourism and even suffered a devastating blow.

Although China does not have data on the operation of enterprises during the pandemic released by national departments at the national level, some think tanks have conducted surveys and published relevant data. For example, according to TianYanCha's[5] national enterprise big data for the first quarter of 2020, more than 460,000 enterprises have closed down in China. The business dilemma under the influence of the pandemic directly led to a sharp rise in the unemployment rate, which rose sharply in the first half of 2020. The number of new jobs has dropped sharply by about 1.37 million year-on-year, and the national urban survey unemployment rate in April and May 2020 were 6 and 5.9% respectively, an increase of 1 and 0.9% year-on-year. Among them, the urban surveyed unemployment rate in 31 large cities was 5.8 and 5.9%, an increase of 0.8 and 0.9% year-on-year. As of the end of May, the cumulative number of new jobs was 4.6 million, a year-on-year decrease of 22.95%.[6]

The pandemic has had a great impact on China's labor market, but the impact on various occupational sectors is heterogeneous. Some sectors have relatively small "pressure-bearing areas," while others have very large "pressure-bearing areas." For example, the data center of the Ministry of Culture and Tourism, a subsidiary of the China Tourism Research Institute, released the analysis of tourism economic operation in 2021 and the development forecast in 2022, which showed that China's tourism industry was hit particularly hard by the unprecedented pandemic. The report shows that among the respondents, the unemployment rate is as high as 68.1%, and only 13.8% are stably employed in the industry. Nearly 60% of the employees have been unemployed for more than one year, 76.1% of the total respondents have been unemployed for more than half a year, and more than 10% have been unemployed for three to six months. Nearly 80% of the respondents admitted that long-term unemployment had a great impact on their lives, including affecting the repayment of debts such as housing loans and car loans, increasing the economic pressure on their lives, and some respondents were facing bankruptcy.[7]

In Rural Spaces

The development of relative poverty in rural spaces during the pandemic has some unique characteristics. First, a large number of rural migrant workers working in cities suddenly lost their jobs during the pandemic, and many small and micro enterprises laid off a lot of short-term and temporary employees due to economic pressure, many of whom are rural migrant workers. During pandemic, millions of migrant workers from rural areas were forced to return to their hometowns, and agriculture was unable to absorb so many returning laborers, which led to an increase in short-term relative poverty. Second, due to the implementation of community quarantines and city-wide lockdown during the pandemic, coupled with the implementation of periodic blockades of various transportation lines, these factors have led to the closure of the market, and both online and offline transactions of agricultural products have been greatly restricted. Thus, the income of farmers has also been greatly affected, and the stagnation and decline of farmers' income in the crisis period has also led to the rise of relative poverty in rural areas.

According to a set of data released by the Ministry of Agriculture and Rural Affairs (MARA) of China in 2020, more than 8 million new migrant workers returned to their hometowns in China during the pandemic.[8] These groups have become vulnerable groups of livelihoods, and it is difficult to guarantee basic living and material welfare amidst the coronavirus pandemic. The same dataset from the MARA also shows that most migrant workers still choose to stay in the cities because they think it will be more difficult to earn income after returning to the countryside, so they may fall into poverty after returning home. The floating population from rural areas mainly works in the informal sectors, and most migrant workers are the main labor forces in precarious and low-income sectors. Therefore, their living conditions are particularly worrying during the pandemic crisis, because their work is often temporary, precarious, and unstable, and most of them are not included in the protection scope of the social insurance system. Therefore, in a special crisis such as the coronavirus pandemic, they cannot rely on the regular employment-based social insurance system to provide protection for their livelihood. Since China's official unemployment data only includes those employed in the formal sector, but not those employed in the informal sector, the unemployment rate in China's statistics is usually underestimated, and it does not include the unemployment of urban migrants, especially migrant workers. During the pandemic, a large number of migrant workers returned home from unemployment, which was not reflected in the official unemployment statistics.

Response of Economic Policy, Tax Policy and Social Policy to Relative Poverty During the Pandemic

In the face of the coronavirus pandemic, China's relative poverty has actually experienced an upward trend on the basis of the steady decline of general poverty in the past few years. The continuous impact on the labor market and service sector during the pandemic has also affected the basic livelihood of a large number of people. Like most countries in the world, the Chinese government has also taken some distinct measures to alleviate the social crisis caused by the pandemic. At the same time, some existing institutional arrangements also play an important role in reducing relative poverty. Here, this article will broaden the perspective and comprehensively introduce how China's economic, fiscal, and social policy responded to the social crisis caused by Covid-19. Public policy measures will be mainly linked to the issue of relative poverty, rather than focusing upon medical policy, epidemic prevention policy and public health policy during the pandemic.

Economic, Fiscal and Tax Policy

During the Covid-19, enterprises in all areas and sectors have been greatly affected, among which the micro and small enterprises, the medium-sized enterprises have suffered the most. In order to help difficult enterprises greatly affected by the pandemic and help small, medium-sized, and micro enterprises return to work and production, many Chinese cities require that the loan interest rate is not higher than the one-year loan market quotation interest rate (LPR) plus 50 basis points, and the relevant financial departments will also discount the interest on the loan. In order to help small and medium-sized enterprises get out of their current difficulties and support and encourage them to resume work and production, relevant government departments have given support to the financing needs of enterprises engaged in the production, transportation and sales of living materials through separate credit scale, simplifying the approval process and providing preferential interest rates, especially for enterprises in need of loans, the financial department also offered a 50% discount.

Moreover, for small and medium-sized enterprises and micro-enterprises in difficult circumstances, various local governments in China have also introduced special preferential measures to reduce corporate tax and personal income tax, and some public service institutions and welfare institutions such as nurseries, kindergartens, nursing homes, and welfare institutions for the disabled can be exempted from business tax. In addition, China's central government has also focused on reducing the burden of social security premiums on enterprises. The government requires a periodic reduction or exemption of the employers' contributions on pension, unemployment, work-related injury, and basic medical insurance amidst the pandemic (Lu et al. 2020; ten Brink et al. 2021).

Self-employed workers and various types of flexible employees who participate in the basic endowment insurance for enterprise employees as individuals can voluntarily suspend their premiums payment in 2020–2021, and the purpose of these special policies is to reduce the labor cost of enterprises and enhance their confidence in resuming work and production.

Unemployment Insurance

Amidst the pandemic, China's unemployment insurance system has played an important role in reducing the social problems caused by mass unemployment and in preventing and reducing relative poverty. At the same time, the unemployment insurance has also partially reduced the social pain index caused by relative poverty. China's existing unemployment insurance system has relatively strict application conditions. For example, under normal conditions, employees can receive 12-month unemployment insurance benefits after paying 1–5 years, that is, the insured must pay continuously for at least one year to be eligible for benefits. Insured persons who have contributed for less than 5 years lose their entitlement to receive unemployment insurance benefits after 12 months of benefit receipt.

During the pandemic, the Chinese government has adopted more resilient unemployment insurance measures. For example, in June 2020, the Ministry of Human Resources and Social Security (MHRSS) and the Ministry of Finance (MOF) jointly issued the document "Notice on Expanding the Scope of Unemployment Insurance."[9] It is clarified: From March to December 2020, unemployed persons who have received unemployment insurance benefits and have not yet been employed and insured unemployed persons who do not meet the requirements for receiving unemployment insurance benefits, can apply for unemployment subsidies for 6 months, and the standard does not exceed 80% of local unemployment insurance benefits. At the same time, the document also stipulates that the unemployed migrant workers recruited by the enterprises, who do not pay personal insurance contributions and have worked continuously for one year, shall be paid a one-time living allowance in time. From May to December 2020, unemployed migrant workers who have been insured for less than one year after January 1, 2019, will be granted temporary living allowance for no more than three months on a monthly basis with reference to the Minimum Living Standard Scheme (MLSS) of the local cities. Unemployed migrant workers who have the same insurance payment as urban workers shall be paid unemployment insurance benefits or unemployment subsidies according to the regulations of the insured place. Local governments in China have also designated local measures to expand the coverage and payment of unemployment insurance based on this document, and supplemented local unemployment insurance and employment promotion measures according to local conditions.[10]

Further, during the Covid-19 Pandemic, the Chinese government greatly simplified the complicated procedures for applying for unemployment insurance. The new unemployment insurance policy also stipulates that online application for unemployment insurance should be promoted nationwide. The unemployed can also apply to local employment service institutions or social insurance agencies with their ID card or social security card without providing proof of termination of labor relations or unemployment registration. The reduction of traditional welfare bureaucracy and the establishment of emerging digital bureaucracy have become important "institutional dividends" for millions of unemployed during the crisis period (Sun et al. 2022).

Social Assistance

During the Covid-19 Pandemic, the social assistance scheme, especially China's urban and rural Minimum Living Standard Schemes (MLSS, in Chinese: Dibao), played an irreplaceable role in alleviating relative poverty. It should be noted that the MLSS is the core institutional mechanism for anti-poverty during the pandemic. During the crisis caused by the pandemic, local governments in China have repeatedly raised the standard of Dibao and relaxed the payment restrictions of Dibao, so that people who have suffered income loss and relative poverty during the pandemic can get through the "valley of tears" through the benefits of social assistance.

According to the summary made by China News Network in November 2021, 10 Chinese provinces increased the Dibao-benefits in 2021: for example, the Dibao in Beijing was adjusted from 1,170 yuan to 1,245 yuan per person per month, the urban Dibao in Gansu Province was increased from 6,924 to 7,476 yuan per person per year in 2021, and the urban Dibao standard in Yunnan was increased from 640 to 660 yuan per person per month, From July 1, 2021, Shanghai raised the Dibao standard from 1,240 to 1,330 yuan per person per month, an increase of 90 yuan per month with a growth rate of 7.26%. In addition, the guidance standard of rural Dibao in Hunan has been raised from 4,000 to 4,300 yuan per year, and Zhejiang Provincial Department of Civil Affairs and other departments issued a document in July to strengthen the monitoring, early warning, and dynamic management of low-income households, and reasonably determine the relief standard. In 2021, the Dibao benefit level in the Zhejiang province has exceed 10,000 yuan.[11]

During the pandemic, many provinces and cities in China implemented temporary assistance measures for the Covid-19. These temporary assistance measures are mainly aimed at socially vulnerable groups related to pandemic. For example, low- and middle-income groups infected with Covid-19 and asymptomatic infection can apply for temporary assistance because they are facing temporary difficulties in life, and those who are unable to go out for work or production and operation due to the Covid-19 virus can also apply for temporary assistance. Migrant workers who have lost their jobs because of Covid-19 can also apply for temporary assistance. The special temporary assistance during the Covid-19 Pandemic additionally covers those temporarily stranded due to the implementation of traffic control and other reasons, as well as the foreign population in difficulty due to infection and home-quarantine.

In addition, many cities in China have greatly simplified the application procedures for Dibao allowances, shortened the processing time limit, and reduced the threshold and obstacles for applying for Dibao (ten Brink et al. 2021). Most Chinese cities have promoted the digital way to apply for Dibao and encouraged eligible residents to apply for subsistence allowances from local civil affairs departments through telephone, WeChat, apps, internet, and other contactless means. The Covid-19 has surprisingly accelerated the digitization of Chinese social policy (Liu 2022; Wang et al. 2021).

Secondary Poverty—A Form of Relative Poverty

As far as China's relative poverty is concerned, there are some objective ontological existences independent of the pandemic. This is the "secondary poverty" issue that Chinese scholars often discuss (Ni 2017; Zhao 2021). The notion of "secondary poverty" is a concept beyond the traditional concept of income poverty, because some groups in society do not belong to poor groups from the perspective of income but fall into poverty due to some specific natural and social reasons or natural and social risks, such as the reduction of agricultural production caused by floods and the rise of farmers' relative poverty. Another example is passive poverty caused by physical disability caused by traffic accident injury. There are two kinds of secondary poverty that deserve special attention—namely "poverty caused by medical treatment" (yinyi zhipin) and "poverty caused by care" (yinhu zhipin).

One is the "catastrophic health expenditure" proposed by the World Health Organization. According to the WHO's definition family's compulsory health expenditure is greater than or exceeds 40% of the general consumption of the family, it is considered to have medical catastrophic expenditure. Catastrophic household expenditures often arise in the area of serious diseases. According to the calculations of Ma et al. (2019), the catastrophic medical expenditure of Chinese households dropped from 12.57% in 2010 to 8.94% in 2016, but compared with developed countries, Chinese household catastrophic health expenditure is still high. Since 2000, China has gradually established a medical insurance system covering the entire population. However, due to the fragmentation of the system and the limitation of reimbursement ratios, "paying out of pocket" in medical insurance is still a significant problem. In addition, China's medical insurance also has significant localization characteristics, which is somewhat similar to the federal medical insurance system. Different regions have great differences in the medical insurance deductible amounts, capping line, and reimbursement ratios of hospitals at different levels, especially for major diseases. This leads to the relative poverty phenomenon of many people due to serious diseases even after the establishment of the medical insurance system covering the entire people in

China (Liu 2022). Family catastrophic medical expenditure is still an urgent problem to be solved.

Another area that has a big impact on secondary poverty is the field of long-term care. Generally, if there is a disabled elderly person in a family, for ordinary families, one or two relatives are required to take care of the disabled elderly person full-time, which leads to the family labor force being forced to withdraw from the labor market to take care of their relatives. In urban areas, this often means the sharp drop in family income, and the fact that some working family members in rural areas are required to take care of disabled family members, has resulted in barren farmland and a decline in the output of agricultural products, which has also led to a significant reduction in rural family income, and many care-intensive families have become poor due to the care of elderly family members. This "penalty for caregiving"[12] (Glauber 2019) is a complementary reason for China's rise in relative poverty in an ageing age.

In response to the rising demand for long-term care in Chinese society, the Chinese government has chosen to launch a pilot long-term care insurance in various cities like Shanghai, Nantong, and Qingdao etc. (Liu and Sun 2015). In the first round of pilots, China has chosen to pilot the long-term care insurance in various cities, and since 2021, China has started the second round of long-term care insurance pilots. So far, a total of 49 cities have participated in the long-term care insurance pilot program. Although the Chinese government has implemented a pilot program, the long-term care insurance is still in the experimental stage of local policies and has not risen to the stage of specific policy implementation. The Chinese government has not yet established a specific timetable for establishing an institutionalized, nationwide long-term care insurance system. Due to the lack of a national long-term care insurance system, the withdrawal of family members from the labor market due to family elderly care needs is still an important cause of relative poverty in the contemporary Chinese society. This problem can only be solved by establishing a long-term care insurance at national level.

Conclusion and Discussion

This paper introduces the development of China's relative poverty during the Covid-19 Pandemic. The conclusion is that China's relative poverty in the grand narrative of national anti-poverty originally showed a downward trend year by year. However, this downward trend stopped during the Covid-19 period, and China's relative poverty has risen slightly again. Considering that many households and individuals affected by business closures and unemployment have not applied for Dibao due to the possible "stigma effect," or that many unemployed people who have fallen into relative poverty have not been registered in the country's formal unemployment statistics, so the actual relative poverty rate in China during the pandemic may have been higher.

Different sectors have been affected unevenly during the pandemic. Some specific sectors, such as the service, catering, and tourism sector, have suffered devastating blows under the continuous and long-term stringent lockdown measures. Various small and medium-sized enterprises have gone bankrupt, and a large number of tourism industry personnel have lost their sources of livelihood, while employees who can continue to be employed through the home-office-model are less affected. In addition, the secondary poverty mentioned by some Chinese scholars is also other main manifestations of relative poverty, such as poverty due to serious illness or poverty due to long-term care of family members. These poverty phenomena are not caused by the pandemic itself, but the rise of unemployment rate during the pandemic may also aggravate these relative poverty phenomena, creating a "social multiplier effect" of relative poverty.

China's welfare regime includes a repertoire of economic, fiscal, and social policies that have responded vigorously to the severe consequences of the pandemic crisis. In the field of economic policy and fiscal policy, China has enhanced monetary liquidity in the market through its loose monetary policy, while reducing the pressure on taxation and social insurance premiums for enterprises.

In the field of social policy, in addition to conventional social policy measures, special responsive social policy in times of crisis has played a significant role in restraining relative poverty. This irregular responsive social policy artificially expands the coverage of unemployment insurance and social assistance systems, lowers the institutional threshold for applying for benefits, and extends the payment of social welfare benefits. At the same time, it greatly simplified the application procedures through digital means, making the application of unemployment benefits and minimum living allowances *easier* and "*de-bureaucratic*" compared to the pre-pandemic period.

Notes

1. See UN (2015).
2. See WB (2015).
3. Most OECD countries also use this threshold to define social assistance standards, and households with incomes below this threshold are entitled to receive social assistance (Eardley et al. 1996).
4. The data in Figs. 8.1, 8.2, 8.3, 8.4 and 8.5 are synthesized by the author based on the data published by the Ministry of Civil Affairs (MOC) and government statistical bulletin between 2015 and 2020/2021.
5. TianYanCha is a leading business inquiry platform in China. It has collected information on nearly 300 million social entities across the country, and updated information in more than 300 dimensions in a timely manner.
6. See TianYanCha's report "National Enterprise Big Data in the First Quarter of 2020," retrieved from https://www.douban.com/note.
7. See the report "70% unemployed, most of them change careers! The special investigation report on tourism unemployment during the pandemic revealed the number of tourists under the pandemic," https://wenku.baidu.com/view.

8. See China News citing a report by China's Ministry of Agriculture and Rural Affairs, "More than 8 million people have returned to their hometowns. How can China expand the employment of migrant workers?," https://www.chinanews.com.cn/cj/2020/07-01.
9. See the Notice of the Ministry of Human Resources and Social Security on Expanding the Coverage of Unemployment Insurance, https://m.thepaper.cn/baijiahao_7856060.
10. As an example, please refer to the "Notice of Nanjing Municipal Bureau of Finance on Expanding the Scope of Unemployment Insurance" issued by Nanjing Municipal Human Resources and Social Security Bureau, https://www.ushui.net/law.
11. See the report from China News Network "Up! This year, 10 provinces will raise the minimum living standard, and this province will set the standard more than 10,000 yuan," http://www.hn.chinanews.com.cn/news/cjxx/2021/1117.
12. There are similar expressions in the Chinese semantic environment: if one person is disabled, the whole family will be impoverished (*yiren shineng, quanjia zhipin*); if one person is disabled, the whole family will be out of balance (*yiren shineng, quanjia shiheng*).

References

De Haan, A., and S. Maxwell. 2017. Poverty and social exclusion in North and South. *IDS Bulletin*, 481A.

Eardley, T., J. Bradshaw, J. Ditch, and I. Gough. 1996. *Social assistance in OECD countries: Synthesis report*. https://eprints.whiterose.ac.uk/73427.

Foster, J.E. 1998. Absolute versus relative poverty. *The American Economic Review* 88 (2): 335–341.

Glauber, R. 2019. The wage penalty for parental caregiving: Has it declined over time? *Journal of Marriage and Family* 81 (2): 415–433.

Gustafsson, B., and P.J. Pedersen. 2018. *Poverty and low income in the Nordic countries*. Routledge.

Halleröd, B., and D. Larsson. 2008. Poverty, welfare problems and social exclusion. *International Journal of Social Welfare* 17 (1): 15–25.

Kabeer, N. 2000. Social exclusion, poverty and discrimination towards an analytical framework. *IDS Bulletin* 31 (4): 83–97.

Kangas, O., and J. Palme. 2000. Does social policy matter? Poverty cycles in OECD countries. *International Journal of Health Services* 30 (2): 335–352.

Leisering, L., P. Buhr, and U. Traiser-Diop. 2006. *Soziale Grundsicherung in der Weltgesellschaft: Monetäre Mindestsicherungssysteme in den Ländern des Südens und des Nordens—Weltweiter Survey und theoretische Verortung*. Bielefeld: Transcript Verlag.

Leisering, L., T. Liu, and T. Ten Brink. 2017. Synthesizing disparate ideas: How a Chinese model of social assistance was forged. *Global Social Policy* 17 (3): 307–327.

Liu, T., and L. Sun. 2015. An apocalyptic vision of ageing in China. *Zeitschrift für Gerontologie und Geriatrie* 48 (4): 354–364.

Liu, T., and L. Sun. 2016. Urban social assistance in China: Transnational diffusion and national interpretation. *Journal of Current Chinese Affairs* 45 (2): 29–51.

Liu, T. 2022. Social policy reform driven by crises: Promoting and reshaping social policy during the SARS and Covid-19 pandemics in China. *Social Policy and Administration*. https://doi.org/10.1111/spol.12818.

Lu, Q., Z. Cai, B. Chen, and T. Liu. 2020. Social policy responses to the Covid-19 crisis in China in 2020. *International Journal of Environmental Research and Public Health* 17 (16): 5896.

Ma, X., Z. Wang, and X. Liu. 2019. Progress on catastrophic health expenditure in China: Evidence from China family panel studies (CFPS) 2010 to 2016. *International Journal of Environmental Research and Public Health* 16 (23): 4775.

Madden, D. 2000. Relative or absolute poverty lines: A new approach. *Review of Income and Wealth* 46 (2): 181–199.

Moller, S., E. Huber, J.D. Stephens, D. Bradley, and F. Nielsen. 2003. Determinants of relative poverty in advanced capitalist democracies. *American Sociological Review* 68: 22–51.

Ni, Y. 2017. *Research on secondary poverty of ecological immigrants: Taking village C in W city as an example*. https://kns.cnki.net/kcms.

Notten, G., and C. De Neubourg. 2011. Monitoring absolute and relative poverty: "Not enough" is not the same as "much less." *Review of Income and Wealth* 57 (2): 247–269.

Ravallion, M., and S. Chen. 2011. Weakly relative poverty. *Review of Economics and Statistics* 93 (4): 1251–1261.

Selgin, G. 2021. The fiscal and monetary response to Covid-19: What the great depression has-and hasn't-taught us. *Economic Affairs* 41 (1): 3–20.

Sun, L., T. Liu, and W. Wang. 2022. Working from home in urban China during the Covid-19 pandemic: Assemblages of work-family interference. *Work, Employment and Society* 09500170221080870.

ten Brink, T., Y. Li, and T. Liu. 2021. *China's social policy response to Covid-19: Pragmatic adjustment of existing welfare institutions*. https://media.suub.uni-bremen.de.

UN, United Nations. 2015. *World summit for social development 1995*, chapter 2. https://www.un.org/development/desa.

Van Vliet, O., and C. Wang. 2015. Social investment and poverty reduction: A comparative analysis across fifteen European countries. *Journal of Social Policy* 44 (3): 611–638.

Wang, W., L. Sun, T. Liu, and T. Lai. 2021. The use of e-health during the Covid-19 pandemic: A case study in China's Hubei Province. *Health Sociology Review* 1–17.

WB, World Bank. 2015. *FAQs: Global poverty line update*. https://www.worldbank.org.

WB, World Bank. 2018. *Poverty and shared prosperity 2018*. https://www.worldbank.org.

Zhao, Z. 2021. Old propositions and new challenges for poverty alleviation and development after 2020. *Agricultural Economics* 1: 70–72.

Chapter 9
The Covid-19 Pandemic in Taiwan: With Special Reference to Older People's Problems

Shiau-Fang Chao and Wan-I Lin

Abstract While Covid-19 was ravaging the world and causing millions of deaths, Taiwan was being praised for its highly effective response to the virus. Even though Taiwan was one of the most successful nations in the fight against Covid-19, the older people in Taiwan were still disproportionally affected by the pandemic. Whereas persons aged 60 or over accounted for 16.5% of the confirmed (registered) cases in Taiwan, they accounted for over 88% of related deaths. To prevent the spread of the virus, Taiwan Center for Disease Control established the Central Epidemic Command Center on Dec. 31, 2019. Policy responses were promptly implemented according the development of the pandemic; these involved border control, banning public gatherings, the mandating of wearing face masks and the monitoring of body temperature in public, stay-at-home orders, and the maintenance of social distancing. The Taiwan government Taiwan government distribution resources, ensured information accessibility and made contingency plans for vulnerable groups with limited access to resources and information. This chapter has three aims. Firstly, it will discuss how older people with special needs, including heath care needs, disabilities, residents of long-term care facilities, and those living alone, were affected by Covid-19-related policies. Secondly, it will present policy that have been adopted in response to these impacts. Thirdly, based on the experience of Taiwan, recommendations and suggestions are made to mitigate the effects of disasters associated with virus and to sustain the physical, mental and social well-being of older people.

Keywords Covid-19 Pandemic · Taiwan · Government responses · Policy outcomes · Policy recommendations

---

S.-F. Chao (✉) · W.-I. Lin
Department of Social Work, National Taiwan University, Taipei, Taiwan
e-mail: sfchao@ntu.edu.tw

C. Aspalter (ed.), *Covid-19 Pandemic*,
https://doi.org/10.1007/978-981-99-2497-4_9

Covid-19 Pandemic in Taiwan

While the Covid-19 Pandemic ravaged the world and caused millions of deaths, Taiwan was praised for its highly effective response to the virus. By March 6, 2022, Taiwan had only 20,797 confirmed/registered cases (5,344 imported, 15,453 domestic) and 853 deaths. On January 20, 2020, the level 2 Central Epidemic Command Center (CECC) was established and the first confirmed (registered) imported case of Covid-19 was reported on January 21, 2020 (Taiwan CDC 2020a). In February 15, 2020, the first coronavirus death was announced and on February 27, 2020, the CECC was upgraded to level 1 owing to the rapid increases in the number of Covid cases globally.

Figure 9.1 displays the weekly trends in Covid-19 confirmed/registered cases. Taiwan had experienced four pandemic outbreaks from January 2020 to March 2022 (CPT 2022; Taiwan CDC 2022a). The first outbreak occurred between March and mid-April, 2020, mainly as a result of cluster infection on the Diamond Princess *cruise* ship and a Taiwanese *naval* ship; it comprised 35 domestic cases and 322 imported cases. and was caused by transmission by an international flight crew; that month, a total of 20 domestic cases and 93 imported cases were reported. The third outbreak took place from late April to late July, 2021, resulting from cluster infections of the Alpha variant of the *coronavirus* in hotels for international flight crews, hostess houses, and places for religious gatherings. Because of a surge in domestic confirmed/registered cases, the CECC announced a nationwide Level 3 epidemic alert in mid-May for the first time in Taiwan history. The following mandates were implemented:

(1) Masks had to be worn outside;
(2) Leisure and entertainment facilities were ordered to close;
(3) Dining-in services were prohibited in restaurants and food-vending locations;
(4) All activities and gatherings that involved five or more people indoors and ten or more people outdoors were banned, including at schools, wedding banquets, memorial ceremonies, sports competitions, and exhibitions;

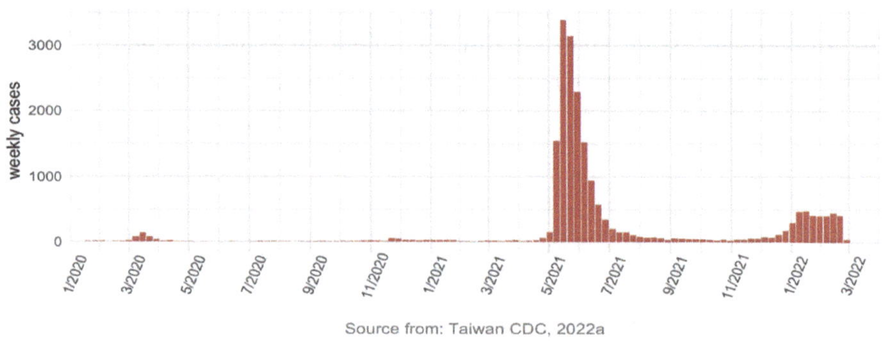

Fig. 9.1 Weekly Confirmed/Registered Covid-19 Cases in Taiwan (Jan. 2020–Feb. 2022)

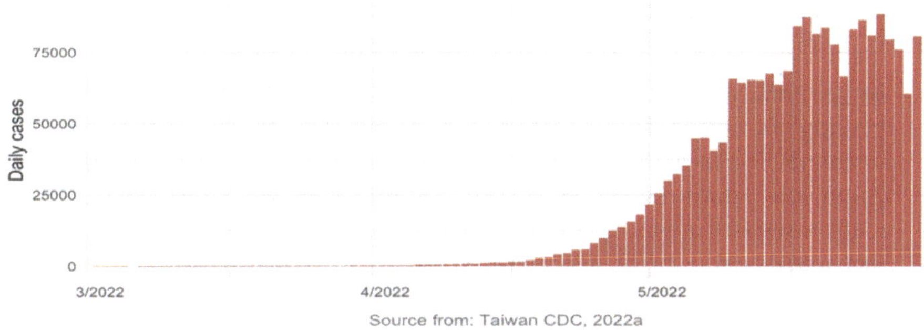

Fig. 9.2 Daily Confirmed/Registered Covid-19 Cases in Taiwan (Mar. 2022–May. 2022)

(5) Epidemic-related prevention guidelines for businesses, schools, and workplaces had to be strictly followed, favoring remote working (Taiwan CDC 2021a).

The epidemic alert was lowered to level 2 in late July, 2021, when 14,286 domestic cases and 333 imported cases were reported. The fourth surge *was of the Omicron* variant of Covid-19, which occurred from late January to early March, 2022 and began with a cluster at Taoyuan Airport. With an uptick in cases in January 2021, 2022, and total of 721 domestic confirmed/registered cases and 2,165 imported cases, restrictions were re-tightened nationwide in that month.

Noting that many Western and Asia countries have gradually returned to normal life, the Taiwan government proposed the "New Taiwan Model" in March 2022. The "New Taiwan Model" is expected to balance epidemic prevention with economic development by gradually relaxing pandemic control mandates and enabling Taiwan to live with Covid-19. The "New Taiwan Model" recognized that "zero confirmed cases" may not be feasible given the fast spread of the *Omicron* variant (Chen et al. 2022). The main means of pandemic prevention was increasing vaccination rates to reduce the incidence of moderate to severe illness after infection, and to maintain healthcare capacity. Therefore, has also been called the "disaster damage reduction and coexistence with Covid-19" period. As seen in Fig. 9.2, the number of confirmed/ registered cases increased rapidly from late April, 2022, reaching a peak of 100,000 every day in mid-May, 2022. At the time of writing, around three million people have been infected in the "disaster damage reduction and coexistence with Covid-19" period and 4,403 deaths have been reported (Taiwan CDC 2022b).

Main Preventive Measures to Control the Covid-19 Spread

Except for the Level 3 epidemic alert specific measures mentioned above, Taiwan has leveraged its experience in combating the 2003 SARS outbreak by rapidly issuing the following general regulations in February, 2020 to reduce the risk of Covid-19 transmission. Regulations were gradually loosened from April, 2022, when Taiwan launched the "New Taiwan Model" (CPT 2022; CVT 2022; Huang 2020; MHW 2022a; Taiwan CDC 2020b, c, d). These included the following:

(1) Border control: With some exceptions, foreign nationals were prohibited from entering Taiwan in March, 2020, and all travelers to Taiwan have had to quarantine for 14 days.
(2) Community transmission prevention: People who have had contact with confirmed cases are forced to isolate at home for 14 days.
(3) Face mask supply and distribution: To secure sufficient provision of face masks for frontline healthcare workers, the exporting of face masks was banned from January 24 to May 31, 2020. Masks thus secured be purchased at designated National Health Insurance (NHI)-contracted pharmacies.
(4) Vaccination: To facilitate vaccination, the "Covid-19 Vaccination Reservation System" was announced. Vaccine eligibility was set according to the supply of vaccines. People were grouped into ten categories that reflected their priority. As of June 14, 2022, 91% of the population had had their first dose of the Covid-19 vaccine, 82.39% the second, and 68.43% their third.
(5) Social distancing: Starting from April 1, 2020, the CECC implemented measures to encourage social distancing. Avoiding close contact and maintaining physical distance from others in public were advised.

Covid-19 Pandemic and Older Adults in Taiwan

Even though Taiwan has been one of the most successful nations in the fight against Covid-19, its older people were disproportionally affected by the pandemic. Table 9.1 presents the number of confirmed/registered cases and deaths by gender and age group from Jan. 1 to June 15, 2022. Persons aged 60 or over accounted for more than 88% of deaths from Jan. 1, 2020 to Dec. 31, 2021 and over 90% of the deaths from Jan. 1 to June 15, 2022. Notably, in the age groups 60–69 and 70–79 years, the death rate for males was nearly double that for females of the same age both from Jan 1, 2020 to Dec. 31, 2021 (60–69 years: 18.6% for males (n = 156), 8.6% for females (n = 72); 70–79 years: 20.3% for males (n = 170), 10.5% for females (n = 88)), and from Jan. 1, 2022 to June 15, 2022 (60–69 years: 8.4% for males (n = 309), 4.0% for females (n = 149); 70–79 years: 13.8% for males (n = 511), 8.1% for females (n = 300)). Of people aged over 60, males consistently accounted for more deaths than females in the same age group, suggesting that older males were more likely to develop Covid-19-associated mortality.

As well as having a disproportionately high infection fatality rate, older adults are more vulnerable to Covid-19 than other age groups because the pandemic threatens their access to health care, disrupts usual home- and community-based services (HCBS), increases internal and external ageism, and reduces opportunities to secure essential income, housing and daily necessities. All of these effects can worsen health-related, social, and financial disparities in aging populations (Chao and Yu 2021; Miller 2020; Morrow-Howell et al. 2020). Although the vulnerability of older populations to the Covid-19 Pandemic has been documented, little work has

Table 9.1 Confirmed/registered cases and deaths by gender and age group from 2020/01/01 to 2022/06/15

	2020/01/01–2021/12/31				2022/01/01–2022/06/15			
	Confirmed		Deaths		Confirmed		Deaths	
Age	Male	Female	Male	Female	Male	Female	Male	Female
0–9	266	242	0	0	170,801	152,940	10	5
10–19	290	270	0	0	148,856	128,669	4	0
20–29	804	670	0	0	258,975	250,717	7	3
30–39	1121	1068	7	1	267,980	294,547	18	7
40–49	1007	1255	7	14	228,342	283,986	64	26
50–59	1215	1465	50	15	155,743	201,882	149	44
60–69	1558	1351	156	72	127,292	162,805	309	149
70–79	769	607	170	88	63,002	72,172	511	300
80–89	264	249	104	82	25,592	34,011	651	595
90 and above	65	67	41	31	6782	8439	390	451
Total	7359	7244	535	303	1,453,365	1,590,168	2113	1580

Source Taiwan CDC (2022b)

addressed how Covid-19-related policies affect the lives of older persons—especially those with special needs.

The section below will firstly list the main preventive measures that have been taken in institutions and services during the Covid-19 Pandemic and are most frequently used by older persons. These include services in hospitals, long-term care (LTC) institutions, and HCBS. They also include the use of foreign care workers. Secondly, the section below will consider how older individuals with special needs, such as those with particular health conditions, dementia, or LTC needs, and those who live alone, were influenced by the mandates. Lastly, based on Taiwan's experience, the following section will consider how the relevant implementations were modified in light of their effects.

Preventive Measures in Hospital and Older People with Health Conditions

Decreases in Numbers of Outpatient Visits and Hospital Admissions

The Covid-19 Pandemic has dramatically reduced the delivery of, and access to, health care globally, including in Taiwan. For patients, the fear of contracting Covid-19 in medical facilities and the implementation of lockdown or stay-at-home orders have inhibited them from seeking medical care. The reduction or termination of standard medical services and changed opening hours have greatly reduced the ability of medical facilities to provide regular health care services, detrimentally affecting the health of patients (Holtz 2021). According to the National Health Insurance Administration (NHIA), overall outpatient visits were 8.1% lower (15.56 million visits) from January to June, 2020 than in the same period in 2019. Outpatient clinics in various settings reported the largest decline (10.7% or 10.5 million visits), followed by hospitals (7.1% or 3.97 million visits), dental clinics (4.8% or 0.85 million visits), and, lastly, traditional Chinese medicine establishments (0.9% or 0.17 million visits) (Li 2020).

Panel A in Appendix A shows the average number of outpatient visits per 0.1 million people in five-year age groups from 2017 to 2020 in Taiwan. Panel B in Appendix A shows change in average number of outpatient visits per 0.1 million people, when number in the earlier year was substituted by the later year (GEC 2022a). According to Panel B in Appendix A, age group 0–4 exhibited the largest decline in the average number of outpatient visits from 2018 to 2019 when the first Covid-19 surge occurred internationally; this decline was −1,138; it was followed by that of age group 75–79 (−1,063 visits), and that of age group 65–69 (−824 visits), representing declines of 1.17, 1.05, and 0.83%, respectively.

The findings suggested that second only to infants and children in early childhood, older adults, and especially the young-old (age 65–69 years) and the middle-old (age 75–79 years) exhibited the greatest decline in average number of outpatient visits in the first year of the pandemic. In 2019 to 2020, when the first Covid-19 outbreak occurred in Taiwan, average outpatient visits per 0.1 million people fell in all age groups except 70–74. The age group 15–19 saw the largest decline, −3,206, in average outpatient visits of, followed by age group 75–79 (−2,583 visits), and then age group 25–29 (−2,521 visits), corresponding to declines of 3.46, 2.57, and 2.75%, respectively. All age groups experienced a substantial decrease in outpatient visits and no obvious difference in this respect between older and younger populations was observed.

However, the impact of Covid-19 on hospital admissions appeared to be more considerable in the older population. Panel A in Appendix B presents the average number of hospital admissions per 0.1 million people for five-year age groups from 2017 to 2020. Panel B in Appendix B exhibits changes in average hospital admissions in each age group (GEC 2022b). As seen in Panel B in Appendix B, age groups 75–79, 85 and above, and 65–69 outnumbered other age groups and saw the largest declines in average hospital admissions per 0.1 million people from 2018 to 2019; these were declines of -304, -203, and -93, or 1.38, 0.52, and 0.67%, respectively. The drop in average hospital admissions was more significant from 2019 to 2020. The age group 80 and above had the largest decline, -2897, in average hospital admissions, and was followed in this respect by age group 0–4 (−2,557 admissions), age group 5–9 (−2,447 admissions), and lastly age group 80–84 (−2280 admissions), representing declines of 3.46, 2.57, and 2.75%, respectively. The very old (age 80 years and above) population consistently ranked as one of the three age groups with the greatest declines in *average* hospital admissions from 2018 to 2019 and from 2019 to 2020.

The results supported the finding that older adults, especially very old adults, were more likely than other age groups to have experienced a reduction in, or disruption to, hospitalization during the Covid-19 Pandemic.

The reduction in hospital admissions for the older population during the Covid-19 Pandemic was greater than that of outpatient visits. Three reasons may contribute to this difference. Firstly, except for children under the age of nine, the average number of hospital admissions per 0.1 million people steadily increases with age, whereas the distribution of average outpatient visits is more equal across age groups. Since older people constituted a larger share of patients who are admitted to hospital, the larger drop in their hospital admissions is expected. A second possible explanation is that the older population, and especially the oldest-old, are at high risk of Covid-19 infection and mortality, so their unnecessary or less urgent hospital admissions are more likely to be delayed or cancelled to *reduce* the *risk of infection.* A third possible explanation is that infection control measures that were announced by the CECC largely focused on hospital wards, so hospital admissions were more likely to be affected than outpatient visits. However, *delays or cancelations of* hospital admissions and reductions in outpatient visits can disrupt routine health services and make standard health care inaccessible, worsening health outcomes. The next section will discuss how older people may be affected by delayed health care services.

Infection Control Measures in Taiwanese Hospitals and Their Effects on Health of Patients

Two major infection control measures were mandated by the CECC for implementation in hospital settings as the Covid-19 Pandemic developed. Firstly, adopting the "divided cabin, divided flow" strategy. This involved confirming Covid-19 cases and suspended cases such as patients who had a history of traveling to high-risk countries and had Covid-19-associated conditions, such as fever or respiratory tract symptoms, and then separating them from other patients in confined areas to prevent potential environmental contamination. Medical staff who were responsible for the patients in the confined areas were forbidden to interact directly with their colleagues at the hospital. If one of the medical staff was infected, all his or her team members were required to quarantine for 14 days (Chang et al. 2020). Second, except under special circumstances, visits to hospital wards were prohibited. Only one person was allowed to accompany each hospital inpatient. Both patients and the accompanying person had to have a negative Covid-19 test result (Taiwan CDC 2021b). Consequently, the ability of hospitals to provide regular health services was reduced owing to medical staff shortages and the designation of some general wards as Covid-19-specific wards or zones.

The fear of Covid-19 increased barriers to access to medical services; this effect came might have come together with reduction in health care capacity to have harmful effects on patients' health. In the pandemic, unnecessary or non-urgent medical care, such as general medical examinations, some surgical operations or occupational or physical rehabilitation, were suspended. Many patients also postponed or cancelled their medical appointments. Consequently, patients with chronic conditions who required the continual use of prescription medications, which include most of the older population, may have had their regular visits to doctors disrupted, directly leading to poor control of their chronic diseases and indirectly increasing their risks of severe complications. Moreover, medical adherence and compliance dropped significantly in the outbreak stage of the pandemic in Taiwan (Lang 2021). Consider stroke cases as an example. Rodrigues et al. (2021) suggested that the Covid-19 epidemic increased the time from an onset of symptoms to the making of an emergency call, waiting times, and the time from the onset of symptoms to arrival at a hospital (in Portugal, based on a Portuguese sample). These findings may apply to Taiwan because the fear of being infected might have made patients more hesitant to go to hospital, even when potential mortality was involved (Lang 2021).

Visiting restrictions and policies regarding confinement have made dying in a hospital even more dreadful. Since visiting restrictions apply to all hospital wards, including those of terminally ill persons and hospice wards, patients have died in hospital with very few family members with them. Furthermore, families of patients with confirmed Covid-19 may not be allowed to enter confined areas and so can only say goodbye to their loved one via video (Chen 2020). Since Covid-19 is listed as one of the fifth type of notifiable diseases in Taiwan, patients with confirmed Covid-19 (are expected to TRY must) be cremated within 24 h of their demise (MOJ 2019). Traditionally, Taiwanese older adults greatly value returning home to die, surrounded by all family members, seeing and saying farewell face-to-face to them as they near death as part a "good death" or "successful dying." Also, being unable to follow traditional funeral rites is considered to fail to bring good fortune for their offspring. For family members, failure to complete a 49-day mourning process may cause the deceased to "leave" unpeacefully with hindrances, causing lifelong regret to the bereaved family members. Hence, the visiting restrictions and policies regarding confinement in the Covid-19 Pandemic clash with traditional rites and beliefs as patients approach death, creating a state of affairs that is unacceptable for both older persons and their families.

Adaptive Strategies in Government and Hospitals

To address patients' hesitation to make outpatient visits in the pandemic and the potential risk of worsening health as a result of delayed or irregular medical treatment, the NHIA, MHW in Taiwan expanded the range of clinics that were eligible for operation under the existing "Regulations of Treatment using Telemedicine," enabling them to provide "video diagnosis and treatment clinics." In May, 2021, it also expanded the range of patients who were qualified for such services. Patients with chronic health conditions who require the persistent use of long-term medications as well as older persons who are concerned about going to hospitals or clinics are expected to benefit most from this relaxation of rules (Deng 2021).

From August 2021, when the epidemic alert was lessened from Level 3 to Level 2, visiting restrictions have been modified according to the type of patients and type of hospital ward. Visiting policies for certain hospital wards, including intensive care, hospice, respiratory care, psychiatric, and children's wards, as well as wards for patients with disabilities or in critical condition, have been loosened and made more flexible. The allowed number of persons who can accompany patients below 12 years old, above 65 years old, with disabilities, or requiring such accompaniment as assessed by the medical institution, has been increased. Visiting restrictions may be adjusted by counties and cities based on their particular pandemic risk level (Taiwan CDC 2021c). All of these efforts have been made to reduce the difficulty of searching for medical care and the impact of infection control measures on inpatient and outpatient care—especially in the older population.

Preventive Measures Affecting Home- and Community-Based Services and Migrant Home Care Workers

(A) Changes in the Use of Home- and Community-Based Services and Migrant Home Care Workers

By the end of 2020, older population of Taiwan was approximately 3.79 million, or 16.07% of the total population. By the end of 2021, the population had increased to 3.94 million or 16.85% (DHR 2022). According to the Long-Term Care 2.0 Plan for Taiwan, approximately 12.7% of the older population reports living with at least one disability in Instrumental Activities of Daily Living (IADL). Taking younger populations into account, including adults of 50–64 years old with disabilities, indigenous people of 50–64 years old with disabilities, adults of 50 years or older with dementia, and adults of 50 years or younger with disabilities, nearly 0.82 million people needed LTC in Taiwan at 2020 and the number is estimated to be increasing by 0.03 million per year since then (MHW 2016).

(B) Use of Home-Based Services

Table 9.2 shows the number of users of home-based services (HBS), the change in the number of users between this year and last, and the percentage change from 2017 to 2020. The number of HBS users was 96,522 in 2018, and the number increased by 72.19% from 2017. While adults aged 65 or older accounted for over 80% of HBS users, the rapid increase in users was consistent with an assumption of rising demand and usage of HBS as a result of the ageing of the population in Taiwan. However, the number of users increased by only 8,948 or 9.27% from 2018 to 2019. This rate of increase was much lower than that from 2017 to 2018. However, the number of HBS users increased by 50.33% from 2019 to 2020, as 53,083 more people used HBS. Unlike health care utilization, which is relatively predictable and stable, a decision to use HBS can be very complicated and influenced by various interrelated factors concerning caregivers and care recipients.

The fast expansion of HBS providers and relaxation of the rules that govern eligibility for service when the Long-Term Care 2.0 Plan was firstly implemented in 2017 has led to a rapid increase in the number of HBS users from 2016 to 2017, so the rate of increase was lower from 2017 to 2018. The increase of 50.33% in the number of HBS users from 2019 to 2020 might have been caused in part by two Covid-19-related measures that affected the LTC service system. The first was the closure of adult day care centers during lockdowns, which forced adult day care recipients to turn to HBS (Hsu 2021). The second was border control measures during the pandemic, which made international movement difficult and reduced the number of migrant workers who were allowed to enter Taiwan (Wu 2021a, b). Thus, some people who needed LTC might have turned to HBS. The shift in users from migrant workers to HBS is evident in the decline in the number of migrant home care workers from 2019 to 2020 (Table 9.3).

(C) Change in the Importation of Migrant Home Care Workers

Table 9.3 presents the number of migrant home care workers in Taiwan, the change in the number of workers from last year to this, and the percentage of change thereof from 2017 to 2021. As a result of the increase in the number of persons with LTC needs, the number of migrant home care workers has increased steadily from 2017 to 2018 and from 2018 to 2019. However, since the four major migrant worker exporting countries, including Indonesia, Vietnam, Philippines, and Thailand, were listed by the Taiwan government as high-risk countries at the end of 2020, the entry of foreign workers, including migrant home care workers was terminated until November 2021 (MOL 2021). As seen in Table 9.3, the number of migrant home care workers decreased by 4.05% from 2019 to 2020, partly as a result of boarder control and international travel restrictions. A sharp decline of 10.35% from 2020 to 2021 was caused by the suspension of the importation of foreign labor.

(D) Change in the Use of Adult Day Care Services

Table 9.4 provides the number of adult day care users, the change in the number of users from last year to this, and the percentage of change from 2017 to 2020. The rate of increase in the number of users varied with the year; it was 76.15% from 2017 to 2018, 11.71% from 2018 to 2019, and 35.95% from 2019 to 2020. At first glance, the Covid-19 Pandemic had no obvious effect on the number of adult day care users, except perhaps for a slowing of growth. However, it would be too early to conclude that adult day care users were less likely to be affected by the pandemic. In contrast, we should be aware that changes in the number of such users may not alone reveal how the epidemic has influenced the lives of those users.

(E) Change in Number of Visits to Community Care Centers

By the end of 2016, Taiwan had 2,593 community care centers, and this number increased by approximately 20% annually to reach 4,610 in April, 2022 (SFAA 2022). Table 9.5 presents the number of visits for four types of services that are provided by community care centers; these are greeting and visit, telephone greeting and referral service, catering services, and health promotion activities. The table also shows the change in the number of visits for these services from last year to this, as well as the rate of change from 2017 to 2020. According to Table 9.5, the number of visits in greeting and visit service decreased by 2.14% from 2018 to 2019, in phone greeting and referral service increased by 2.31%, in catering services increased by 30.38%, and in health promotion activities increased by 49.13%. The number of visits for all the four types of services increased by 6.66 to 100.38% from 2019 to 2020. However, the increase was mainly caused by an amendment of subsidy standards from 2018, encouraging part time community care centers to transition to full time operation and to increase their range of service provided (Chang 2018). Therefore, the number of visits to phone greetings and referral services, and catering services increased markedly from 2019 to 2020. The rate of increase in users of health promotion activities was much lower than those of users of the other three types of services that are delivered in community care centers. *The variation of growth rate with service type reflects how* community care centers were affected by the pandemic. *The frequency of use of* health promotion activities, the number of users thereof and the number such activities performed, have increased only slightly, despite *the increase in the number of* community care centers and speedy development of the other three types of services.

Table 9.2 Number of home-based services users from 2017 to 2020

Year	Number of users	Change in number of users compared to last year	Change rate (%)
2017	56,056	–	–
2018	96,522	40,466	72.19
2019	105,470	8,948	9.27
2020	158,553	53,083	50.33

Source Gender Equality Committee, Executive Yuan (2022c)

Table 9.3 Number of migrant home care workers from 2017 to 2021

Year	Number of workers	Change in number of workers compared to last year	Change rate (%)
2017	233,368	–	–
2018	241,000	7632	3.27
2019	244,379	3379	1.4
2020	234,476	−9903	−4.05
2021	210,208	−24,268	−10.35

Source Labor Statistics Inquiry Network (2022)

Table 9.4 Number of adult day care users from 2017 to 2021

Year	Number of users	Change in number of users compared to last year	Change rate (%)
2017	5091	–	–
2018	8968	3877	76.15
2019	10,018	1050	11.71
2020	13,619	3,601	35.95

Source Gender Equality Committee, Executive Yuan (2022)

Effects of Infection Control Measures on Home- and Community-Based Services and the Termination of the Entry of Migrant Home Care Workers on Community-Dwelling Older Adults

Several infection control measures for local government, service-providing organizations, and staff that deliver HCBS were announced by the Taiwan CECC or CDC in 2020 and subsequently revised according to the progress of the pandemic. These included "Covid-19 Epidemic Prevention Advice and Precautions for Home-based, Community-based, Long-term Care Stations, Community Care Centers and Dementia Care Centers" in Februray 2020, and "Covid-19 Epidemic Prevention for Community Workers Guidelines" in March, 2020 (MHW 2022b). These measures mostly regulated the behavior of HCBS providers to improve health monitoring, to improve the management of staff, and to meet the demands of residents in the community.

(A) Closure of Community Care Centers: Disruption of Daily Routine and Social Isolation

Of all infection control measures, the suspension of community-based services (CBS) may have been most impactful on the lives of older persons with LTC needs and on their caregivers. During the Level 3 epidemic alert in mid-May, 2021, all adult day cares and community care centers were closed. When the epidemic alert was lowered to Level 2, all HCBS were expected to provide but local government was

Table 9.5 Number of Community Care Center Visits from 2017 to 2020

	No. of visits				Change in No. of users compared to last year				Change rate (%)			
	Visit and greeting	Phone greeting	Catering service	Health promotion activities	Visit and greeting	Phone greeting	Catering service	Health promotion activities	Visit & greeting	Phone greeting	Catering service	Health promotion activities
2017	82,565	76,905	77,316	4,975,711	–	–	–	–	–	–	–	–
2018	82,985	77,958	110,493	8,697,399	420	1,053	33,177	3,721,688	0,51	1,37	42,91	74,8
2019	81,211	79,756	144,057	12,970,338	−1,774	1,798	33,564	4,272,939	−2,14	2,31	3,38	49,13
2020	128,235	144,220	288,664	13,833,917	47,024	64,464	144,607	863,579	57,9	80,83	100,38	6,66

Source Gender Equality Committee, Executive Yuan (2022)

authorized to impose additional restrictions and controls if needed (MHW 2022b). Cheng et al. (2021) investigated the effect of the shutdown of community care centers on older persons between July and August, 2020. They found that the percentage of participants in community care centers who ceased visiting community care centers increased significantly since the outbreak of the pandemic in March, 2020, regardless of whether they were directly affected the shutdown of community care centers or not. Moreover, approximately 15% of the participants who had stopped attending community care centers following the outbreak of the pandemic decided not to return to the service providers afterward. The study found that the closure of community care centers has both short-term and long-term effects on the participation in community care centers. In the short-term, the cessation of community care centers can lead to immediate interruption in participants' daily routine. In the long term, this disruption can reduce older adults' tendency to remain continuously involved in services even after the epidemic.

In addition to changing participation patterns, the closure of community care centers can also harm the emotional well-being and social relationships of older participants. According to Cheng et al. (2021), older adults cited not being lonely, being cared about, and having more opportunities to interact with others as the most common benefits of engaging in community care centers. The termination of services can significantly limit older individuals' from meaningful social activities and interactions, increasing their feelings of loneliness. Additionally, the threat that is posed by the closure community care centers to the mental health of older adults can also manifest in a significant increase in their expression of feelings of jumpiness, nervousness, and worry about family and friends. Older participants who experienced the shutting down of their community care center were more likely to feel hopeless than those who did not (Cheng et al. 2021).

(B) Closure of Adult Day Care Centers: Impact on Older Persons with Dementia and Their Caregivers

The closure of adult day care centers posed serious risks to the physical, mental, social, and economic well-being of older adults with dementia and their caregivers. Adult day care can be considered to be an illness prevention and health promotion program for older people, and especially for those with dementia, but it also critically offers family caregivers respite from caregiving duties or enables them to continue working, minimizing the physical, emotional, and financial burdens of family members. Therefore, the closing of adult day care centers as a result of the Level 3 epidemic alert in mid-May, 2021 forced working caregivers to leave their jobs to take care of their family members. Caring for persons with dementia, especially those with severe *psychological* symptoms and behavioral disturbances, all day at home alone can be very stressful and difficult for caregivers, exhausting them both physically and mentally (Chang 2021; TADA 2021).

Unlike users of community care centers, who are relatively healthy and capable of self-care, care recipients at adult day cares typically suffer from, on average, a moderate level of dementia. They rely greatly on a regular daily routine to increase social interaction and cognitive stimulation. Being unable to go to adult day care centers can worsen their *psychological* and behavioral symptoms owing to the disruption of their daily routines and also increase their risk of becoming a victim of elder maltreatment (TADA 2021). Another major concern is that the physical and cognitive deterioration thus caused may be irreversible. Accordingly, the physical and mental health status of adult day care participants can degenerate very fast during a lockdown. Consequently, the Level 3 epidemic alert made some of them no longer eligible for day care services, requiring that they are moved into more intensive care, such as institutional care, earlier than expected (Chang 2021). Therefore, the cutting off of adult day care services can be very harmful for their users.

(C) Worries of Home-Based Services Users and the Effect of Prohibiting the Entry of Migrant Home Care Workers to Taiwan

As mentioned in an earlier section, participants at adult day care centers who needed care when those centers were shut down and persons with LTC needs who were unable to benefit from migrant care workers due to the prohibition of their entry into the country were encouraged to turn to home services. However, the use of home services is not without cost during a pandemic. Chao and Yu (2021) interviewed 592 disabled community-dwelling older adults in Taiwan between April and July, 2020, in Taiwan. They found that HBS users experienced significantly more Covid-19-related worries and more depressive symptoms than non-HBS users. Additionally, HBS users also exhibited significantly more Covid-19-related worries and more depressive symptoms than CBS users.

These findings revealed that disabled older adults are more vulnerable with respect to mental health than their healthier counterparts. The pandemic differently affects the mental health of older adults with disabilities, among whom HBS users are more defenseless against negative mental health conditions that are induced Covid-19 than CBS users. One possible reason is that HBS users depend on hands-on care to support them at home and are cared for by front-line home-care professionals who are at high risk of infection but have no way to avoid the threat, triggering more worries about Covid-19 (Chao and Yu 2021; Cohen and Tavares 2020).

The burden on family caregivers has been exacerbated by the prohibition against the entry of migrant home care workers to Taiwan during the pandemic, as a result of which the number of arrivals has dropped sharply since 2020, causing a shortage in the migrant workforce in all industries, including healthcare. Employers who wanted to hire a foreign care worker had to wait longer than usual and pay a higher salary than was paid before the epidemic. Even worse, the shortage of migrant workers has caused different industries to compete for them. The care industry normally involves long working hours, low wages, and intense labor, and so it is commonly less favored by migrant workers than other industries, such as manufacturing (Wu 2021a, b).

In Taiwan, to be eligible for help from a migrant care worker, an applicant must have a Barthel Index of lower than 35 if younger than 80 years or lower than 60 if aged 80 years or older. Eligible applicants usually have severe impairment and need extended supervision and intensive care (WDA 2022). The caregivers of such recipients are also at high risk of having to leave work for the purpose of caregiving, making them more likely to have to live in poverty. The prohibition of the entry of migrant home care workers has worsened the insufficiency of the supply of migrant care workers, leaving families of persons with severe LTC needs with high caregiving burdens. Also, the competition among industries for the migrant workforce has become more serious. Families of persons with severe LTC needs must pay more to acquire assistance with care work, considerably increasing their financial burden and risk of falling into poverty.

(D) Adaptive Strategies for Delivering Home- and Community-Based Services and the Entry of Migrant Home Care Workers into Taiwan

Based on the "2021 Covid-19 Vaccination Program" that was announced by the Taiwan CDC (Taiwan CDC 2021d), users and direct care workers in HCBS were in the category that was ranked fifth for vaccination, after health care professionals, frontline epidemic prevention, high-risk frontline workers, and persons sent abroad for diplomatic purposes, in order to maintain the functioning of institutional and social care systems. By prioritizing users of, and workers in, HCBS for vaccination, CBS was reopened as quickly as possible after the Level 3 epidemic alert expired, to provide older adults with at least one dose of vaccine, and achieving an overall staff vaccination rate of 80% by July, 2021 (Yang and Yang 2021). Appropriate protective equipment and fully vaccinated direct care workers allowed the delivery HBS to be continued.

In response to the termination of CBS, most community care centers and adult day care offered online courses to healthy and sub-healthy older adults who were cognitively and physically capable of taking video lessons. These service providers also offered online care and online group lessons to support the mental health of older persons and facilitate their social interaction during the lockdown. HBS were provided to older persons who did not have internet access or unable to use virtual services (Huang 2021).

The MHW subsidized a portion of the wages of CBS providers who followed the orders of CECC and provided no services during the lockdown. These bailouts sustained CBS providers throughout the epidemic. Also, caregivers of family members with LTC needs could apply for unpaid care leave. Compensation was given for the subsistence of caregivers whose care recipients were infected or quarantined (Jian et al. 2021). When the epidemic situation had become stable and the epidemic situation in various source countries had eased, to alleviate industrial labor shortages and fulfill meet the demand for care manpower, the migrant workers were allowed again to enter the country from November, 2021; the first to reenter were from Indonesia, which was followed by Thailand, the Philippines and Vietnam (WDA 2021).

Infection Control Measures in Long-Term Care Facilities

Number of Residents of Long-Term Care Facilities

As seen in Table 9.6, at the end of 2020, Taiwan had a total of 1,059 LTC institutions with 52,244 residents and 552 nursing homes with 31,705 residents aged 65 years and above. In Taiwan, LTC institutions provide residential services for older adults with LTC needs and are administered by the Social and Family Affairs Administration, MHW. Nursing homes offer both short-term care and LTC to people who cannot be cared for at home or in the community; they are supervised by Department of Nursing and Health Care, MHW. Thus, people aged 60 or older with LTC needs can be placed in both LTC institutions and nursing homes, but nursing homes have fewer age restrictions. By the end of 2020, 2.216% of the older population lived in residential care settings, including LTC institutions or nursing homes (DHR 2022; GEC 2022c). Herein, "LTC facilities" refers to both LTC institutions and nursing homes.

Residents in LTC facilities have been considered to be at the greatest risk of infection among all older people. Residents in LTC facilities are older and have more severe health conditions than community-dwelling older people. Their movement is usually restricted within the institutions and resident population densities are typically high (Lin et al. 2022). Moreover, frontline and hands-on care are necessities in LTC facilities and cannot be omitted or terminated. Every operation involves close-contact and the number of staff is the minimum required, leaving no slack when replacements must be found (Wu 2022). Therefore, from January to May, 2022, when Taiwan entered the "disaster damage reduction coexistence" period, 1,018 LTC facilities reported infections of 10,724 residents and 4,020 staff. The peak in this period ran from May 23 to May 29, 2022, when the number of confirmed/registered cases in Taiwan exceeded 570,000, of which residents in LTC facilities accounted for 1.75%. However, of the 660 deaths in this period, residents in LTC facilities represented nearly 30% (Yang et al. 2022), indicating that the fast spread of the virus in institutional settings and the disproportionally high mortality of this population.

Table 9.6 Number of residential care users by years

	Long-term care institution	Nursing home	
	60 above	Total	65 above
2017	48,295	37,466	25,846
2018	49,575	39,713	27,167
2019	50,966	43,095	29,920
2020	52,244	45,283	31,705

Source Gender Equality Committee, Executive Yuan (2022)

Infection Control Measures in Long-Term Care Institutions

As required by "Enhanced Covid-19 Control Measures for Residential Long-Term Care Facilities," announced by CECC, several infection control measures were implemented and adjusted over time. The main control measures included restricted visits and over 90% of the staff and the full vaccination of over 90% of staff and 80% of residents (MHW 2022c). Also, the staff at LTC facilities had to monitor their health status, divide into groups, and separate their work and rest areas from each other to avoid cluster infection (Jian et al. 2021). During the Level 3 epidemic alert, residents in LTC facilities were prevented from going out except to seek necessary medical care or for mourning; visits were suspended (DOH 2021).

For residents and their families, the most impactful measures might have been the suspension or restriction of visits. Visitation restriction required families and friends to reduce their frequency of, or even stop, seeing their relatives in institutions. Most people in LTC facilities are very senior with both physical and cognitive impairment. They may not be able to comprehend what is happening with the virus or the pandemic, and so feel "abandoned" by their families (Lin et al. 2022). The families of the residents had to face various fears, such as being "forgotten" by their loved ones, or being informed that their relatives were infected or deceased (Jiang 2022).

LTC facilities faced several challenges, which made coping with the epidemic very difficult. Specifically, the long-standing problem of workforce shortages in LTC facilities made supplementary manpower unavailable. Additionally, separating work places, rest areas and working groups was not feasible for all small institutions because they had a limited number of staff and little space. Lastly, LTC facilities that complied with the epidemic prevention policy and temporarily closed or delayed opening might have suffered economic hardship and would have needed support to alleviate their financial burden and avoid bankruptcy.

Adaptive Strategies in Long-Term Care Facilities

In response to the challenges above, visitor management measures for LTC facilities were modified as the epidemic developed and exceptions were made. For example, since April 2022, visits in cities and counties with high infection rates, such as Taipei City and New Taipei City, remained suspended, but exceptions have been made for patients who are severely ill or have been assessed as necessary by the institutions as requiring visits. In cities and counties that were not listed as having high risk, visits can be arranged with no more than three visitors per resident per visit and only one resident can receive visits within a room at a time (Taiwan CDC 2022c).

The MOL determined that the epidemic is an "incident" that meets the criteria set by the "Labor Standards Act," forcing staff at LTC facilities to work overtime as necessary. Thus, staff in LTC facilities were exempted from the "working for seven days with one day off" mandate, and their daily working period could exceed 12 h.

Their monthly overtime working hours could also exceed the 46-h upper limit (DSA 2020). The financial losses, and salaries of employees, of institutions that were facing financial losses and business interruptions as a result of the order of the CECC were subsided when their average monthly income dropped by at least 15% for any three consecutive months during the pandemic (DSA 2020).

Effects of Infection Control Measures on Older Adults Who Live Alone

Number of Older Adults Who Live Alone in Taiwan

Based on the 2017 Survey on the Living Conditions of Older People (SLCOP) in Taiwan, of the 3,745 community-dwelling participants who were aged 65 years and over, 8.94% of them lived alone, and 20.38% resided with a spouse or partner only. The percentage of the Taiwanese older population who lived alone or with a spouse or partner was lower than in the West, including Europe and North America, but was close to that in countries in the Asia–Pacific region (Ausubel 2020).

Living alone may be associated with poorer physical health, including more cardiovascular disease, lower physical functioning, higher incidence of frailty, and poorer mental health, manifesting as more depressive symptoms, reduced cognitive function, and greater anxiety and loneliness. Living alone is also associated with poor quality of life and higher mortality. However, the above associations are inconsistent across studies and results concerning the effects of living alone on physical, mental health and well-being are inconclusive (Hsu 2020). As suggested by Hsu (2020), living alone can be merely a living arrangement, and not necessarily a determinant of loneliness or isolation. However, living alone may be especially harmful when it comes with other risk factors, such as low education, low income and high disability. Therefore, Taiwan has developed a unique system for serving) older adults who live alone in the community. The system identifies persons aged 65 or over who live alone and need a watch, or have coresident(s) who are unable to provide care. Local government is responsible for providing visits, telephone calls, food, and accompaniment to hospital. By the end of 2021, a total of 42,929 older individuals were identified by the system, comprising 17,621 males and 25,308 females (DOS 2022).

Effects of Infection Control Measures on Older Adults Who Live Alone

As mentioned earlier, the Taiwan government had launched several systems to facilitate the distribution of pandemic-related resources and to support the implementation of infection control measures, such as vaccination reservation, name-based mask and

Covid-19 rapid test kit distribution, and the making of appointments for video diagnosis and treatment. Also, people largely rely on delivery platform to order food and have groceries delivered, especially during the Level 3 alert and quarantine. However, according to the 2017 SLCOP in Taiwan, 73.48% of older adults had never used the internet or had no device to access it. Thus, without assistance or adequate guidance, most older people could not complete the pandemic-related registration or application online. Li et al. (2021) found that found that older adults in Taiwan who lived alone experienced a significant decline in social participation and life satisfaction as well as an increase in depression after the Level 3 epidemic alert. Additionally, the infection control measures most severely impacted the social participation and psychological well-being of those who were both illiterate and older (over 85 years and above).

These findings suggest that owing to a lack of an informal support network and limited ability to access information technology, older adults who lived alone might have suffered from a shortage of daily necessities, were unable to seek medical treatment, and feared having an accident or being sick alone at home, making their lives more stressful than the lives of older adults with coresidents during the Covid-19 Pandemic (Ye 2021). Moreover, the combination of living alone, social isolation, advanced age and low social economic status made the epidemic especially detrimental, and sometimes even deadly, for older people.

Adaptive Strategies for Older Adults Who Live Alone

In response to threat to living conditions that was posed by the pandemic, a special program to support the lives and health of older adults who live alone was developed during the Level 3 epidemic alert. It focused on strengthening available services and enhancing multidisciplinary cooperation (MHW 2021b). Local government was responsible for integrating resources from departments that dealt with social affairs, health, civil affairs, and policing, and from non-governmental organizations, to deliver food, HBS, daily necessities and epidemic prevention materials to listed older adults who lived alone. Phone calls were made on a daily basis and messages from public were conveyed. For older persons who had no contact with another person for 24 h, emergency responses were provided and visits were arranged. These efforts and prompt policy responses ensured that older adults who lived alone were taken care of relatively well in communities, as reflected by the low mortality in this vulnerable population throughout the pandemic.

Suggestions for Future Policy Responses for Older Persons in a Pandemic

From the beginning of the Covid-19 Pandemic, Taiwan has been widely heralded for its successful control of the spread of the virus and effective government response to it. At the time of writing this paper, Taiwan is going through the "disaster damage reduction and coexistence" period and new challenges continue to emerge. Drawing on the experience of Taiwan and other countries, the actions or policy responses listed below should be considered in the future to address more comprehensively the impact of Covid-19 Pandemic on older people in Taiwan.

(1) Ensure the Accessibility of Services and Support for Older Adults with Covid-19 Infection

Little information on the experience of older adults who have been treated for Covid-19 in Taiwan is available. According to Pel-Littel et al. (2022), older adults experienced physical symptoms and emotional responses to the diagnosis in the first phase of the disease. In the second phase, when they were hospitalized, they suffered from an inability to participate in decision-making about their healthcare, frustration and confused communication with health professionals, and a feeling of isolation throughout the process. After recovery from Covid-19, most older adults still regarded their health as worsened, so their social interaction and opportunities for activities were still limited. Drawing from older adults' experiences of infection in the West, more effort should be made to facilitate communication about healthcare decisions during treatment and to improve the accessibility of rehabilitation services, meaningful activities, and social support during recovery. Also, older persons who are diagnosed with Covid-19 should be classified by degree of vulnerability, which is related to their ability to comprehend information and communications, their ability to follow instructions for rehabilitation, and their potential to resume social relationships and social activities.

(2) Consider the Demands of Stakeholders Who Serve Older People in Various Settings

As discussed above, Covid-19 affects not only older people, but also all involved stakeholders. Those stakeholders include professional providers of services for healthy, sub-healthy and disabled older adults, such as HCBS and the services that are provided in community care centers and at LTC facilities. The stakeholders include not only professional but also semi-professional and non-professional service providers, such as domestic and migrant workers who provide hands-on care and family caregivers. Responsive and adequate policy support, including financial subsidies, flexible management mandates and clear guidelines, should be developed in a timely manner and within budget. Additionally, adaptability and interchangeability across stakeholders in various setting to ensure the continuous provision of social and health support as well as LTC, and to prevent burnout or the overloading of service resources.

(3) Address the Health and Social Resource Disparities in the Pandemic

Older people are a heterogeneous population that can be variously impacted by Covid-19. More effort should be made to understand how older people in different contexts are affected by the pandemic. Effects vary with, for example, gender, living area, living arrangement, type of residence, health and cognitive status. The effect of outbreaks on health and social resource disparities occur should also be understood (Chao and Yu 2021). When technology, including that used in remote health care, the video diagnosis and treatment of Covid-19, and virtual care or group activities, is regarded as an effective means of combating the effects of physical distancing and restrictions in the pandemic, older people's needs and abilities regarding the use of technology must be considered more thoroughly and hands-on training should be offered to make the use of technology easier for them (Jaffe et al. 2020). Notably, older adults who are unable to use technology and online resources may be more unprotected than others in the older population in the pandemic owing to their restricted health, cognitive or social status. Special attention should therefore be paid to these susceptible older adults and more practical support than simply virtual services should be designed and delivered for them.

(4) Combat Social Isolation and Loneliness and Ensure Quality of Life in the Epidemic

The lockdowns and Covid-19-related control measures had a great impact on the mental health of older people globally, including in Taiwan. Older people are more likely to report difficulties in managing their loneliness, social isolation, and prolonged grief that follows the loss of, or separation from, families and loved ones. They are thus them at a higher risk of depressive symptoms and loss of quality of life (Chao and Yu 2021; Marzo et al. 2022). According to Horn et al. (2021), in the pandemic, older persons in certain disadvantaged groups owing to their health or social condition, including being female, having a chronic illness, having children, and living alone, were more likely to experience reduced well-being, which manifests in a depressed mood and a lack of social contact. Therefore, more services must be developed to sustain the mental health, well-being, and quality of life of older people, and especially those with limited health and social resources.

(5) Counter Ageism and Sustain Engagement in Meaningful Activities and a Desired Lifestyle

The third outbreak that occurred in the middle of 2021 was caused in part by a cluster infection in hostess teahouses in Wanhua District, which is the old town *of Taipei City*. Although hostess teahouses have been stigmatized as pornographic, especially in the mainstream media, their presence represents an unmet need for social interaction for lonely older males, who have no one to talk and no place to go for leisure (Hsieh 2021). After the third outbreak, the older population has been unreasonably blamed as the reason for lockdowns and a burden on both society and the healthcare system, intensifying prevailing ageism. Then, a kind of benevolent ageism, involving viewing older people as homogeneous and weak, offering unwanted help without considering individual differences, and rationalizing the imposition of stricter guidelines on older people, has been rationalized and widely accepted (Kornadt et al. 2021). However, when the end does not justify the mean, unexpected and irreversible negative consequences may overcome the benefits of the pandemic control measures; these negative consequences include increased self-isolation and the reinforcement of internal and external ageism against older people. Drawing on Taiwan's experience, policymakers and practitioners should counter ageism to avoid the unequal treatment of older persons in the pandemic, regardless of whether it is benevolent, hostile or of any other kind. The other lesson of the experience of Taiwan is the need for a reasonable balance among engagement in culturally meaningful activities, maintaining a desirable lifestyle, and pandemic control as the core of any policies and the delivery of services for older people: one-size-fits-all policies cannot suit everyone.

(6) Cultural Competence When Working with Older People

Relatively little attention has been paid to the cultural competence of professionals who serve older adults. Older adult cultural competence refers to the integration of behaviors and attitudes that meet the needs and preferences of older adults in various situations into a system, organization or professional operation (AIDS Community Research Initiative of America 2022). Cultural competence can also facilitate an understanding of older individuals' decisions about healthcare or service utilization, their beliefs and coping strategies with respect to Covid-19, and their preferences about how to be cared for while ill and dying in difference cultural contexts (Periyakoil 2019). Cultural competence enables professionals in different fields to work and communicate effectively with older persons, meeting their needs in a respectful and dignified way. It should be therefore be at the core of the training and education of human services professionals.

(7) Improve Data Collection and Promote the Use of Data to Support Policy-Making

One of the keys to successfully combating the spread of the virus in Taiwan was its fast adoption of numerous novel digital technologies and prompt utilization of big data analytics to support Covid-19-related policy-making. These included the use national health insurance and immigration databases to generate on-time alerts in clinics based on patients' travel histories (Wang et al. 2020). More timely data collection and the integration of numerous datasets to support policy-making will be needed in the future. For instance, the use of data from healthcare and social services systems, enables policymakers to evaluate the distribution and utilization of health care, LTC, HCBS, and other social resources. Accordingly, inequity in the utilization of services by the older population in different areas and different subgroups can be assessed. The integration of databases on clinical visits, elder abuse, LTC, and labor insurance and a systematic comparison of changes that occur before during, and after the pandemic, enables much important information to be extracted. This may include how Covid-19 affects older people of different backgrounds and conditions, including of income and employment; the incidence of elder abuse, the use of LTC and health care, and their interrelationships. Thus, continuous data collection, data integration, and the consideration of the implications of data will be require to promote the effectiveness of governance, resource distribution and policy-setting. Big data analytics can help to identify ways of sustaining the well-being of older population in the pandemic and help them develop their resilience against adverse experiences.

In conclusion, older persons in Taiwan have faced numerous challenges as a result of the Covid-19 Pandemic. The Taiwan government has implemented various measures to prevent the spread of the virus, and these measures have had a great impacted on the life of older individuals in different settings and with various needs. Although these measures have been loosened or adapted to mitigate their most damaging effects, several issues should be considered to improve the quality of governance as well as to ensure the well-being of older persons with heterogeneous backgrounds.

Firstly, the needs of older individuals before, during, and after infection should be understood and the resources that are required to sustain their physical, mental, social, and financial well-being should be delivered on time. Secondly, in addition to older persons, all stakeholders that are involved in providing informal and formal services to the older population should be supported to avoid burnout and the collapse of the service system. Thirdly, maintaining the continuum of care and services for older individuals with different physical and cognitive statuses is critical in the pandemic to maintain their dignity and quality of life. Fourthly, the facilitation of communication with, and rights advocacy for, older adults should be put at the center of the training and education of human service professionals, allowing better methods of policy implementation and practice to be identified. Finally, seniors who are marginalized or disadvantaged for reasons of gender, economic status, cultural context, and social relationship, should be closely monitored by obtaining relevant information using more advanced technologies to reduce the disproportionately negative impacts of Covid-19 on some groups. Taiwan's experience and the aforementioned methods can be used to mitigate the effects of the Covid-19 Pandemic on older people in Taiwan and other countries, and to protect their well-being.

Appendix A: Panel A—Average Outpatient Visits in Every 0.1 Million People from 2017–2020

	Total visits/ years	0–4	5–9	10–14	15–19	20–24	25–29	30–34	35–39	40–44
2017	94,524	94,962	99,871	95,449	92,192	93,772	93,370	90,394	92,871	92,415
2018	94,689	96,986	98,324	96,022	93,555	91,893	92,799	91,886	92,179	93,285

(continued)

(continued)

	Total visits/ years	0–4	5–9	10–14	15–19	20–24	25–29	30–34	35–39	40–44
2019	94,816	95,848	99,463	96,468	92,787	92,539	93,797	91,689	91,862	93,885
2020	93,467	94,378	99,955	94,466	89,581	91,465	91,276	91,274	89,680	91,666

	Total visits/ years	45–49	50–54	55–59	60–64	65–69	70–74	75–79	80–84	85 above
2017	94,524	91,121	91,508	94,348	95,526	100,574	99,794	101,482	104,497	110,853
2018	94,689	91,097	91,915	94,191	95,909	99,600	100,901	101,383	104,521	110,576
2019	94,816	91,428	92,148	93,624	95,748	98,776	102,194	100,320	104,762	110,788
2020	93,467	89,909	91,008	92,369	94,354	97,752	102,811	97,737	104,481	110,715

Source Gender Equality Committee Executive Yuan (2022a).

Appendix A: Panel B—Changes Between Years in Average Outpatient Visits in Every 0.1 Million People from 2017–2020

	Visits change/ years	0–4	5–9	10–14	15–19	20–24	25–29	30–34	35–39	40–44
2017	–	–	–	–	–	–	–	–	–	–
2018	165	2,024	−1,547	573	1,363	−1,879	−571	1,492	-692	870
2019	127	−1,138	1,139	446	−768	646	998	−197	−317	600
2020	−1,349	−1,470	492	−2,002	−3,206	−1,074	−2,521	−415	−2,182	−2,219

	Visits change/ years	45–49	50–54	55–59	60–64	65–69	70–74	75–79	80–84	85 above
2017	–	–	–	–	–	–	–	–	–	–
2018	165	−24	407	−157	383	−974	1,107	−99	24	−277
2019	127	331	233	−567	−161	−824	1,293	−1,063	241	212
2020	−1,349	−1,519	−1,140	−1,255	−1,394	−1,024	617	−2,583	−281	−73

Source Gender Equality Committee, Executive Yuan (2022a)

Appendix B: Panel A—Average Hospital Admissions in Every 0.1 Million people by Age Group from 2017–2020

	Total visits/years	0–4	5–9	10–14	15–19	20–24	25–29	30–34	35–39	40–44
2017	8,558	14,330	5,191	2,415	2,701	3,868	5,458	7,299	6,738	5,787
2018	8,637	14,612	5,188	2,515	2,815	3,806	5,264	7,115	6,495	5,872
2019	8,821	14,765	5,790	2,824	2,960	3,881	5,300	7,060	6,534	5,962
2020	8,262	12,208	3,343	2,060	2,833	3,894	5,055	6,874	6,281	5,765

	Total visits/ years	45–49	50–54	55–59	60–64	65–69	70–74	75–79	80–84	85 above
2017	8,558	6,184	7,163	8,654	10,645	14,059	17,734	22,043	27,996	38,851
2018	8,637	6,205	7,218	8,700	10,735	13,919	17,836	22,108	27,887	38,739
2019	8,821	6,368	7,341	8,786	10,807	13,826	17,875	21,804	27,814	38,536
2020	8,262	6,175	7,057	8,320	10,174	12,937	16,876	19,975	25,534	35,639

Source Gender Equality Committee, Executive Yuan (2022b)

Appendix B: Panel B—Changes in Average Hospital Admissions by Age Group from 2017–2020

	Visits change/years	0–4	5–9	10–14	15–19	20–24	25–29	30–34	35–39	40–44
2017	–	–	–	–	–	–	–	–	–	–
2018	79	282	−3	100	114	−62	−194	−184	−243	85
2019	184	153	602	309	145	75	36	−55	39	90
2020	−559	−2,557	−2,447	−764	−127	13	−245	−186	−253	−197

	Visits change/ years	45–49	50–54	55–59	60–64	65–69	70–74	75–79	80–84	85 above
2017	–	–	–	–	–	–	–	–	–	–
2018	79	21	55	46	90	−140	102	65	−109	− 112
2019	184	163	123	86	72	−93	39	−304	−73	−203
2020	−559	−193	−284	−466	−633	−889	−999	− 1,829	− 2,280–	−2,897

Source Gender Equality Committee, Executive Yuan (2022b)

References

AIDS Community Research Initiative of America. 2022. *Older adult cultural competence*. https://www.nursesinaidscare.org.

Ausubel, J. 2020. *Older people are more likely to live alone in the U.S. than elsewhere in the world*. https://www.pewresearch.org.

Chang, T. W. 2021. Many families can't hold it anymore! Community-based services were closed due to the epidemic, making it even more difficult to take care of persons with dementia. *The Reporter*. https://www.twreporter.org.

Chang, Y. M. 2018. *Long-term care 2.0 promotes the overall care service system in the community*. https://ms-community.azurewebsites.net.

Chang, Y.T., C.Y. Lin, M.J. Tsai, C.T. Hung, C.W. Hsu, P.L. Lu, and M.F. Hou. 2020. Infection control measures of a Taiwanese hospital to confront the Covid-19 pandemic. *The Kaohsiung Journal of Medical Sciences* 36 (5): 296–304.

Chao, S.F. and M.S. Yu. 2021. Covid-19-related worries, social disruptions, and depressive symptoms among community-dwelling older adults with disabilities: What makes the difference? *Journals of Gerontology: Series B: Psychological Sciences and Social Sciences*. https://doi.org/10.1093/geronb/gbab157.

Chen, J., et al. 2022. The era of coexistence with viruses—Omicron's new challenge. *The Reporter*. https://www.twreporter.org/topics.

Chen, W. T. 2020. The regret of the victims of the epidemic, missed the last chance to see the mother under restricted visits. *Central News Agency*. https://www.cna.com.tw/news.

Cheng, C.W., S.F. Cheng, and C.Y. Hung. 2021. Preliminary study on the impact of the closure of community care centers on the elderly under the prevention of Covid-19. *Community Development Quarterly* 175: 87–100.

Cohen, M.A. and J. Tavares. 2020. Who are the most at-risk older adults in the Covid-19 era? *It's not just those in nursing homes. Journal of Aging and Social Policy* 32 (4–5): 380–386.

CPT, Covid-19 Pandemic in Taiwan. 2022. *Website*. https://en.wikipedia.org.

CVT, Covid-19 Vaccination in Taiwan. 2022. *Website*. https://en.wikipedia.org.

Deng, G.F. 2021. Epidemic explosion and nosocomial infection, chronic patients can choose "video diagnosis and treatment" for remote follow-up. *For a Better life*. https://www.commonhealth.com.tw/article/84251.

DOH, Department of Health, Taipei City Government. 2021. *In response to the central epidemic command center raising the Covid-19 epidemic alert level to level 3 on May 15, 2021, residents of long-term care institutions suspend unnecessary going out*. https://health.gov.taipei.

DHR, Department of Household Registration, Ministry of the Interior. 2022. *Demographics by age structure indices*. https://www.ris.gov.tw.

DSA, Department of Social Affairs, Taipei City Government. 2020. *Preparing for the worst, long-term care institutions deploy anti-epidemic in advance*. https://homecare.gov.taipei.

DOS, Division of Statistics, Ministry of Health and Welfare. 2022. *Number of listed older people living alone who need care and an overview of services*. https://dep.mohw.gov.tw.

GEC, Gender Equality Committee, Executive Yuan. 2022a. *Average outpatient visits every 0.1 million people by 5-year age group (2017–2020)*. https://www.gender.ey.gov.tw.

GEC, Gender Equality Committee, Executive Yuan. 2022b. *Average hospital admissions every 0.1 million people by 5-year age group (2017–2020)*. https://www.gender.ey.gov.tw.

GEC, Gender Equality Committee, Executive Yuan. 2022c. *Important gender statistics database*. https://www.gender.ey.gov.tw.

Holtz, L. 2021. *Covid-19's impact on overall health care services in Africa: Africa in focus*. https://www.brookings.edu/blog/africa-in-focus/2021/10/12.

Horn, V., M. Semmler, and C. Schweppe. 2021. Older people in Germany during the Covid-19 pandemic: The least, the more, and the most affected. *Journal of Population Ageing* 1–22. https://doi.org/10.1007/s12062-021-09352-4.

Hsieh, M.Y. 2021. *Unknown "lonely old man:" Just want to find someone to talk to.* https://today.line.me/tw.

Hsu, C.W. 2021. *Care attendants: Internships interrupted during the epidemic.* https://health.udn.com/health/story.

Hsu, H.C. 2020. Typologies of loneliness, isolation and living alone are associated with psychological well-being among older adults in Taipei: A cross-sectional study. *International Journal of Environmental Research and Public Health* 17 (24): 9181. https://doi.org/10.3390/ijerph17249181.

Huang, H.C. 2021. *Schools are suspended for the elderly, community care does not close during the epidemic.* https://ms-community.azurewebsites.net.

Huang, I.Y.F. 2020. Fighting Covid-19 through government initiatives and collaborative government: The Taiwan experience. *Public Admission Review* 80 (4): 665–670.

Jaffe, I., R. Hayashi, and M.R. Hassan. 2020. *Responding the needs of older people during the Covid-19 pandemic—Sharing lessons learned.* https://www.jcie.org/programs/healthy-aging.

Jian, H.J., T.R. Du, C.Y. Yang, and Y.T. Wu. 2021. Social affairs department's response to the Covid-19 epidemic. *Community Development Quarterly* 175: 8–22.

Jiang, W.Y. 2022. *New Taipei announced that long-term care institutions were prohibited from visiting: She was worried that her mother would forget hers.* https://udn.com/news/story.

Kornadt, A.E., I. Albert, M. Hoffmann, E. Murdock, and J. Nell. 2021. Perceived ageism during the Covid-19-crisis is longitudinally related to subjective perceptions of aging. *Frontiers in Public Health* 9: 679711. https://doi.org/10.3389/fpubh.2021.679711.

LSIN, Labor Statistics Inquiry Network. 2022. *Number of industrial and social welfare migrant workers by projects.* https://statdb.mol.gov.tw.

Lang, H.C. 2021. The impact and reflection of Covid-19 pandemic to health care industries and patients' health. *Humanities and Social Sciences Newsletter Quarterly* 22 (4): 31–36.

Li, H.M., C.Y. Hsu, M.L. Chen, and B.J. Jeng. 2021. Social participation and mental health of elderly people living alone before and after the Covid-19 level 3 alert. *Bulletin of Chung Hwa University of Medical Technology* 55: 92–111.

Li, P.C. 2020. *Covid-19's impact on health care utilization in Taiwan.* https://ibmi.taiwan-healthcare.org.

Lin, C.L., J.Y. Hsu, H.Y. Wang, and M.C. Pu. 2022. *Long-term care residents are the most vulnerable group.* https://health.udn.com/health/story/120950/6350254.

Marzo, R.R., et al. 2022. Quality of life of the elderly during the Covid-19 pandemic in Asian countries: A cross-sectional study across six countries. *Life (Basel, Switzerland)* 12 (3): 365. https://doi.org/10.3390/life12030365.

Miller, E.A. 2020. Protecting and improving the lives of older adults in the Covid-19 era. *Journal of Aging & Social Policy* 32: 297–309.

MHW, Ministry of Health and Welfare. 2016. *The long-term care 2.0 plan.* https://1966.gov.tw.

MHW, Ministry of Health and Welfare. 2021a. *2017 survey on the living conditions of older people.* https://dep.mohw.gov.tw.

MHW, Ministry of Health and Welfare. 2021b. *Enhanced care services for the elderly living alone during the Covid-19 alert level 3.* https://www.mohw.gov.tw.

MHW, Ministry of Health and Welfare. 2022a. *Major policies.* https://covid19.mohw.gov.tw.

MHW, Ministry of Health and Welfare. 2022b. *Epidemic prevention measures and related guidelines from the central epidemic command center*. https://1966.gov.tw.

MHW, Ministry of Health and Welfare. 2022c. *Adjustment of visitor management measures for residential long-term care institutions nationwide from March 1.* https://www.mohw.gov.tw.

MOJ, Ministry of Justice. 2019. *Laws & regulations database of the republic of china: Law on the prevention and control of infectious diseases.* https://law.moj.gov.tw.

MOL, Ministry of Labor. 2021. *The epidemic in the origin countries of migrant workers have risen to level 3, and the ministry of labor has introduced measures to strengthen epidemic prevention and management*. https://www.mol.gov.tw.

Morrow-Howell, N., N. Galucia, and E. Swinford. 2020. Recovering from the Covid-19 pandemic: A focus on older adults. *Journal of Aging & Social Policy* 32: 526–535.

NCHPC, National Center for High-Performance Computing. 2022. *Covid-19 dashboard: Vaccination.* https://covid-19.nchc.org.tw.

Pel-Little, R.E., D.E. Stekelenburg, H.C. Willems, S. Jansen, J. Festen, and van der Linden, C. 2022. Lessons learned from the Covid-19 pandemic as experienced by older adults treated for Covid-19 *Gerontology & Geriatric Medicine* 8. https://doi.org/10.1177/23337214221086831.

Periyakoil, V.S. 2019. Building a culturally competent workforce to care for diverse older adults: Scope of the problem and potential solution. *Journal of the American Geriatrics Society* 67: S423-432.

Rodrigues, M., M. Grunho, A. Rachão, E. Silva, A. Cordeiro, M. Guilherme, and L. Pereira. 2021. The impact of Covid-19 pandemic in stroke code activation and time from symptom onset to hospital arrival in a Portuguese comprehensive stroke centre. *Revue Neurologique* 73 (3): 89–95.

SFAA, Social and Family Affairs Administration, Ministry of Health and Welfare. 2022. *Service sites statistics.* https://www.sfaa.gov.tw.

TADA, Taiwan Alzheimer's Disease Association. 2021. *Taiwan Alzheimer's disease association calls for quick restoration of community-based dementia services.* https://homecare.gov.taipei.

Taiwan CDC. 2020a. *Press releases.* https://www.cdc.gov.tw.

Taiwan CDC. 2020b. *Prevention and control of Covid-19 in Taiwan.* https://www.cdc.gov.tw.

Taiwan CDC. 2020c. *Press releases.* https://www.cdc.gov.tw.

Taiwan CDC. 2020d. *CECC announces social distancing measures for Covid-19.* https://www.cdc.gov.tw.

Taiwan CDC. 2021a. *Nationwide level 3 epidemic alert extended to June 28; related measures remain effective to fight against Covid-19 in community.* https://www.cdc.gov.tw.

Taiwan CDC. 2021b. From August 24, 2021a, *Press release for hospitals across the country will be open to visiting patients with conditions.* https://www.cdc.gov.tw.

Taiwan CDC. 2021c. *Press release for hospitals in north areas and long-term care facilities.* https://www.cdc.gov.tw.

Taiwan CDC. 2021d. *Publicly funded vaccinations.* https://www.cdc.gov.tw.

Taiwan CDC. 2022a. *Area, age, and gender statistical table.* https://data.cdc.gov.tw.

Taiwan CDC. 2022b. *Statistics on the number of confirmed cases and deaths of Covid-19 in the country since 2020: Statistics by age and gender.* https://www.cdc.gov.tw.

Taiwan CDC. 2022c. *Adjustment of visitor management measures for residential long-term care institutions across the country with immediate effect.* https://www.cdc.gov.tw.

Wang, C.J., C.Y. Ng, and R.H. Brook. 2020. Response to Covid-19 in Taiwan: Big data analytics, new technology, and proactive testing. *JAMA* 323 (14): 1341–1342.

WDA, Workforce Development Agency, Ministry of Labor. 2021. *Since November 11, 2011, the introduction of migrant projects has been opened, and the first wave will be opened to Indonesia.* https://www.wda.gov.tw.

WDA, Workforce Development Agency, Ministry of Labor. 2022. *Qualifications and regulations for migrant workers.* https://www.wda.gov.tw.

Wu, H.Y. 2021a. The lack of migrant workers leads to the problem of labor shortages, and the burden on employers is heavier. *Central News Agency.* https://www.cna.com.tw.

Wu, H.Y. 2021b. *The lack of migrant workers leads to labor shortages, and the burden on employers becomes heavier.* https://www.cna.com.tw.

Wu, M.D. 2022. *Covid-19 epidemic and the stability of community care—Taking long-term care institutions as an example.* https://www.ankecare.com.

Yang, Y.T., Y.C. Chiu, S.C. Tsou, and S.J. Li. 2022. *Covid-19 Adds 145 deaths and long-term care institutions account for 30%.* https://udn.com.

Yang, Y.Y. and Yang, M.J. 2021. *Considering that people over 65 can get the vaccine, day care centers and community long-term care sites are expected to be unblocked.* https://news.ltn.com.tw.

Ye, G.Y. 2021. *Don't dare to go out: lack of face-to-face interaction, elders are forced to live more "alone" under the epidemic.* https://health.udn.com

Chapter 10
The Covid-19 Pandemic in Thailand: With Special Reference to Informal Workers' Problems

Wannaphong Durongkaveroj

Abstract Thailand has been internationally praised for avoiding a Covid-19 disaster. Throughout 2020, Thailand has relatively low number of Covid-19 cases and fatalities compared to many Western and developing countries. This success would not have been possible without stringent measures including the continued state of emergency, a nationwide nightly curfew, and border restrictions. All these measures have come at the expense of the economy. The Thai economy has been the hardest hit among ASEAN countries as the economy contracted by 6.1% and the poverty rate rose by 0.6 percentage points in 2020. However, these aggregate statistics underestimate the true cost of the pandemic. Thailand has a very large informal sector, which accounted for more than 50% of the workforce and most of them work in low-paying services sectors such as hotel, restaurant, and construction. These sectors suffered sharp contraction. The available data indicate that between 2019 and 2020, informal workers saw their monthly income drop by 4%, a notably larger decline than formal counterparts. Without proper social protection and job contract, informal workers are more prone to losing job and declining living standards. Falling quality of life among informal workers is the driving force of rising poverty rate during the pandemic. Key mitigating policies include undertaking targeted policies focusing on income and health inequity, and reducing the levels of informal employment.

Keywords Covid-19 Pandemic · Thailand · Informal workers · Income losses · Unemployment · Poverty · Social protection

Introduction

The Covid-19 Pandemic has affected almost all sectors of our society. However, the impact of the pandemic is uneven primarily because the majority of informal workers are employed in the hardest-hit sectors (e.g., accommodation and food services and

W. Durongkaveroj (✉)
Faculty of Economics, Ramkhamhaeng University, Bangkok, Thailand
e-mail: wannaphong@ru.ac.th

C. Aspalter (ed.), *Covid-19 Pandemic*,
https://doi.org/10.1007/978-981-99-2497-4_10

wholesale and retail trade) and they have less access to health services and social protection (Narula 2020; Webb et al. 2020). At the onset of the pandemic, the ILO (2020) estimated that about 1.6 billion workers in the informal economy are expected to be severely affected by lockdown and other containment measures to curb infections such as border closures, cancellation of public events, and restrictions of size of gatherings. To examine the lives of informal workers during the pandemic is thus key to understand how the pandemic affects our society.

Thailand is an excellent case study to analyze the impacts of the Covid-19 Pandemic on the informal economy because, among developing countries, Thailand stands out in terms of the large size of the informal sector. In 2021, 19.6 million people work informally in Thailand, accounting for 52% of total workforce (NSO 2022). This group of workers is vulnerable since they lack of income security and comprehensive social protection measures. An early study by Komin et al. (2020) using a survey of 384 informal sector workers shows that these workers saw dramatic decrease in their monthly income. On average, informal workers made about one-fourth of their average monthly income before the pandemic. Massage therapist was found to experience the largest monthly income drop (96%), followed by hairdresser (93%) and general employment (82%). Note however that this severe economic impact occurred during the first wave of the pandemic in Thailand when the government used a 75-day national lockdown as a key tool to contain the coronavirus. Even though the government of Thailand provided a monthly cash handout to informal workers as mentioned in previous section, less than 50% of the survey respondents received cash assistance. Reasons for missing this scheme are, for example, they could not complete the online registration and they were listed as farmers which made them ineligible for the program.

A recent report by WIEGO (2022) deserves attention. The report aims to examine the impacts of the Covid-19 Pandemic on informal workers in different countries. For Thailand, the analysis is drawn from two rounds of survey: (1) June-July 2020 and (2) July–August 2021. The sample covers 293 informal workers across different occupations such as domestic workers, street vendors, and massage therapists. It is found that the impacts of the pandemic are uneven even among informal workers. While average days worked per week among motorcycle and taxi drivers and domestic workers did not change much for the period under study, massage therapists experienced about 4-day decline in their days worked. The study also suggests that gross earnings among informal workers reduced significantly between 2019 and 2020. On average, informal workers in all occupations except domestic workers received less than 40% of their pre-pandemic median incomes. Street vendors; massage therapists; and home-based workers experienced a large drop in their incomes. Even though motorcycle and taxi driver can operate during the pandemic, they suffered significantly due to low demand from passengers who started working from home.

The purpose of this chapter is to document the lives of informal workers in Thailand before and during the pandemic. It contributes to an increasingly expanding literature on the Covid-19 Pandemic. While previous studies (e.g., Komin et al. 2021; Chen et al. 2022) focus on specific period (e.g., during the first wave of the pandemic in Thailand), this chapter compares the economic lives of informal workers before and during the pandemic. While previous research (i.e., Finnegan and Singh 2004; Mehrotra 2009; Horn 2010) on informal workers explore how economic impact of economic crisis on informal workers, this study looks at changes in real income and other indicators (e.g., occupations and medical expenses) driven by both the pandemic itself and the measures used to contain the spread of the disease. They also demonstrate how effective policy responses are in response to the pandemic. If the Covid-19 measures are well designed and implemented, informal workers should be protected and their economic conditions should not be downgraded significantly during the pandemic. Therefore, this analysis aims to shed light on a comprehensive impact of the Covid-19 Pandemic.

This chapter is structured as follows: Sect. 10.2 describes the Covid-19 outbreak in Thailand and its impact on the Thai economy. In Sect. 10.3, I outline the informal economy in Thailand. Section 10.4 provide policy responses for informal workers. A final section concludes with policy recommendations.

The Covid-19 Pandemic in Thailand and Its Impact on the Economy

Thailand has been internationally praised for avoiding a Covid-19 disaster in 2020. Despite recording the first case of the virus outside of China on 13 January 2020, the country managed to avoid its first death until early March 2020. On 26 March 2020, the State of Emergency was declared, and it has served as a legal emergency power in response to the pandemic through health and economic measures. Throughout 2020, Thailand had 7,000 confirmed/registered cases with merely 61 deaths, a low figure compared to other Western countries. This stellar achievement in containing the coronavirus is mainly due to several stringent measures implemented between March and June 2020 such as border control, closure of schools and universities, and work-from-home scheme. According to Hale et al. (2021), Thailand's stringency index, a composite measure based on nine response metrics such as workplace closures and travel bans, was highest in early April 2020. Most of the strict measures were lifted about June 2020.

Even though these government policies seemed to be effective in preventing the spread of the virus, the economy fell in recession for the first time since the 2008 Global Financial Crisis. The Thai economy was the second hardest hit among ASEAN countries in 2020, after the Philippines. Its economy contracted by 6.2% in 2020 (WB, 2022). As shown in Fig. 10.1, the Thai economy experienced the four consecutive quarters of negative GDP growth. In particular, the economy in the second quarter of 2020 decreased by 12.3%, which was closed to the contraction in the second quarter of 1998 (NESDC 2022). During this quarter, private consumption expenditure declined by 6.6% while exports of goods and services fell by 28%. Growth in government consumption reinforced by government programs during the pandemic was not enough to offset sluggish demand from private sector.

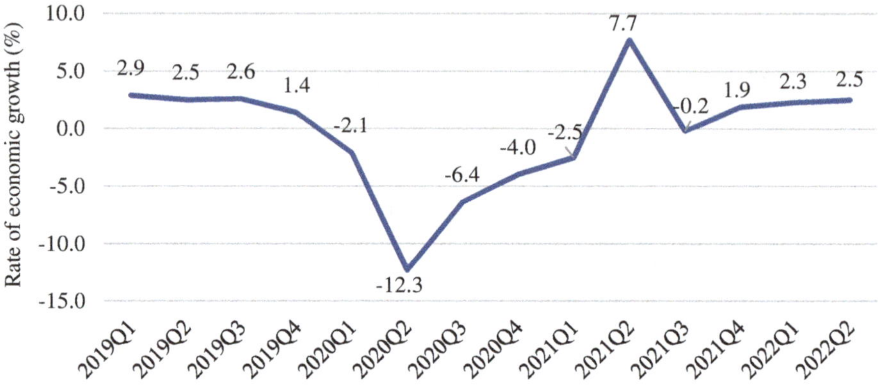

Fig. 10.1 Real GDP growth (chained volume measure) between 2019 Q1 and 2022 Q2. *Source* Author's compilation based on data from NESDC (2022)

This is because the Thai economy heavily relies on tourism and travel-related services. In 2019, about 40 million foreign tourists visited Thailand which helped generate revenue from tourism of 60 billion USD, accounting for about 11% of GDP (World Tourism Organization 2022). Before the pandemic, accommodation and food services tourism alone accounted for 6% of the country's GDP, a larger share compared to agriculture, construction, and education. Yet, as shown in Fig. 10.2, this sector fell by 37.5% between 2019 and 2020 (NESDC 2022). Other sectors also saw a pronounced decrease in output such as transportation and storage (-22.91%) and manufacturing (−5.56%).

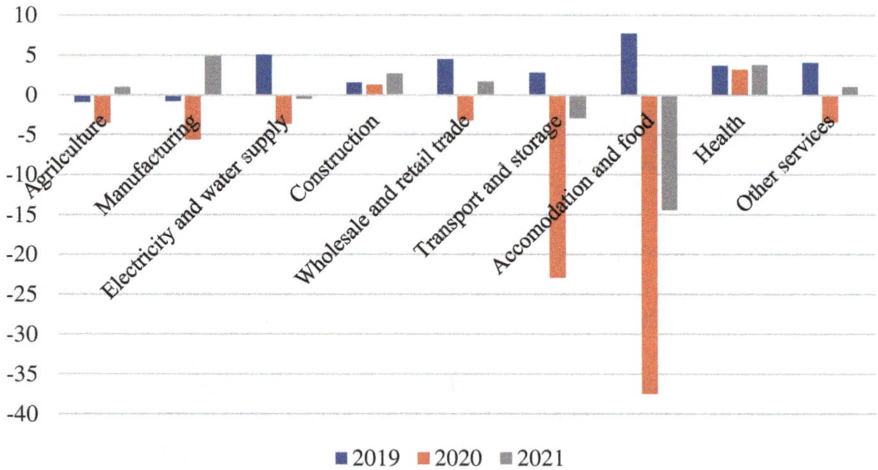

Fig. 10.2 Real output growth (chained volume measure) by sector between 2019 and 2021. *Source* Author's compilation based on data from NESDC (2022)

Unsurprisingly, economic recession in 2020 has resulted in a significant increase in unemployment rate. Unemployment rate rose from 1% in the fourth quarter of 2019 to 2% in the second quarter of 2020. Unemployment rate stood at 1.9% for the two subsequent quarters. Due to the large informal sector and agriculture remaining a big employer, Thailand's unemployment rate is always low before the pandemic. A surge in unemployment rate in 2020 is the highest rate seen in a decade.

In addition, the decrease in income caused by the pandemic translated into an increase in poverty. Thailand's national poverty rate increased from 6.24% in 2019 to 6.84% in 2020. About 500,000 more people lived on less than the national poverty line set at 2,762 Baht (US$88.24) per month. Nevertheless, poverty-increase effect of the Covid-19 Pandemic is not even across regions. While the Northeast of Thailand saw a higher increase in poverty between 2019 and 2020, the poverty rate fell in Bangkok and the Central. This demonstrates differences in the Covid-19 measures and policy responses during the pandemic in across provinces. The data from NESDC (2022) also reveal that the pandemic affected poorer people than richer counterparts. The poorest 10% saw a decline in their consumption expenditure by 1.59% in 2020. However, other groups of population, who are richer, saw a small increase in their expenditure. This indicates that an increase in poverty incidence during the first year of the pandemic is primarily driven by lower living standard among the poorest of the country.

Rising unemployment results in higher demand for social security services. An insured worker under Section 33 of the Social Security Act BE 2533 (1990)—a formal worker—can claim their unemployment benefit from Social Security Fund (SSF). During 2020 and 2021, there was an increase in unemployment benefit. As shown in Table 10.1, dismissed workers receive compensation of 70% of their monthly salaries for a period not exceeding 200 days, an increase from pre-pandemic compensation of 50% with a maximum period of 180 days. Unemployed persons due to resignation or termination of the contract receive 50% of their monthly salaries for up to 90 days, an increase from compensation of 30% before the pandemic. Those who were affected from the Covid-19 measures, effective from 19 December 2020, receive compensation of 50% of their monthly salaries for up to 90 days. Note that the maximum amount of monthly salary being calculated is 15,000 Baht (US$429.23), meaning that the maximum amount of unemployment benefit is 7,500 Baht (US$160) for all cases. Insured and formal workers therefore enjoy higher protection during the pandemic in terms of higher amount of compensation and longer period of payment.

From Table 10.2, there was a significant increase in the number of unemployed workers who claim unemployment benefit from the social security office (SSO).

About one-fifth of formal employment claimed their unemployment benefit from the Social Security Office in 2020, a high figure compared to previous years. Of two million unemployment claims, half of them was caused by the Covid-19 measures such as lock down and closures of restaurants. Insured workers who were laid off and claimed their unemployment benefit increased significantly from 66,358 cases in 2019 to 340,143 cases in 2020. This illustrates economic hardship faced by

Table 10.1 Unemployment benefit for formal workers under Section 33

	Dismissal		Resignation/Expiry of contract		COVID-19 measures	
	Benefit (% of monthly salary) (%)	Period (days)	Benefit (% of monthly salary) (%)	Period (days)	Benefit (% of monthly salary)	Period (days)
Before 2020	50	180	30	90	N/A	N/A
2020–2021	70	200	50	90	50%	90
2022	50	180	30	90	N/A	N/A

Source Author's compilation based on data from Social Security Office (2022)
Note Maximum amount of monthly salary being calculated for unemployment benefit is 15,000 Baht in all cases

Table 10.2 Number of unemployment benefit claims by formal workers under Section 33

	Causes of being unemployed				Total unemployment claims	Total workers under Sect. 33 (Millions)	Share of unemployment claim in total workers (%)
	Dismissal	Resignation	Expiry of contract	COVID-19 measures			
2017	60,850	601,753	34,816	N/A	697,419	10.84	6.43
2018	59,579	547,541	34,709	N/A	641,829	11.60	5.53
2019	66,358	604,314	44,316	N/A	714,988	11.69	6.12
2020	340,143	813,461	58,703	945,587	2,157,894	11.12	19.40
2021	148,716	728,127	48,060	628,699	1,553,602	11.14	13.95

Source Author's compilation based on data from cocial security office (2022)

formal employment at the onset of the pandemic. However, unknown is how uninsured workers went through economic crisis without comprehensive social protection measures.

Like other countries in the world, the number of confirmed/registered Covid-19 cases and deaths spiked in 2021 as the delta variant (B.1.617.2) became a main variant since July 2021. Bangkok and other provinces were declared 'a red zone,' meaning that the Covid-19 measures were stricter (i.e., take-away services, early close of shopping mall, and construction being closed). Educational institutions, bars, sport centers remained closed. This is the fourth wave of the Covid-19 outbreak. The Covid-19 cases reached their peak in August 2021. The country recorded more than 2 million coronavirus cases between July and December 2021. Daily severe and ventilated Covid-19 cases (bed occupancy) also rose sharply in this wave, reaching its peak of 5,000 cases in the mid of August 2021. Hospital bed occupancy stood at 80,000 during the same period (WHO 2022). From July to December 2021, the country reported a cumulative total of 20,000 deaths from Covid-19, a sharp increase compared to 2020.

However, 2021 is the first year of Covid-19 vaccination. Thailand started its Covid-19 vaccination campaign in the late February 2021 as Mr. Anutin Charnvirakul, Public Health Minister, received first Covid jab in the country. The first 200,000 doses of Covid-19 vaccine came from China (Sinovac). Healthcare professionals, the elderly, and persons with comorbidities were given priority. Daily number of Covid-19 vaccine doses administered rose from about 12,000 doses per day in early April 2021 to 100,000 doses per day in late May 2021. The country began Covid-19 vaccine rollout using Astrazeneca in June 2021, resulting in an increase in its capability to rollout vaccines to other groups of population. Daily Covid-19 vaccine doses reached its maximum of 800,000 doses per day in mid-October 2021. At the time, about 60% of Thai population received at least one does of the Covid-19 vaccine. mRNA vaccines (Pfizer BioNTech and Moderna) arrived in Thailand in the fourth quarter of 2021.

Given the debate on slow vaccine rollout in 2021 and types of Covid-19 vaccine being imported (Kitro et al. 2021; Kategaew et al. 2022; Wongnuch et al. 2022), the Thai economy saw a recovery in 2021 but is yet to reach its pre-pandemic level. The economy grew at 1.6% in 2021, a lower rate of growth compared to other countries in the region such as Indonesia, Malaysia, and the Philippines (WB, 2022). Since its economy depended significantly on tourism sector, reopening the country to foreign visitors played a key role in resuscitating the economy. The country only welcomed vaccinated tourists without any quarantine requirements from November 2021. The number of international visitors jumped from 20,272 in October 2021 to 427,869 in December 2021 (Ministry of Tourism and Sports, 2022). As shown in Fig. 10.2, accommodation and food services activities in 2021 declined by 14.4% compared to 2020. The contribution of this sector of national GDP was lowest since 2011. However, several sectors started to revive. Manufacturing expanded 4.89% from 2020, thanks to strong global demand. Financial and insurance activities and construction also saw promising growth.

Official statistics on poverty and income inequality for 2021 are yet to be released but they are expected to perform better due to economic recovery. However, unemployment rate was still high. On average, unemployment rate stood at 1.93% in 2021, 0.3 percentage points higher than that in 2020. Total workforce decreased from 37.93 million to 37.71 million between 2020 and 2021. This decline was because a significant decrease of informal employment by 766,329. Bangkok alone saw a fall in informal employment by 225,541, accounting for one-third of decreased informal employment.

Informal Sector in Thailand

Over the past few decades, Thailand has transformed from an agricultural-based economy to industry- and services-led economy. From one of the poorest countries in the world in 1950s, Thailand is currently an upper-middle income country, thanks to its sustained economic growth through export-oriented industrialization development strategy (Warr 2019).

It is, however, widely known that Thailand has a sheer size of informal economy. Thailand's labor market comprised 37.7 million workers in 2021. Of total workforce, formal sector employment is 18.1million (48% of the workforce) while informal sector employment is a19.6 million (52% of the workforce). Table 10.3 summarizes formal and informal employment in Thailand from 2017 to 2021.

Over the past five years, the share of informal employment in total workforce declined constantly, from 55.2% in 2017 to 52% in 2021. During this period, the number of informal workers fell by 1.2 million. Between 2020 and 2021, the number of formal employment increased from 17.5 million to 18.1 million while the number of informal worker decreased from 20.4 million to 19.6 million. With a fall in total workforce, the figure suggests that there were a significant number of informal workers who were unemployed during the pandemic and not actively seeking employment and willing to work.

Table 10.4 shows differences in educational attainment between formal and informal workers. There exists a striking difference in educational level between these two groups of workers. About one-third of informal workers in Thailand do not complete primary school or do not have formal education. The figure is low (8.8%) among formal workers. In addition, only 10.7% of informal workers achieve higher education while 35.4% of formal workers are college or university graduates.

Table 10.5 reports the distribution of formal and informal employment by age. It reveals that informal workers are in general older. Informal workers aged greater than 40 years accounted for more than 70% of total informal employment in 2021.

Table 10.3 Formal and Informal Employment in Thailand (million)

	2017	2018	2019	2020	2021
Formal	16.9 (44.8%)	17.1 (44.7%)	17.1 (45.7%)	17.5 (46.2%)	18.1 (48.0%)
Informal	20.8 (55.2%)	21.2 (55.3%)	20.4 (54.3%)	20.4 (53.8%)	19.6 (52.0%)
Total workforce	37.7	38.3	37.5	37.9	37.7

Source Author's compilation based on data from NSO (2022)
Note: Percentage in total workforce in parenthesis

Table 10.4 Percentage of formal and informal employment by level of educational attainment in 2021

	Formal worker	Informal workers
Below primary or no education	8.8	28.9
Primary	15.9	27.6
lower-secondary	17.2	17.2
Upper-secondary	21.4	15.4
Higher education	35.4	10.7

Source Author's compilation based on data from NSO (2022)

Table 10.5 Formal and informal employment by age in 2021

Age	Number (Million)	
	Formal	Informal
15–24	1.8 (10.0)	1.5 (7.7)
25–39	7.9 (43.9)	4.2 (21.4)
40–59	7.7 (42.8)	9.6 (49.0)
60 +	0.6 (3.3)	4.3 (21.9)
Total	18 (100.0)	19.6 (100.0)

Source Author's compilation based on data from NSO (2022)
Note: Percentage in total employment in each group in parenthesis

This indicates that informal sector can provide job opportunity for the elderly while such opportunity in formal sector is limited due to an official retirement age. Another interesting point is the share of workers aged between 15 and 24 years old. We may expect to see a smaller number of workers aged less than 25 years old to work in formal sector due to minimum education requirement. This does not seem true in the case of Thailand since the number of formal workers aged between 15 and 24 years old is almost 1 million greater than those in informal sector.

Table 10.6 shows the distribution of formal and informal employment by economic sector between 2019 and 2021. Before the pandemic, agriculture, forestry, and fishing employed 56.3% of informal workers. Wholesale and retail trade (16.1% of informal workers) also had a high share of informal workers. About 9% of informal workers is in accommodation and food services activities. However, most of formal employment work in services sector including financial sector, business services, and public sector. Manufacturing also has a large number of formal workers (27% of formal workers).

During the pandemic years, the figure is roughly the same for formal employment. Several sectors saw an increase in the share of formal employment such as wholesale and resale trade; agriculture, forestry, and fishing; and transport storage. There is a significant increase in the percentage of informal workers in agriculture, forestry, and fishing. The share of informal employment in manufacturing and accommodation and food services declined, suggesting a sluggish demand from the world economy.

According to Fig. 10.2, accommodation and food service activities were the most hit by the pandemic since its real output declined by 37.5% between 2019 and 2020 and this sector employed about 10% of informal workers, this suggests that informal workers in hotel and restaurant sectors experienced severe economic hardship at the onset of the pandemic. While a large number of informal workers was concentrated in agriculture, its output fell relatively less compared to other sectors.

Table 10.7 shows the distribution of formal and informal workers by occupation in 2019 and 2021. Before the Covid-19 Pandemic, formal workers were employed

Table 10.6 Percentage of formal and informal employment by economic sector in 2019 and 2021

	2019		2020		2021	
	Formal	Formal	Formal	Informal	Formal	Informal
Agriculture, forestry, and fishing	6.4	56.3	7.0	55.6	7.3	58.1
Manufacturing	27.0	6.0	26.0	5.8	26.4	5.6
Construction	6.5	4.4	7.2	4.4	6.7	4.1
Wholesale and retail trade	15.7	16.1	16.0	16.9	16.7	16.5
Transportation storage	4.6	2.6	4.8	2.5	5.7	1.9
Accommodation and food services	6.3	8.8	5.7	9.2	5.4	8.3
Activities of household as employers	1.2	0.1	1.3	0.0	1.1	0.1
Others	32.3	5.7	32.0	5.6	30.7	5.4

Source: Author's compilation based on data from NSO (2022)

as service workers and shop sales workers (17.2% of formal workers); plant and machine operators (16.1%); and elementary workers (13.1%). There is no obvious change during the pandemic except legislators, senior officials, and manager and skilled agricultural and fishery workers which saw a moderate decline in number and percentage of total formal employment. For informal workers, about 53.9% were hired as skilled agricultural and fishery workers in 2019. Also, about one-fourth of informal workers were employed as service workers and shop sales workers. In 2021, there was a smaller share of informal workers who worked as legislators, senior officials, and managers. Of 0.7 million informal workers who were out of the workforce, services workers and shop sales workers were most affected, followed by plant and machine operators and skilled agricultural and fishery workers.

Tables 10.8, 10.9 report health conditions and welfare among informal workers. From Table 10.8, the number of informal employment who got hurt or had accident in 2020 was 3.82 million, rose from 3.15 million in 2017. About one-third of informal workers did not receive medical treatment because either hurt or accident was minor. Less than one-fourth of them bought medicine from drug store. In addition, less than 1% had to stay in hospital longer than three days. Note however that there is no statistics for formal employment so that comparison is not applicable in this issue.

Table 10.9 shows percentage of informal employment by the benefits paid for medical expenses. The percentage of informal workers without medical benefit decreased from 31.9% in 2017 to 27.0% in 2019. However, there was a big jump in this figure in 2020. The data also reveal that own payment for medical expenses increased significantly between 2019 and 2020. This indicates that informal workers experienced a higher cost of medical expenses during the Covid-19 Pandemic. Interestingly, it is also found that the percentage of informal workers who used universal health insurance fell from 62 to 53.7% during the pandemic. It suggests that an attempt to cover universal health to informal workers was interrupted by the pandemic.

Table 10.10 compares the real monthly income between formal and informal workers in three economic sectors: Agriculture, manufacturing, and services. The

Table 10.7 Occupation by formal and informal employment in 2019 and 2021

	Number				Percentage			
	2019		2021		2019		2021	
	Formal	Informal	Formal	Informal	Formal	Informal	Formal	Informal
Legislators, senior officials, and managers	0.91	0.46	0.8	0.4	5.3	2.3	4.5	1.8
Professionals	1.89	0.14	1.9	0.1	11	0.7	10.6	0.7
Technicians and associate professionals	1.47	0.14	1.5	0.1	8.6	0.7	8.5	0.7
Clerks	1.59	0.06	1.7	0.1	9.3	0.3	9.2	0.4
Service workers and shop sales workers	2.94	4.58	3.1	4.4	17.2	22.5	17.3	22.4
Skilled agricultural and fishery workers	0.87	10.94	1.1	10.8	5.1	53.8	5.8	55.2
Craft and related trades workers	2.27	1.7	2.4	1.6	13.3	8.3	13.1	8.1
Plant and machine operators	2.77	0.76	3.1	0.6	16.1	3.7	17.1	3.1
Elementary occupations	2.36	1.56	2.5	1.5	13.7	7.7	13.8	7.6
Other	0.07	0	0.01	0	0.4	0	0.1	0
Total	17.14	20.34	18.11	19.6	100	100	100	100

Source: Author's compilation based on data from NSO (2022)

data do not allow us to look at real income among workers in more disaggregated fashion. It is found that real income of informal employment is always lower than that of formal employment. The largest difference in real income is seen in services sector. Informal workers in services and manufacturing have the same wage level of formal workers in the agriculture sector.

Before the Covid-19 Pandemic, formal workers experienced a faster rate of growth in monthly real income. This growth was driven by real income growth in services sector. The pandemic affected real income differently. In 2020, only formal workers in agriculture saw a decrease in real income (a decrease by 0.5%). However, real income of informal employment on average fell in all sectors, especially those in the services sector. On average, real income among formal workers increased by 4.44% between 2019 and 2020. During the same period, informal workers saw a decrease

Table 10.8 Number and percentage of informal employment by medical treatments

	Number				Percentage			
	2017	2018	2019	2020	2017	2018	2019	2020
No medical treatment	2,288.9	2,701.0	2,060.1	2,635.3	72.7	71.8	66.6	68.9
Buy medicine from drug store	727.2	899.5	770.3	838.1	23.1	23.9	24.9	21.9
Stay in hospital for less than 3 days	80.8	119.4	58.8	86.6	2.6	3.2	1.9	2.3
Stay in hospital for at least 3 days	49.5	39.2	29.4	28.8	1.6	1.1	1	0.8
Lose some organs	0.8	1.2	0.5	0.1	0	0	0	0
Unknown	–	–	173.7	234.9	0	0	5.6	6.1
Total	3,147.2	3,760.3	3,092.8	3,823.8	100	100	100	100

Source: Author's compilation based on data from NSO (2022)

Table 10.9 Percentage of informal employment by the benefits paid for medical expenses

	2017	2018	2019	2020
Without medical benefit	31.8	31.7	27.0	38.6
Employer's payment	0.8	1.8	1.5	1.6
Parents, relatives, friends	0.3	0.9	0.1	1
Own payment	30.7	29	25.4	36
With medical benefit	68.2	68.3	73	61.4
Universal health insurance	59.7	61.1	62	53.7
Social security/compensation fund	0	0	0	0
Welfare from official/state enterprise	3	1.1	1.7	0.9
Private health insurance	4.5	5.3	6.3	6.5
Others	1	0.8	3	0.3

Source: Author's compilation based on data from NSO (2022)

of 2.52% in their real incomes. This indicates that only informal workers seem to experience economic disadvantage and lower level of living standard during the first year of the pandemic.

In 2021, the economy was again hit hard but not equally. Real income among formal workers fell in all sectors between 2020 and 2021. When comparing with 2020, it is found that formal employment saw a fall in average wage in all sectors, except services. Informal workers experienced a larger decline in real income. Those informal workers who worked in the services sector saw a decrease in real income by -4.36%, which is larger than the average fall in real income. This indicates that informal workers were more affected in terms of decreased real income in 2021.

Uneven impacts on informal workers are not surprising since numerous studies suggest that this group of workers is vulnerable to economic crisis (Doane et al. 2003;

Table 10.10 Real income between formal and informal workers before and after the pandemic

		Total	Agriculture	Manufacturing	Service
2018	Formal	14,845.44	6,003.07	13,132.96	16,790.40
	Informal	6,446.28	5,307.59	7,204.08	7,132.85
2019	Formal	14,969.48	6,265.83	13,366.77	16,808.51
	Informal	6,813.97	5,547.89	7,596.45	7,659.01
2020	Formal	15,633.77	6,234.55	14,038.32	17,552.94
	Informal	6,641.98	5,439.85	7,424.58	7,462.90
2021	Formal	14,967.61	6,207.69	13,304.32	16,838.31
	Informal	6,768.71	5,361.24	7,467.01	7,324.78
Δ 2019–2020 (%)	Formal	4.44	−0.50	5.02	4.43
	Informal	−2.52	−1.95	−2.26	−2.56
Δ 2019–2021 (%)	Formal	−0.01	−0.93	−0.47	0.18
	Informal	−0.66	−3.36	−1.70	−4.36

Source: Author's compilation based on data from NSO (2022)

Mehrotra 2009; Baker and Phongpaichit 2021). One of possible reason for informal workers experiencing larger real income loss during the pandemic is because they are concentrated in the hard-hit sector such as accommodation and food services and wholesale and retail trade. However, as seen from Table 10.6, these sectors employ a roughly the same amount of both formal and informal workers before the pandemic. This suggests that uneven impact of the Covid-19 Pandemic, which such impact is larger among informal workers, is because the lack of comprehensive social protection which is expanded for insured persons. The next section outlines support to workers during the pandemic.

Policy Response for Informal Employment

After strict Covid-19 measures being implemented, the government of Thailand has provided additional social assistance to informal workers.

The Thai government introduced the first policy measure named "Rao Mai Ting Gun" (or "No One Will Be Left Behind"), a monthly transfer worth of 5,000 Baht (US$160) for six months for informal workers. The first payment began in April 2020. This stimulus package reached about 15 million recipients, which is lower than the total number of informal workers as shown in Table 10.3. Note that the maximum amount of cash assistance to informal workers is lower than that to unemployed formal workers (5,000 Baht vs. 7,500 Baht). The period of compensation for informal workers is also shorter (90 days vs. 200 days).

In 2021, the government of Thailand also provided financial relief to workers affected by the pandemic. This relief was limited to nine occupations: construction;

accommodation and food services; art, entertainment, and recreational activities; wholesale and retail; transportation and warehouses; business, administration and service support; science and academic activities; information and communication; and other services as stated by the SSO. Formal workers under Section 33 received 2,500-cash handouts per person. If unemployed, they received compensation equal to half of salary but not greater than 7,500 baht. Informal workers must register under Section 40 of the Social Security Act BE 2533 (1990) within July were subject to receive 5,000-bath cash handouts per person.

Informal workers also registered for the half-half co-payment subsidy scheme. This scheme was first introduced in mid-2020 and it has continued until recently. Essentially, government pays half of consumption spending (e.g., food, drink, and necessary goods) for up to 150 Baht per person per day. There were 10 million recipients of this scheme in Phase I. The total amount of cash subsidy was 3,000 Baht. Those who are currently receiving other monthly cash assistance programs such as the State Welfare Card are not eligible for this scheme. In 2022, about 26.5 million people, including both formal and informal employment, can register for the fifth phase of this scheme. The total amount of subsidy for this phase was 800 Baht.

Other than cash handouts, the Bank of Thailand issues financial rehabilitation measures to support debtors affected by the pandemic. Policy measures include lower minimum percentage paid on credit card loans and increasing credit limit.

Conclusion

The world has known the Covid-19 Pandemic for about two years. Scholars and policymakers have realized the economic and health impacts brought by the pandemic and policy measures aimed to contain the spread the infection are uneven across populations. Among people with vulnerable health conditions and low-income earners, informal workers are severely affected.

This chapter aims to examine how the Covid-19 Pandemic impacts on informal workers in the context of Thailand. While its economy has been hard hit due to its great reliance on tourism and tourist-related sectors, it is informal worker, an uninsured person being excluded of expanding comprehensive social protection before the pandemic, who has seen a large drop in real income during the pandemic. Those who work in accommodation and food service activities seem to face larger negative economic impact because of large decline in economic activities and relatively high share of informal employment. Despite experiencing larger economic hardship, temporary cash assistance to informal workers is lower compared to unemployed formal worker, and the period of compensation for informal workers is shorter.

For policy recommendation, the government of Thailand should expand social assistance to informal workers in terms of cash handouts and period of compensation. This is not only because they lack of social protection but also because they are central to the Thai economy. The Thai economy could not resuscitate and rebound to its pre-pandemic level unless informal workers are more protected and prioritized. While transition from the informal to the formal economy is a key development challenge of the country, to maintain the quality of life among informal workers during economic and health crisis is second to none.

References

Baker, C., and P. Phongpaichit. 2021. Thailand and the Covid-19 pandemic in 2020. *Southeast Asian Affairs* 2021: 356–378.

Chen, M.A., E. Grapsa, G. Ismail, M. Rogan, M. Valdivia, L. Alfers, J. Harvey, A.C. Ogando, S.O. Reed, and S. Roever. 2022. Covid-19 and informal work: Evidence from 11 Cities. *International Labour Review* 161 (1): 29–58.

Doane D., S. Ofreneo, and D. Srikajon 2003. Social protection for informal workers in the garment industry: Philippines and Thailand, in: F. Lund and J. Nicholson (eds.), *Chains of production, ladders of protection*, University of Natal Press: Durban.

Finnegan G., and Singh A. 2004. *Role of the informal sector in coping with economic crisis in Thailand and Zambia*, https://www.ilo.org.

Hale, T., N. Angrist, R. Goldszmidt, B. Kira, A. Petherick, T. Phillips, S. Webster, E. Cameron-Blake, L. Hallas, S. Majumdar, and H. Tatlow. 2021. A global panel database of pandemic policies (Oxford Covid-19 government response tracker). *Nature Human Behaviour* 5: 529–538.

Horn, Z.E. 2010. The Effects of the global economic crisis on women in the informal economy: Research findings from WIEGO and the inclusive cities partners. *Gender and Development* 18 (2): 263–276.

ILO. 2020. *Impact of Lockdown Measures on the Informal Economy*, https://www.ilo.org.

Kategaew, W., S. Youngkong, S. Taychakhoonavudh, S. Techathawat, and N. Chaiyakunapak. 2022. Potential changes in vaccine access and policy landscape in Thailand post Covid-19 pandemic. *Human Vaccines and Immunotherapeutics* 18 (6): 2095823. https://doi.org/10.1080/21645515.2022.2095823.

Kitro, A., W. Sirikul, C. Piankusol, P. Rirermsonthorn, M. Seesen, K. Wangsan, P. Assavanopakun, V. Surawattanasakul, A. Kosai, and R. Sapbamrer. 2021. Acceptance, attitude, and factors affecting the intention to accept Covid-19 vaccine among Thai people and expatriates living in Thailand. *Vaccine* 39 (52): 7554–7561.

Komin, W., R. Thepparp, B. Subsing, and D. Engstrom. 2021. Covid-19 and its impact on informal sector workers: A case study of Thailand. *Asia Pacific Journal of Social Work and Development* 31 (1–2): 80–88.

Mehrotra, S. 2009. The impact of the economic crisis on the informal sector and poverty in East Asia. *Global Social Policy* 9: 101–118.

MTS, Ministry of Tourism and Sports. 2022. *Tourism statistics 2021*, https://www.mots.go.th.

Narula, R. 2020. Policy opportunities and challenges from the Covid-19 pandemic for economies with large informal sectors. *Journal of International Business Policy* 3: 302–310.

NESDC, National Economic and Social Development Council. 2022. *Economic and social indicators*, https://www.nesdc.go.th.

NSO, National Statistical Office of Thailand. 2022. *Informal worker survey*, http://www.nso.go.th/sites/2014.

SSO, Social Security Office (2022), *Statistics of Social Security Fund*, https://www.sso.go.th.

Warr P.G. 2019. Economic development of post-war Thailand, In: *Routledge handbook of contemporary Thailand*, ed. P. Chachavalpongpun, Routledge: Oxon.

Webb, A., R. McQuaid, and S. Rand. 2020. Employment in the informal economy: Implications of the Covid-19 pandemic. *International Journal of Sociology and Social Policy* 40 (9/10): 1005–1019.

WHO (2022), Covid-19 situation, Thailand, *WHO Thailand Weekly Situation Update*, No. 248, https://cdn.who.int.

WIEGO. 2022. *Covid-19 crisis and the informal economy in Bangkok, Thailand: Lasting impacts and an agenda for recovery*, https://www.wiego.org/resources.

Wongnuch, P., T. Mulikaburt, T. Apidechkul, P. Srichan, R. Tamornpak, A. Udplong, S. Suratana, and S. Kitchanapaibul. 2022. Acceptance and accessibility to the early phase Covid-19 vaccination among the healthcare workers and hill tribe population in Thailand. *Scientific Report* 12 (1): 11035. https://doi.org/10.1038/s41598-022-15149-y.

World Bank. 2022. *World development indicators*, https://databank.worldbank.org.

World Tourism Organization. 2022. *Tourism statistics database*, https://www.unwto.org/statistics.

Chapter 11
The Covid-19 Pandemic in Italy: With Special Reference to the Effects on Women and Families

Isabella Crespi, Sara Mazzucchelli, and Maria Letizia Bosoni

Abstract The Italian Government implemented different containment measures at the various phases of the pandemic. This has profoundly transformed people's lives, both from the point of view of family and significant relationships, and at work, substantially modifying the relationship between these two significant areas. In this chapter, we will first present an overview of the containment measures implemented to tackle the spreading of the virus and outline their main policies, their contents, aims, and underlying focus. Then we will focus on consequences for women. With the emergence of the Covid 19 emergency in the early 2020s, the media immediately started to highlight the likely future increase in cases of violence against women in the home due to the increased risk of lockdown and the difficulties for victims living with their abuser to report and seek support services. A second theme is the impact on family and work responsibilities integration. Several studies in Italy, including a longitudinal survey conducted by the authors, have shown how the emergency and containment measures impacted both personal/parental and work spheres, producing adverse effects on the specific group of working parents, especially women. Using a longitudinal approach, with data collected in three waves (April, July, and December 2020), we assess the consequences of the *Working From Home policy*, showing that wellbeing decreased and work-life conflict increased with time and that working parents found the first lockdown particularly challenging.

Paragraph attribution: The text is written jointly by the authors, however, Crespi wrote "Introduction", "Violence Against Women in Interpersonal and Family Relationships" ; Mazzucchelli "Government Response and Evaluation of It", "Work-Family Reconciliation Strategies in Italy in 2020: Longitudinal Evidence"; Bosoni "The Development of the Pandemic in Italy", "The Emergency Phase", "The Coexistence Phase", "Impact on Mortality and Births", "Impacts on Work and Schooling", "Impact on Family and Work Integration: An Overview".

I. Crespi (✉)
University of Macerata, Macerata, Italy
e-mail: isabella.crespi@unimc.it

S. Mazzucchelli · M. L. Bosoni
Catholic University of Milan, Milan, Italy

C. Aspalter (ed.), *Covid-19 Pandemic*,
https://doi.org/10.1007/978-981-99-2497-4_11

Keywords Covid-19 pandemic · Italy · Women · Violence against women · Family and work responsibilities

Introduction

In Italy, as in many countries, the Covid-19 Pandemic declared by the WHO first emerged in a significant way in February 2020. Italy was one of the first European countries to be severely affected by the virus. Health and emergency responses included the closure of schools and childcare, the scaling back of non-essential activities, an increase in *working from home* (WFH) arrangements, and the confinement of people to their homes. All of this had some specific, and some ambiguous, effects on the social sphere.

This chapter will first present an overview of the development of the pandemic in Italy, including the progression of the virus's transmission, its impact on population groups and the containment measures implemented to tackle its spread. The central policies introduced by the Italian government will then be presented and discussed, with an emphasis on their contents, aims and underlying foci. We will then examine the consequences of the pandemic for women and families. The pandemic has highlighted some ambiguities and risks with regard to gender relations, in particular, the relationship between men and women, which is often characterised by cohabitation and therefore proximity. Social distancing on a collective level has had a counterpart in greater closeness in the personal sphere.

Taking this gendered perspective in examining the consequences of the pandemic, we will focus, particularly, on violence against women in interpersonal relationships. Covid-19 brought about the likelihood of an uptick in cases of violence against women in the home, due to the increased risk of lockdowns and the difficulties for victims who live with their abusers in reporting and seeking support services. We will also take into consideration the integration of family and work responsibilities. In particular, we look at the impact of working from home on the care-work balance from a gender perspective. Several studies in Italy, including a longitudinal survey conducted by the authors, have shown how the emergency and containment measures implemented as a result of the pandemic impacted both personal/parental and work spheres, producing adverse effects on specific groups of working people, especially parents and women.

The Development of the Pandemic in Italy

The Covid-19 Pandemic has been described as unprecedented, not only because of its health and socioeconomic impacts, but also because it triggered containment measures and policies that had never been used before, including the closure of schools and childcare, the curtailment of non-essential activities and *working from home* (WFH) directives (Dayal and Tiko 2020). Italy was one of the first European countries to be severely affected by the virus.

We can identify two different periods of the pandemic in Italy: an emergency phase (2020) and a phase of coexistence with the virus (late 2020 and onwards). Table 11.1 summarises the main phases of the pandemic and the measures introduced.

Table 11.1 Development of the Pandemic in Italy (2020–2021)

Date	Contagion waves	Main policies and measures
Emergency phase		
31 January 2020	First two cases of Covid-19	Italy declares a state of emergency
4 March 2020	First phase of the infection (first wave)	First rigid lockdown, all schools and services closed
17 March 2020	–	***Cura Italia Decree***
7 April 2020	Contagion rate decreases	***Liquidity Decree***
26 April 2020	Contagion rate decreases again	Partial reopening (not schools)
18 May 2020	–	***Relaunch Decree***
June 2020	Low contagion rate	All restrictions are dropped
Coexistence phase		
September 2020	Schools and kindergartens reopen	–
October 2020	Contagion rate increases (second wave)	***Ristori Decree***
November 2020	Infections still high	Colour system introduced with partial lockdown
December 2020	–	Vaccination campaign begins
February 2021	Contagion rate increases again (third wave)	Partial lockdown in some regions – vaccinations continue
19 March 2021	–	***Support Decree***
April–May 2021	Contagion rate decreases (vaccine effect)	Vaccines for adolescents
July 2021	–	Green Pass introduced for some activities and trips
October 2021	–	Green Pass mandatory for all private and public workers
November 2021	Contagion rate increases (but less than 2020) (fourth wave)	–
April 2022	Complete vaccination cycle: 89.96% of the population over 12 years	End of the state of emergency

The Emergency Phase

The pandemic response went through various stages during 2020, driven by a need to manage the emergency linked to the rapid increase in SARS-CoV-2 infections and an overloaded health system. On 31 January 2020, the first two cases (Chinese tourists) of Covid-19 were found in Italy. A nationwide state of emergency was declared. On 21 February, the first Italian Covid-19 case was registered. Partial lockdowns were instituted in the most severely affected territories.

However, contagion rates increased, and on 4 March the Italian government announced the suspension of school and university activities and the first rigid lockdown. Italy was the first Western country to adopt such stringent measures. After a few days, the government introduced further measures: all non-essential activities were suspended and leaving the home was prohibited except for reasons such as obtaining health assistance or food supplies. All parks were closed. Working from home—not a common practice in Italy—became mandatory for private companies and the public sector in March 2020. Infections continued to rapidly increase. On 27 March, Italy recorded 86,000 cases and 969 deaths—at the time the highest number recorded since the beginning of the pandemic. From then on, however, cases declined. In summer 2020 almost all restrictions were removed: parks, summer centres for children, cinemas and theatres were reopened, albeit with stringent protocols. However, there were still localised lockdowns. Additionally, new variants of SARS-CoV-2 from other countries contributed to the extension of the state of emergency until October 2020. In August 2020 trials of the first vaccines (Sputnik and Pfizer) were announced, generating hope among the populace. Thus, the emergency phase was characterised by the need to face an exponential increase in infections, which required drastic measures and a rapid change in habits and daily routines.

The Coexistence Phase

The phase of coexistence with the virus started in September 2020: schools and childcare services reopened, with some restrictions and rigid health protocols. However, in early October infections started to grow again (second wave) and the pressure on the health system increased. Gyms and swimming pools closed and schools partly returned to distance learning. In November 2020, the colour zone system was introduced in Italy[1] (white = no restrictions, yellow = partial restrictions, orange = some activities closed, red = total lockdown). At the same time, positive results about the efficacy of Pfizer and Moderna vaccines were announced. The vaccination campaign began in Italy at the end of December 2020. First in line were healthcare workers, then vulnerable groups (elderly, disabled) and then the rest of the population by age group. At the end of February 2021, a third wave of infections exploded in Italy. Restrictions were imposed based on the colour zone system. Schools and educational childcare services were closed in high-risk areas (orange and red regions) in March 2021.

With the implementation of the vaccination campaign, infections began to gradually decline from April: 639 cases were registered on 30 June. This was the best day since the start of the second wave in October 2020. In July 2021 the European Green Pass was introduced for travel. It was able to be obtained by those who had had at least one dose of the vaccine or who had recovered from Covid-19. From 15 October the Green Pass became compulsory in Italy for all public and private employees (leading to many protests). In November 2021, due to the development of numerous variants of the virus, the fourth wave started, although there were limited cases compared to the same period in the previous year (vaccine effect). The new cases seemed to be spreading mainly among children—including infants—and the non-vaccinated segment of the population. In April 2022, 89.9% of the population over 12 years completed the vaccination cycle, and the state of emergency ended.

The phase of coexistence, with infections going up and down, led to a slow adaptation to new routines, with the awareness that even with the end of the pandemic in sight, there would not be a simple return to the past.

Impact on Mortality and Births

From the beginning of the pandemic (March 2020) to January 2022, the total excess deaths,[2] compared to the 2015–19 average, was 178,000, with most of these in 2021 (Istat 2022a). 60% of these were attributable to Covid-19 (29,210), 10% to pneumonia and 30% to other causes. The elder citizens were severely affected by the virus: of the total deaths from Covid-19, about 85% were over 70 years of age, and most of them were in residential care (Istat 2020a). From the start of the pandemic (March 2020) to January 2022, the total excess mortality, compared to the 2015–19 average, was 178,000 deaths, with most of the deaths in 2021 being observed in the first quarter, when vaccination coverage was still very low (Istat 2022a).

The vaccination campaign that commenced at the end of 2020 attracted high levels of coverage starting from May 2021, especially in the over-60 age group. As the vaccination campaign progressed, mortality significantly decreased, particularly in the over-80 age group, despite the spread of new and more transmissible variants.

The Covid-19 emergency had a significant impact on the relationships between generations: the elderly population was the most greatly affected, especially those in residential centres. In addition, there was also a strong contraction in births: in 2020 there were 404,892 births (15,000 fewer than in 2019), and the average number of children of Italian women stood at 1.17. The decrease in births continued in 2021, and the number of births with at least one foreign parent also decreased (19,000 fewer). However, it must be noted that this was an accentuation of a phenomenon that already existed in Italy (Istat, 2020b).

Impacts on Work and Schooling

The restrictions introduced to deal with the pandemic in Italy changed over time. Specifically, the rules relating to work and schools varied a great deal throughout 2020. During the first wave of the pandemic (March–July 2020) all work that was not deemed essential (i.e. distribution and logistics, health services, pharmacy work, logistics, production of basic goods) became remote. Working from home was extended until the end of 2020 for at least 50% of public employees. At the same time, the 'right to WFH' was granted to parents of children under 14, or who had at least one child with a severe disability or family members with severe disabilities or chronic illnesses.

During the first wave of the pandemic, all schools and universities were closed and distance learning (DL) was introduced. Thus, the daily lives of the young people radically changed. According to data for 2022 from the Italian National Institute of Statistics, social distancing caused a drop in face-to-face socialising and an increase in the use of chat and social media to communicate with friends. However, children were found to prefer face-to-face teaching to distance learning, while foreign children experienced greater difficulty in accessing the distant learning and they often reported a worsening of family economic conditions (Istat 2022b). This situation caused considerable inconvenience for families with a lack of access to suitable IT equipment or an inadequate internet connection, as well as for teachers with poor digital skills (Pavolini et al. 2021).

The Covid-19 Pandemic has disrupted experiences essential to children's growth and development, including attendance at early childcare and schools, thus depriving children of precious learning opportunities.

With regard to childcare services for children under 6 years of age, a study carried out by the government[3] between April and June 2021 reported high levels of stress in teachers and educators and families' fears about using early childcare services. Moreover, because of health protocols, there was a reduction in opening hours and the number of children accepted, as well as an increase in costs, especially in the private sector. Consequently, there was a decrease in the number of children enrolled in early childcare compared to the previous year, particularly in private services (45%) and in childcare in the centre and south of the country.

There are still few studies on the consequences of this pandemic for children. A survey conducted by IRCCS Gaslini[4] to monitor the impact of the pandemic on the psychological state of children and families showed that in the early stages of the pandemic, 65% of children under the age of 6 and 71% of those over the age of 6 (up to 18) had behavioural problems and symptoms of regression. As for children under the age of 6, the most frequent complaints were increased irritability, sleep disturbances and anxiety disorders (restlessness, separation anxiety).

Government Response and Evaluation of It

Across the various phases of the pandemic emergency, the Italian government has implemented different measures to support families, workers and businesses. Here, we attempt to detail the path taken and conclude with a summary judgement. The provisions introduced by Decree-Law 2 March 2020, No. 9 aimed to ensure necessary initial economic support to citizens and businesses facing financial liquidity problems due to the spread of Covid-19.

The Cura Italia Decree (Decree-Law 17 March 2020, No. 18) contained new measures to limit the adverse effects of the Covid-19 emergency on the national socioeconomic fabric. It included measures to strengthen the National Health Service, civil protection and security, as well as support for public and private work in favor of families and businesses. It contained provisions for justice, transport, the agricultural and sports sectors, entertainment and culture, and schools and universities, allowed for the suspension of payment obligations for taxes and contributions, and provided tax incentives.

The Liquidity Decree (Decree-Law 8 April 2020, No. 23) introduced urgent measures regarding access to credit and the postponement of obligations for companies and special powers in sectors of strategic importance and justice. The decree intervened to support companies in difficulty with specific measures in five main areas: access to credit and support for liquidity; exports and internationalization; investments and business continuity; the strengthening of special powers in sectors of strategic importance and transparency of obligations in financial matters; and fiscal and accounting measures.

On 13 May the Council of Ministers approved a decree law (Relaunch Decree) that introduced urgent measures in the field of health, support for work and the economy, and social policies. The decree intervened in various areas in a transversal way to ensure the unity, coherence and completeness of the measures aimed at protecting families and workers, and to safeguard and support businesses, artisans and freelancers. The measures also included initiatives for the consolidation, streamlining and speeding up speeding up of procedures and process of the institutions of protection and social cohesion. This decree was extended by Decree-Law 16 June 2020, No. 52, which introduced further urgent measures with regard to wage integration treatment. Decree-Law 14 August 2020, No. 104 introduced urgent measures to support and revive the economy. With this last decree, the government allocated an additional 25 billion euros to be used to continue the recovery from the negative consequences of the pandemic and to support workers, families and businesses in disadvantaged areas of the country. With this decree, the total resources deployed to react to the emergency reached 100 billion euros, equal to 6 percentage points of GDP.

This investment continued with the Ristori Decree (Decree-Law 28 October 2020, No. 137), which introduced further urgent measures for the protection of health and the support of workers and production sectors, as well as the areas of justice and safety as they related to pandemic. The text stated there would be an allocation of 5.4 billion euros in terms of net debt and 6.2 billion in terms of balance to be financed, to be allocated to the restoration of economic activities affected, directly or indirectly, by the restrictions, with the aim of protecting health, as well as supporting the workers employed in the affected businesses (restaurants, bars, pizzerias, pastry shops, ice-cream parlors, theatres, cinemas, gyms and swimming pools). This decree was marked by rapidity of implementation, simplicity and effectiveness and by a close and constant comparison with the trade associations most closely involved in this very delicate phase. The decree noted that the health restrictions had forced many operators and areas of the economy to suddenly change their plans.

The Ristori Decrees (Ristori of November 7, 21 and 29 of 2020) introduced further urgent measures to deal with the consequences of the pandemic. They allowed for a further allocation of resources intended for the restoration of the economic activities affected by the health restrictions and support of workers employed in industries, as well as further measures related to the continuing emergency. Among the main measures introduced were non-repayable contributions; the establishment of a fund for new contributions; tax credit on commercial rents; suspension of tax payments; suspension of social security contributions; a babysitter bonus; extraordinary leave; an 'extraordinary fund' for support to the third sector; support for the agricultural, fishing and aquaculture supply chain; support to strengthen the health system, an increase in local public transport funding; and the establishment of a fund with an endowment of 400 million euros to be disbursed to municipalities for the adoption of urgent food security measures.

With the same intention, the Council of Ministers of 18 December 2020 approved a decree law that introduced further urgent provisions to deal with the health risks associated with the spread of the virus and provided for the allocation of 645 million euros to the immediate restoration of food and drink administration activities, which had seen a drop in turnover due to the measures taken to protect health.

2021 began with a series of restrictive measures relating to travel, dictated by the need to contain the spread of a second wave of the virus throughout the nation (starting from autumn 2020) with a risk of exponential increase predicted during the Christmas holidays.

Following repeated periods of partial or regional lockdowns, Decree-Law 13 March 2021, No. 30 introduced support interventions for workers with children with regard to distance learning or quarantine. Decree-Law 22 March 2021, No. 41 (Sostegni Decree) provided for an allocation of around 32 billion euros to strengthen tools to combat the spread of Covid-19 and to contain the social and economic impact of the health measures. The planned interventions were divided into five main areas: support for businesses and third sector operators; working and fighting against poverty; health and safety; support for local authorities; and further sectoral interventions.

With the same purpose, on 25 May, Decree-Law 73/2021 stated that it would provide for the allocation of around 40 billion euros to strengthen and extend tools to combat the spread of the virus and to contain the social and economic impact of the health measures. The planned interventions were divided into seven main lines of action: support for businesses, the economy and reduction of fixed costs; access to business credit and liquidity; health protection; work and social policies; support to local authorities; young people, school and research; and sectoral measures.

In late spring, a new phase of intervention was inaugurated where—in light of scientific data that demonstrated that the spread of the virus was slowing—a schedule was outlined relating to the progressive elimination of restrictions. There were three pillars of the country's relaunch strategy: the vaccination campaign, the introduction of measures to support the economy and businesses, and the encouragement of growth through investment. Investment in the vaccination campaign was supported by the vision of Decree-Law 23 July 2021, No. 105, with the introduction of the Green Pass measure and a progressive extension of the state of emergency, first until 31 July 2021 and then until 31 March 2022.

Decree-Law 10 September 2021, No. 122 made the Green Pass compulsory in schools, higher education and social health assistance, while Decree-Law 21 September 2021, No. 127 obligated all workers, public and private, to use a Green Pass to access the workplace. These workers included consultants, volunteers and external staff, as well as workers in the home (electricians, housekeepers, babysitters).

Decree-Law 26 November 2021, No. 172 outlined a series of containment measures for the fourth wave of the pandemic in four areas: the obligation to be vaccinated and to have a third dose; extension of the vaccination obligation to new categories; establishment of a reinforced Green Pass; and the strengthening of vaccination controls and promotional campaigns. Decree-Law 24 December 2021, No. 221 introduced a validity of 6 months for the Green Pass (down from 9 months) starting from 1 February 2022, the obligation to wear masks in all situations, including outdoors, and to wear FFP2-type masks on or in all transport and at live performances, sporting events and competitions. The revised Green Pass also covered at-the-counter consumption.

In 2022, the government began to scale back use of the super Green Pass[5] (Law 21 January 2022, No. 3) and modified the rules for the management of the pandemic (Decree-Law 4 February 2022, No. 5) to dedicate itself to interventions to contain the effects of price increases in the electricity sector (Decree-Law 27 January 2022, No. 4). The Covid-19 state of emergency ended on March 31; a new state of emergency was proclaimed until 31 December 2022 to deal with the Russia-Ukraine war and the repercussions for Italy.

It is clear when looking at the different measures adopted by the government over the various phases of the emergency that from a structural point of view (resources at stake, rules of action) there was a disequilibrium in monetary interventions ad hoc (cash) (Donati 2009, 2011), dictated by the need to face the negative impact of the emergency. From a cultural point of view (broader objectives, values underlying the policies) we can see that these measures were underpinned by a short-term logic; they have the true character of emergency measures. Thus, there is close alignment between the structural axis and the cultural axis.

The recipients of the government's monetary support were individuals, but were also recognized as breadwinners, or at least as being responsible for a family unit. However, there is a lack of an overall view of how families fared during the pandemic, including the most fragile families.

The cash measures presented in the Cura Italia Decree were expanded in the subsequent decrees, and included measures to support or protect work, investment in parental leave, babysitting bonuses and support for agile work. These measures were guided by an understanding of people's varying life situations: temporary interruption of work to dedicate oneself to care (leave), outsourcing of care to dedicate oneself to work (babysitting bonus), and acknowledgement of the coexistence of the working and care dimensions (agile work). These interventions were guided by a medium-term logic in which the dimension of emergency, albeit mitigated, was always present.

However, overall, the measures implemented across the pandemic, while supporting families indirectly, implicitly or broadly, demonstrated Italy's inability to truly recognize family relationships and foster a positive integration between work and family responsibilities. This inability negatively impacted personal, family and economic well-being (Cusinato et al., 2020).

In this complex framework—and in light of in-depth analyses of the Italian welfare system and the policies implemented by the government during the pandemic (Mazzucchelli et al. 2020)—it is clear that there is a need to rethink socio-health, family and work policies. The perspective needs to be one of integration and acknowledgement of complexity in order to provide effective and flexible solutions capable of responding according to a comprehensive—but not standardized—logic, and to protect and promote personal and relationship health, as well as family needs and the needs of the production sector.

Consequences of the Pandemic for Women and Families

The pandemic has led to a range of consequences for families. One phenomenon has been an increased risk of domestic violence against women. The second issue is a difficulty in integrating family and work responsibilities, in particular for women and mothers.

Violence Against Women in Interpersonal and Family Relationships

According to various data sources, both international and national, it is estimated that one in three women has experienced some form of violence in her lifetime and that this violence is mostly perpetrated by partner or former partner (Istat 2015a; EU 2014; WHO 2014). The Covid-19 Pandemic and resultant restrictive measures introduced by governments to limit the spread of the virus created a worrying scenario with regard to domestic or couple violence (Simonovic 2022; Piquero et al. 2021). The WHO and other international authorities warned about the increased risk of gender-based violence resulting from more time spent indoors and isolation from social and protective networks, and greater social and economic stress related to both the pandemic and the response measures (Galea e al. 2020; UN 2020).

Women have been more exposed to the risk of abuse and violence as they have been forced to cohabit with their abusers due to the health restrictions. According to data from the WHO, violence against women tripled during months of confinement in the home (WHO 2020). The fact that abused women were living in close proximity to their abusers made it more difficult for them to seek help and report their violent partner. Thus, for some women, the home, far from being a place of protection and well-being, became a site of discomfort and violence.

Scholars have referred to this issue as an 'emergency within an emergency,' and UN Women (2020a,b) has called it a 'shadow pandemic' or 'shadow crisis.' Additionally, children living in violent situations also suffer, and there are increased difficulties for particularly vulnerable populations, such as foreign women, women with disabilities, and those from disadvantaged social and economic backgrounds. The pandemic has led to several possible scenarios: an increase in the number of victims of violence (new cases), an increased severity of pre-existing violence and an increase in requests for help for pre-existing violence. These scenarios could also be concurrent and interrelated in different ways.

We will explore how gender violence has been dealt with during the Covid-19 lockdowns, and how gender-based violence was one of the first social issues that came to light as a result of wide-scale lockdowns. In particular, we focus on the issue of gender violence in intimate and couple relationships during Covid-19 lockdowns and the level of government responsiveness in Italy (Brink et al. 2021; D'Ambrosio and Barba 2021; Lundin et al. 2020).

In the first months of 2020, the media started to highlight a likely future increase in violence against women in the home due to lockdowns and the difficulties victims living with their abuser would have in reporting violence and using support services. The dramatic increase in violence against women related to the pandemic crisis is now well known, and exists among other phenomena that contribute to worsening inequalities and social exclusion (Battistelli and Galantino 2020), in particular gender discrimination (Donato 2020; Fornari et al. 2020; Moffa and Chirivì 2020; Nocenzi and Crespi 2022). Many women with causal jobs that they lost during lockdown were more exposed, as they were forced to stay at home for long periods and be more economically dependent on their partners, making it more difficult to escape violence. In addition, legal provisions for social distancing introduced to contain the virus proved to be an obstacle for victims wanting to access domestic violence shelters.

In the first lockdown (beginning end of March 2020), requests via phone call and chat to the 1522[6] emergency number increased by 79.5%, with a peak occurring in April 2020 (+176.9% compared to April 2019) and May 2020 (+182.2% compared to May 2019) (Istat 2021a). Comparing the first three quarters of 2020 with the first three quarters of 2021, we can see interesting differences in the severity of violence. In the first nine months of 2021, there were 12,305 requests for help made to 1522 via phone call or chat (15,708 in 2020 and 8,647 in 2019). The scaling back of restrictive pandemic measures in 1522 number calling meant that compared to the same period in 2020, reports of violence by partners decreased (from 58.6 to 53.4%) and reports of violence perpetrated by ex-partners, other family members or those outside the family increased.

The data show that the mobility-restricting measures adopted to contain the virus increased women's fears for their own safety. Indeed, the first nine months of 2020 saw an increase in reports of violence in which the victim felt her own life or loved ones' lives were in danger (3,583 compared to 2,663 in 2019). In contrast, the scaling back of restrictions in the same months of 2021 led to a decrease in reports of violence where the victim perceived imminent danger (2,457 in 2021). Istat data concerning the survey on the use of anti-violence centres (CAVs) indicated that in 2020 more than 15,000 women started using centres that adhered to the State-Regions Agreement. More than 90% of the women—about 13,700—went to a centre for the first time in 2020. 5.6% of them started their path out of violence in March, and 15% did so between April and May, overcoming the restrictions imposed by the health emergency. Emergency interventions were, in fact, more frequent in these three months. 19.9% (more than 3,000 women) required an emergency intervention; the need for this type of intervention increased in the months of March, April and May, when the highest percentages of emergency interventions were recorded, equal, respectively, to 21.6, 22.9 and 21.2% (cf Istat 2021b).

Considering the cases where information on the duration of the violence is available (about 10,400), it emerges that for 74.2% of the women—about 7,700—the violence did not start with the pandemic but predated it: 40.6% of the women had suffered violence for more than 5 years and 33.6% for 1 to 5 years. The response of the CAVs was efficient: 12.6% of the women were offered emergency intervention and safety, 14.2% the pathway of removal from the situation of violence and 18% support for autonomy. The services most commonly offered by the centres in 2020 were listening (97.1%) and welcoming (82.8%). In 59.8% of cases, the perpetrator of the violence was the cohabiting partner, in 23% an ex-partner and in 9.5% another family member or relative. Violence suffered outside the family/couple constituted only 7.7%.

As a signatory to the Council of Europe Convention (COE 2011) on preventing and combating violence against women and domestic violence—known as the Istanbul Convention—Italy recognises gender-based violence as a violation of human rights. The national government should fully address violence against women in all its forms and take measures to prevent it, protect its victims and prosecute perpetrators (Cimagalli 2014). The state should also collect relevant disaggregated statistical data at regular intervals on cases of all forms of violence against women, and support research in the field in order to study its root causes and effects and incidence and conviction rates, as well as the efficacy of measures taken to implement the Convention (COE 2011).

This upturn in requests for help was influenced by the activities of public institutions, such as social campaigns promoted by the Department for Equal Opportunities and, in particular, the efforts of anti-violence centres and shelters to reshape their operating methods in order to continue welcoming women and their children (Demurtas et al. 2020). Both the D.i.Re.[7] Network and the national government rolled out advertising campaigns on social and traditional media early in the Covid-19 Pandemic, which may have increased awareness of their services, although both had consistently advertised their services in the past.

In the meantime, after the introduction of lockdowns, some international bodies, such as UN Women, European Institute for Gender Equality (EIGE), the United Nations and WHO, following an increase of incidents of violence in several countries, started to issue recommendations aimed at combating violence against women during the period of the emergency. As a result, the Italian government undertook several measures to support and protect women victims of violence during the pandemic. Among these, the most relevant in Italy were:

- Decree-Law No. 19, on March 17, 2020, which became Law No. 27, April 4, 2020. The law encompassed measures to strengthen the National Health Service and economic support for families, workers and businesses. It allocated 3 million euro in additional funds for anti-violence centres and shelter homes; called for the removal of the abusive man rather than the woman and any minors; and protected the interests of minors by replacing meetings in a neutral setting with remote meetings.
- The Circular Letter of 21 March 2020 of the Ministry of the Interior concerning the reception of women victims of violence. The document highlighted the difficulty for CAVs and shelter homes in accommodating women due to governmental measures requiring social distancing. In order to cope with this difficulty, the Ministry for Equal Opportunities and Family identified new accommodation solutions, including temporary ones, that could provide women victims of violence with refuge.
- The 'Libera puoi' social campaign launched on 24 March 2020 and promoted by the Department for Equal Opportunities. This aimed at promoting the 1522 number, active 24 h a day, and the associated app that allowed women to chat with the operators of anti-violence centres in safety, without the risk of being intercepted by aggressors.
- The Circular of March 27, 2020, of the Ministry of the Interior containing information about the Office for the Coordination and Planning of the Police Forces with regard to gender-based violence and domestic violence and awareness-raising actions. The document highlighted the danger of violence in the home due to pandemic restrictions and reiterated that the National Police and Carabinieri were still operating despite the emergency. In addition, it encouraged maximum awareness of police about the issue and called for compliance with first intervention procedures in order to act promptly to protect the victims.
- The Memorandum of Understanding of April 2, 2020, between the Minister for Equal Opportunities and Family and the presidents of the Federation of the Order of Italian Pharmacists (FOFI) and Assofarm to improve information for women victims of violence and stalking during the health emergency period. In April 2020, the Minister for Family and Equal Opportunities, Elena Bonetti, released 30 million euros to combat male gender-based violence. However, there were difficulties with the funds provided in 2021 by the Department for Equal Opportunities

reaching the regions that did not apply any action plan to combat gender-based violence.

As can be seen from this list, the intention of all these initiatives was to promote close cooperation between bodies that traditionally deal with the fight against violence and increase the number of actors involved. This is interesting to us, because rarely have there been such precise paths towards moral responsibility and action.

It is clear, therefore, that some of the measures adopted during the pandemic (easier access to services and simplified reporting) should be made structural in order to support specialised services such as CAVs, particularly with regard to an increase in beds for women in accommodation and strengthening of actions to respond to requests for help.

Social service and private social workers have previously experienced a need to readjust their operating methods to cope with collective emergencies, such as natural disasters (Di Rosa and Argento 2013; Calbucci, 2016). However, the challenges posed by the pandemic are unprecedented in Italy's recent history. With natural disasters, there is an initial violent and ruinous impact, leading to a massive initial mobilisation of relief, and then a gradual move back to normality. However, the pandemic emergency started with relatively contained episodes, which then developed at an exponential rate that affected both potential victims and potential rescuers—everyone was equally unprepared (Gui, 2020). Also unprecedented was the obligatory upheaval of relational practices—personal relationships were completely disrupted by the need for precautionary physical distancing.

As far as the Italian anti-violence system is concerned, a process of regulation and reorganisation is currently underway to provide adequate support to women in risky. The debate is open, both within the networks of the anti-violence centres and in the institutional seats of power where these changes are discussed, contested and negotiated. At the centre is the tension between the need for standardised criteria for the interventions and the need to personalise them—the various actors in the field often take opposing positions in terms of the approaches and methodologies adopted.

Impact on Family and Work Integration: An Overview

The pandemic has negatively impacted the labour market and employment. The stability and regularity of, and remuneration for, work in Italy has always been a critical issue, and the situation was further exacerbated by the pandemic, with an increase in unemployment beginning in 2020. In this section, we provide some contextual data to highlight the difficulty of balancing work and care responsibilities during the pandemic, then we move into the results of an extensive Italian longitudinal research study.

Widespread working from home has contributed to altering work and family routines. In Italy, before Covid-19, working from home was not of great interest to most workers. Italy held the third last place in Europe with regard to working from home. Interestingly, there was a similar proportion of women who worked from home (4.3%) and who were employed and had a child under 6 years of age (4.5%). In other European countries, such as the Netherlands and Finland, women with pre-schoolers rated at least 6 percentage points higher than the average when it came to those employed. In spring 2020, the share of employed who have worked from home at least one day a week reached 19.3% (up from 4.6% in the second quarter of 2019), rising to 23.6% among women (Istat 2021a).

Recent studies have revealed the negative impact on personal well-being of the long pandemic, social distancing, and working and caring from home. In 2021, the European Union documented[1] (EF 2022) that the well-being and mental health of citizens had reached an all-time low, especially among those who had never experienced working from home before, women and those with other care commitments (Adams-Prassl et al. 2020; Del Boca et al. 2020). Studies showed that the increase in the burden of care and the difficulty in reconciling it with working from home, and anxiety about the pandemic and the resulting uncertainty, increased symptoms of anxiety and burnout in both male and female workers around the world, especially those with children (Mehta 2021). The unprecedented closure and limitation of childcare services and schools across the world increased concern about the risk of social exclusion, growing social inequalities with regard to children's educational opportunities, and growing work-family conflicts and gender inequalities (Blum and Dobrotić 2021; OECD 2020).

Despite this, restrictions continued into 2021. They were fewer compared to summer 2020 and working from home gradually became less prevalent. Pirani and Guetto (2021) highlighted the effect of the pandemic on the well-being and living conditions of Italian parents. The pandemic has worsened psycho-emotional well-being, in particular that of single parents; however, people were optimistic about the future, believing that the pandemic is a setback rather than a structural and definitive reversal of life as we knew it. Pirani and Guetto also underlined the need for more incisive and targeted policies to meet families' different needs, especially families that are more exposed to the risks of economic deprivation and social exclusion. These recommendations are in line with those of other scholars, who have agreed that parents with school-age children and single parents are a group particularly affected by the restrictions, as they are forced to take care of their children without the help of babysitters or grandparents, and also have to supervise their children in distance learning and respond to requests related to their job (Cameron et al. 2020; Naldi et al. 2021).

Covid-19, working from home and the closure of schools have had greater negative consequences for mothers' work than for fathers' (Petts et al. 2020). While these studies have confirmed the widening of the gender gap as a result of the pandemic from an employment point of view, it is interesting to observe that there is increasing international debate about the role that fathers can play in countering the reduced participation of mothers in work. The issue is, however, very complex and

[1] https://www.eurofound.europa.eu/sites/default/files/ef_publication/field_ef_document/ef21064en.pdf

contentious: an Italian qualitative study conducted during the first lockdown (2020) highlighted that although some fathers considered the pandemic (and working from home) an opportunity to be more involved with their children, for most of them a rethinking of their commitment to paid work was not something they could imagine, unlike mothers, who were more inclined to consider job requests as negotiable and perceived a pervasive interference of work in family life. The authors, therefore, concluded that remote work did not allow the redefinition of work models and did not improve the balance between work and private life for the couples interviewed (Cannito and Scavarda 2020; Lagomarsino et al. 2020).

Del Boca et al. (2021) showed that the gender gap in household care-related activities was widest during the first wave of the pandemic, in 2020, and although it was less pronounced during the second wave, it was still higher than pre-Covid-19, suggesting that the time spent by women on housework, childcare and assisting their children with distance learning did not depend on their partners' working arrangements. Conversely, men spent fewer hours helping with the housework and distance learning when their partners were at home. It is interesting, however, that although men who worked remotely or not at all did devote more time to domestic chores and childcare, the increased time they spent at home did not seem to lead to a fundamental reallocation of couples' domestic and childcare roles.

Work-Family Reconciliation Strategies in Italy in 2020: Longitudinal Evidence

In order to better understand the impact of pandemic restrictions on work-family balance, we report data from a mixed-method longitudinal study conducted in Italy during the different waves (T1 = April 2020; T2 = July 2020 and T3 = December 2020),[8] which focused on the impact of reconciling family responsibilities and work, with a specific focus on women working from home.

In particular, the study investigated the following: stress, post-traumatic growth (PTG), work-family balance (WLB), reconciliation strategies, impact on family, working from home (WFH) evaluation and satisfaction with educational services. The analysis was carried out to determine the effect of the pandemic on individuals and their families. The results showed different levels of impact.

At the individual level, stress[9] and post-traumatic growth (PTG)[10] were measured across time and gender. Analysis showed that women reported higher levels of stress and that their stress increased over time. The highest levels of stress were reported at T3. Further, women showed higher levels of PTG—that is, the ability to positively manage the stressful event—but unfortunately, women also showed a significant decrease in this dimension from T2 to T3.

Regarding reconciliation strategies,[11] families were deeply challenged by the forced isolation. Without the support of primary networks during the first wave of the pandemic, the nuclear family found itself facing the challenge of taking care of non-self-sufficient family members (38% personally managed the care load), and looking after children, supporting them in homeschooling and managing their own workload from home. During T2, the reopening of schools, kindergartens and summer camps led to a better situation for parents: 28.6% indicated that they personally took care of their children, 19.7% indicated grandparents took care of them and only 9.1% of children went to a summer camp. Although helped by the opening of schools in T3, the management of children still falls to parents even if this was less than during T1 (27% personally and 12% partner). Parents could rely very little on external help (babysitter 3%, grandparents 12.7%). Children mainly attended school in person (27%). Moreover, the conflict between work and family[12] increased, especially between T1 and T2 and specifically for women. At T2 (post lockdown) and T3 (when schools reopened) the conflict remained quite stable, and still significant.

Considering that most of the sample was working from home, a focus on them seemed important. The most important advantage of WFH[13] was saving the time devoted to and cost of travel ($M_{T2} = 4.32$; $M_{T3} = 4.35$), followed by a sense that one was protecting oneself from the virus ($M_{T2} = 3.92$; $M_{T3} = 4.05$). The possibility of better managing work and private life obtained lower rates.

Regarding the disadvantages of WFH, respondents indicated that they stayed at the PC for a long time ($M_{T2} = 3.46$; $M_{T3} = 3.53$) and worked longer hours ($M_{T2} = 3.43$; $M_{T3} = 3.41$). At T3, respondents indicated that they missed being in touch with their colleagues ($M_{T2} = 3.38$; $M_{T3} = 3.71$).

Particularly for families with young children, childcare services and schools are considered an important partner in educational tasks. The interviewees gave generally positive responses regarding satisfaction with the educational services.[14] However, people were less satisfied with the possibility for families to express disagreement and make proposals (both $M = 2.99$), while they were most satisfied with the attention that educational services gave children ($M = 3.76$) and the educational services' ability to cope with difficulties ($M = 3.45$). Thus, while school and childcare services were attentive to children's well-being and dealt effectively with the crisis, there still needs to be even more dialogue with families.

Finally, government policies and measures[15] were not evaluated positively. Regarding T2 and T3, interviewees were asked about their opinion on the decisions taken by the government during the emergency and the impact of policies on their families. Overall, a negative judgement emerged: people felt that the government did not listen to families when making decisions ($M_{T2} = 2.01$; $M_{T3} = 1.96$) did not consider the different needs of families and did not provide suitable support for different situations ($M_{T2} = 2.22$; $M_{T3} = 2.03$). The policies did not help families to balance the needs of all members ($M_{T2} = 2.29$; $M_{T3} = 2.25$) and did not prevent internal conflict ($M_{T2} = 2.36$; $M_{T3} = 2.38$). This response was particularly negative in families with small children and women, while it was less negative for those who had adult children or no children.

The experience of working parents during the pandemic has been further explored through focus groups[16] in order to deeply understand the impact of this long emergency on parents' lives. Group discussion made it possible to understand in depth the challenges of the parents' transition to a different way of life during the pandemic. Parents have been supported by their employers, in terms of welfare, flexible and suitable working from home schemes, and the presence of a supportive and family-friendly corporate culture. The strength and resilience of family relationships has also been a support, in particular for mothers working from home.

Furthermore, many participants had a child during the emergency. Mothers reported that, in general, the forced isolation and the possibility of working from home after maternity leave resulted in a more positive experience for them: they enjoyed being able to strengthen their bond with their baby, and had a reduced sense of guilt about leaving the baby to work outside the home. Thus, closeness with the baby, even when mothers restarted work (from home) after their maternity leave ended, was associated with positive feelings and a sense of security.

However, parents also reported a sense of loneliness and a lack of both primary relationships and face-to-face relationships with work colleagues. A common issue, highlighted by all the participants, was connected to the uncertainty regarding the end of working from home and the return (total or partial) to the office and the consequent need to reorganise work and family life. The return to the office was in fact talked about with a sense of fear and stress because of this.

A lexical analysis using T-LAB software[17] highlighted some interesting points. The software conducts content analysis and text mining using automatic and semi-automatic processes that allow the user to quickly highlight significant patterns regarding words, themes and variables. The software creates radial diagrams in which the selected word is placed in the center. The other words are distributed around it, each at a distance proportional to its degree of association. The relationships between the central word and those selected by the program are therefore all significant. The word *home*—in the center—was very strongly associated with *child* and with *work*, two aspects that need to be *kept* together; *job, kindergarten and school* must be *managed* and organised. This kind of organisation started during the *lockdown* and persisted and will require a new articulation with the *return* to the office; this strongly engages parents (*woman and husband*). The word *child* was closely associated with *working* from home and with *mum* and *dad*, as reference adults and sole interlocutors during the lockdown and the closure of educational services (kindergarten) and school. The word *alone* (concerning mothers) referred to the sense of loneliness that mothers felt in reconciling family life and working, even with their partner's (*husband*) and *company* support. Associations with *work* confirmed the strong ties to the home space and family dimension (*child, husband*), which required management. *Time* was dedicated to this, using *tools (smart working, phone*) and involved working and relationships with colleagues.

Conclusion and Outlook

The Covid-19 Pandemic has generated social, family and gender-related impacts that will continue into the future. The pandemic has had a large negative effect on the female workforce and has led to a dramatic gender imbalance that does not seem to be healable with the current modest interventions.

The pandemic has had a very significant impact on Italy: over a short time there was a rapid increase in cases and the government needed to introduce very severe containment measures, such as rigid lockdowns, the closure of schools and childcare, restrictions on non-essential activities, and working from home. These restrictions on individual freedom (in particular not being able to leave the house unless it was a necessity) or changes in daily routines (work and care from home) has seen people's lives completely and suddenly turned upside down.

Even in the coexistence phase of the pandemic, with the start of the vaccination campaign and the government's commitment to loosening rigid lockdowns, the climate of stress remained, due to the situation always changing rapidly and the resultant difficulty in making long-term plans (such as travel, work, care duties). Thus, the pandemic has brought about huge and lasting impacts for families and women, who were inadequately supported by government policies.

Several studies in Italy have confirmed these data. The data were also confirmed by a mixed-method study carried out in Italy during 2020. Using a longitudinal approach, with data collected over three waves—April, July and December—we assessed the effects and consequences of working from home (WFH), showing that well-being decreased, work-life conflict increased over time and that working parents found the first lockdown particularly challenging. A second qualitative analysis conducted in 2021, with focus groups of men and women and parents and caregivers working from home, provided a better understanding of the experience of working parents during the pandemic. Alongside relational and economic resources and positive aspects (such as the strength and resilience of family relationships) parents also reported a sense of loneliness and a lack of primary relationships and face-to-face relationships with work colleagues. A common issue, highlighted by all the participants, concerned returning to the office and having to again reorganise daily and family routines.

As in previous emergencies, the Covid-19 Pandemic led to an increase in gender-based violence and domestic violence cases. During the pandemic, social services, anti-violence centres and shelter homes continued to guarantee the reception of women (often accompanied by minors) fleeing violent situations. This was initially done at distance and every possible channel of communication with users was activated. Normal operating methods involve a focus on establishing face-to-face relations to create a climate of trust and cooperation with the victims. In carrying out their work, these services faced numerous critical issues, some contingent on or linked to the disastrous effects of the pandemic, others endemic but exacerbated by this particular moment of crisis. In order to avoid serious violations of human rights, measures that genuinely support women, through the provision of a package of substantial resources, rather than ad hoc 'bonuses,' need to be adopted.

The results invite us to think about future challenges. Various actors have put in place alternative strategies to cope with women's and family's needs and claims in different situations, and one wonders how and to what extent above mentioned practices will turn into lasting change. The ever-looming risk is that good and efficient initiatives to face the emergency are implemented but that the policies, such as those aimed at supporting women and families, are not embedded structurally and that cultural change to eradicate inequalities and imbalances.

Notes

1. Those regions deemed 'orange,' in addition to the curfew from 10 pm to 5 am, forbade any movement outside the municipality of residence except for essential travel to/from work or proved health or emergency reasons. Commercial activities such as restaurants, bars, cafés, etc. were suspended. Schools remained accessible only to and including the second year of middle school (12-year-old pupils). Regions categorized as 'red' applied further restrictions, including the prohibition of unsubstantiated movements within the municipality of residence, the closure of non-food retail activities, and remote schooling from primary school upwards.
2. The excess mortality associated with the Covid-19 Pandemic is the difference between overall deaths from any cause since the beginning of the pandemic and the expected level of deaths calculated on the basis of the average for the period 2015–2019, assumed to be representative of the pre-Covid mortality situation. This indicator allows us to measure both the direct and indirect impact of the pandemic by providing an overall measure of the impact of the pandemic on mortality, in particular of deaths directly associated with Covid-19.
3. https://famiglia.governo.it/media/2690/l-effetto-della-pandemia-sui-servizi-educativi-per-l-infanzia-slide.pdf.
4. https://www.quotidianosanita.it/allegati/allegato8041000.pdf.
5. While the Green Pass can be obtained with a negative molecular (valid for 72 hours) or rapid swab (valid for 48 hours), vaccination is required for the Super Green Pass.
6. 1522 is the toll-free number provided by the DPO-PdCM to support and help victims of gender-based violence and stalking, in line with the Istanbul Convention. Victims of gender-based violence and stalking, in line with the provisions of the Istanbul Convention. It is free of charge, guarantees anonymity and covers different forms of violence 24 hours a day and in 4 different languages besides Italian (English, French, Arabic and Spanish), French, Arabic and Spanish). This helpline provides first aid information in case of emergency or useful services and anti-violence centres active at territorial level to which victims of violence or other users can turn to.

7. D.i. Re-Donne in Rete Contro la Violenza (2020), Covid-19: 2867 Women Approached D.i.Re Anti-Violence Centres During the Lockdown, *press release*, April 14, https://www.direcontrolaviolenza.it.
8. The sample is composed by 306 workers that answer to three wave of data collection (T1=April 2020; T2=July 2020 and T3=December 2020). Specifically, 83.3% were women, 66.7% were married or engaged and 70.9% had children; 61.3% were employed people.
9. 9 Measured by the Perceived Stress Scale (Cohen et al. 1994).
10. Measured by the short version of the Tedeschi et al. 1988 scale.
11. 1 Assessed by ad hoc questions that asked how respondents manage their family load during the three phases of the emergency.
12. Measured using the Agha et al. (2017) Work-Life Balance Scale.
13. Working From Home (WFH) evaluation was assessed by ad hoc questions that asked how respondents were satisfied by their work from home and how they rate their performance, and which were the advantages.
14. By an ad hoc set of questions, respondents were asked to indicate how much they were satisfied with their relationship with the educational services.
15. The FamILens® assessed the impact of the different measures on the family dynamics, relationship, and conflict.
16. Focus groups with a total of 18 parents (mainly mothers and a few fathers).
17. There are several valuable elements of this program: its interface is particularly user-friendly and allows the application to very different fields and objects as well as used in different languages (Italian, English, French, German, Spanish, and Portuguese); all software processes are finally transparent and can be easily customized using a wide and flexible range of analysis tools.

References

Adams-Prassl, A.; Boneva, T.; Golin, M., and Rauh, C. 2020. The impact of the coronavirus lockdown on mental health: Evidence from the US, *Report*, No. 2020-030. Human Capital and Economic Opportunity Working Group, http://humcap.uchicago.edu.

Agha, K., Azmi, F.T., and Khan, S.A. 2017. Work-life balance: Scale development and validation, In: *The work-family balance in light of globalization and technology*, eds. M.L. Heras, N. Chinchilla, M. Grau., Newcastle Upon Tyne: Cambridge Scholars.

Battistelli, F., and M.G. Galantino. 2020. *Sociologia e politica del coronavirus: Tra opinioni e paure*. Milan: FrancoAngeli.

Blum, S., and I. Dobrotić. 2021. Childcare-policy responses in the Covid-19 pandemic: unpacking cross-country variation. *European Societies* 23 (S1): S545–S563.

Brink, J., P. Cullen, K. Beek, and S.A. Peters. 2021. Intimate partner violence during the Covid-19 pandemic in Western and Southern European countries. *European Journal of Public Health* 31 (5): 1058–1063.

Calbucci, R., M. Deidda, M. De Santi, R.T. Di Rosa, A. Fiorentini, E.M. Giuliano, L. Gui, S. Mordeglia, S. Pelosio, F. Sartori, R. Ticchiati, and A. Zannoni. 2016. *Servizio sociale e calamità naturali: Interventi di servizio sociale*. Rome: Edizioni EISS.

Cameron, E.E., K.M. Joyce, C.P. Delaquis, K. Reynolds, J. Protudjer, and L.E. Roos. 2020. Maternal psychological distress & mental health service use during the Covid-19 pandemic. *Journal of Affective Disorders* 276: 765–774.

Cannito, M., and A. Scavarda. 2020. Childcare and remote work during the Covid-19 pandemic: Ideal worker model parenthood and gender inequalities in Italy. *Italian Sociological Review* 10 (3S): 801–820.

Cimagalli, F. 2014. *Le politiche contro la violenza di genere nel welfare che cambia: Concetti, modelli e servizi*. Milan: FrancoAngeli.

COE, Council of Europe. 2011. *Convention on preventing and combating violence against women and domestic violence*, https://www.coe.int.

Cohen, S., T. Kamarck, and R. Mermelstein. 1994. Perceived stress scale. *Measuring Stress: A Guide for Health and Social Scientists* 10 (2): 1–2.

Cusinato, M., S. Iannattone, A. Spoto, M. Poli, C. Moretti, M. Gatta, and M. Miscioscia. 2020. Stress, resilience, and well-being in Italian children and their parents during the Covid-19 pandemic. *International Journal of Environmental Research and Public Health* 17 (22): 8297.

D'Ambrosio, M., and D. Barba. 2021. Violenza intrafamiliare e violenza di genere al tempo del Covid-19: L'indagine sociologica nel conflitto della famiglia e della coppia. *Rivista Italiana Di Conflittologia* 42: 35–73.

Dayal, H.C., and L. Tiko. 2020. When are we going to have the real school? A case study of early childhood education and care teachers' experiences surrounding education during the Covid-19 pandemic. *Australasian Journal of Early Childhood* 45 (4): 336–347.

Del Boca, D., N. Oggero, P. Profeta, and M. Rossi. 2020. Women's and men's work, housework and childcare, before and during Covid-19. *Review of Economics of the Household* 18 (4): 1001–1017.

Del Boca, D., Oggero, N., Profeta, P., Rossi, M. 2021. Did Covid-19 affect the division of labor within the household? Evidence from two waves of the pandemic in Italy, *CEPR Discussion Paper*, No. DP16257, https://ssrn.com.

Demurtas, P., C. Peroni, and A. Mauri. 2020. I Centri antiviolenza ai tempi del Coronavirus. *La Rivista Delle Politiche Sociali* 2: 1–9.

Di Rosa, R.T., and G. Argento. 2013. *Il servizio sociale nell'emergenza: Esperienze e prospettive dall'Abruzzo all'Emilia*. Rome: Aracne.

Donati, P. 2009. *Ropporto Famiglia 2009 CISF, Il costo dei figli: Quale welfare per le famiglie?* Milan: FrancoAngeli.

Donati, P. 2010. *Il costo dei figli: Quale welfare per le famiglie?* Milan: FrancoAngeli.

Donati, P. 2011. *La politica della famiglia: Per un welfare relazionale e sussidiario*, Siena: Cantagalli.

Donato, S. 2020. Gender-based violence against women in intimate and couple relationships. The case of Spain and Italy during the Covid-19 pandemic lockdown, *Italian Sociological Review* 10(3S): 869–887.

EU. 2014. *Violenza contro le donne: Un'indagine a livello di Unione Europea*, European Union Agency for Fundamental Rights, https://fra.europa.eu.

Fornari, S., M. Nocenzi, and E. Ruspini. 2020. *Violenza di genere: L'agency femminile in linee di intervento e buone pratiche, Sicurezza e Scienze Sociali, Fascicolo 3/2019*. Milan: FrancoAngeli.

Galea, S., R.M. Merchant, and N. Lurie. 2020. The mental health consequences of Covid-19 and physical distancing: The need for prevention and early intervention. *JAMA Internal Medicine* 180 (6): 817–818.

Gui, L. 2020. Spiazzamento e apprendimento dall'esperienza in tempo di Covid. In: *Il servizio sociale nell'emergenza Covid-19*, eds. M. Sanfelici, L. Gui and S. Mordeglia. Milan: FrancoAngeli.

ISTAT. 2015a. *La violenza contro le donne dentro e fuori la famiglia, anno 2014*, https://www.istat.it.

ISTAT. 2015b. *Violence against women, year 2014*, https://www.istat.it.

ISTAT. 2020a. *Prima ondata della pandemia. Un'analisi della mortalità per causa e luogo del decesso, marzo-aprile 2020a*, https://www.istat.it

ISTAT. 2020b. *Natalità e fecondità della popolazione residente, anno 2020b*, https://www.istat.it

ISTAT. 2021a. *Le richieste di aiuto durante la pandemia: I dati dei centri antiviolenza, delle Case rifugio e delle chiamate al 1522, anno 2020*, https://www.istat.it

ISTAT. 2021b. *Rapporto BES 2020*, https://www.istat.it.

ISTAT. 2022a. *Impatto dell'epidemia Covid-19 sulla mortalità totale della popolazione residente*, https://www.istat.it.

ISTAT. 2022b. *Indagine sugli alunni delle scuole secondarie, primi dati, anno 2021*, https://www.istat.it.

Lagomarsino, F., I. Coppola, R. Parisi, and N. Rania. 2020. Care tasks and new routines for italian families during the Covid-19 pandemic: Perspectives from women. *Italian Sociological Review* 10 (3S): 847–868.

Lundin, R., Armocida, B., Sdao, P., Pisanu, S., Mariani, I., Veltri, A., Lazzerini, M. 2020. Gender-based violence during the Covid-19 pandemic response in Italy. *Journal of Global Health*, 10(2), https://doi.org/10.7189/jogh.10.020359.

Mazzucchelli, S., M.L. Bosoni, and L. Medina. 2020. The impact of Covid-19 on family relationships in Italy: Withdrawal on the nuclear family. *Italian Sociological Review* 10 (3S): 687–709.

Mehta P. 2021. Work from home-work engagement amid Covid-19 lockdown and employee happiness. *Journal of Public Affairs*, e2709, https://doi.org/10.1002/pa.2709.

Moffa, G., and M. Chirivì. 2020. La violenza di genere confinata tra le pareti domestiche durante il lockdown. *Culture e Studi Del Sociale* 5 (2): 559–567.

Naldi, A., Vallelonga, F., Di Liberto, A., Cavallo, R., Agnesone, M., Gonella, M., Sauta, M.D., Lochner, P., Tondo, G., Bragazzi, N.L., Botto, R., and Leombruni, P. 2021. Covid-19 pandemic-related anxiety, distress and burnout: Prevalence and associated factors in healthcare workers of North-West Italy, *The British Journal of Psychiatry Open*, 7(1), https://doi.org/10.1192/bjo.2020.161.

Nocenzi, M., and I. Crespi. 2022. Il contrasto alla violenza di genere e la pandemia Covid-19. Rischi e ambivalenze nelle politiche di welfare: Un'introduzione al tema in *La Critica Sociologia*; 223; Pisa, Fabrizio Serra Editore; pp. 41–52.

OECD. 2020. *Combatting Covid-19's effect on children.* https://read.oecd-ilibrary.org.

Pavolini, E., G. Argentin, P. Falzetti, M.T. Galanti, E. Campodifiori, and G. Le Rose. 2021. Tutti a casa: Il sistema di istruzione italiano alla prova del Covid-19. *Politiche Sociali* 2: 255–280.

Petts, R.J., D.L. Carlson, and J.R. Pepin. 2020. A gendered pandemic: Childcare, homeschooling, and parents' employment during Covid-19. *Gender, Work & Organization* 28 (S2): 515–534.

Piquero, A.R., W.G. Jennings, E. Jemison, C. Kaukinen, and F.M. Knaul. 2021. Domestic violence during the covid-19 pandemic—Evidence from a systematic review and meta-analysis. *Journal of Criminal Justice* 74: 101806. https://doi.org/10.1016/j.jcrimjus.2021.101806.

Pirani, E. and Guetto, R. 2021. *I genitori single in Italia e gli effetti della pandemia di Covid-19 sul loro benessere e sulle relazioni familiari*, No. 2021/19, Università degli Studi di Firenze, Dipartimento di Statistica, Informatica, Applicazioni "G. Parenti," https://ideas.repec.org

Simonovic, D. 2020. *Submission to the UN special rapporteur on violence against women, its causes and consequences regarding Covid-19 and the increase of domestic violence against women*, https://www.hrw.org.

Tedeschi, R.G.; Park, C.L. and Calhoun, L.G. 1998. Assessment of posttraumatic growth. In: *Posttraumatic growth*, eds. R.G. Tedeschi, C.L. Park and L.G. Calhoun. Oxon: Routledge.

UN. 2020. *Policy brief: The impact of Covid-19 on women*, https://reliefweb.int.

WHO. 2014. *Global status report on violence prevention 2014*, https://www.who.int.

WHO. 2020. *Covid-19 and violence against women: What the health sector/system can do*, https://apps.who.int.

UN Women. 2020a. *Covid-19: Emerging gender data and why it matters*, https://data.unwomen.org.
UN Women. 2020b. *Covid-19 and ending violence against women and girls*, https://www.unwomen.org.

Chapter 12
The Covid-19 Pandemic in Greece: With Special Reference to Women's Employment

Varvara Lalioti

Abstract This chapter seeks to attain a two-fold aim. Firstly, to provide an overview of the way the Covid-19 pandemic evolved in Greece, including the relevant government responses. Secondly, to outline the main implications of the crisis, triggered by both the pandemic and the restraining measures targeted at mitigating the spread of the virus, for women's employment in the country. The chapter sheds light, inter alia, upon the 'direct' and 'indirect' measures adopted by the Greek government, in order to protect the jobs and the well-being of those employed, to encourage the creation of new jobs and to alleviate the impact of the slowdown in product demand that businesses were faced with. Direct measures included, for instance, job retention schemes and measures to address work-life balance, while examples of indirect measures are repayable advance payments to enterprises and mandatory rent reductions in business properties in the sectors hit by the pandemic. The chapter highlights the effects of the pandemic on women's employment in Greece, as exemplified by the fact that the highest educational level functioned as a shield against unemployment, more in the case of women than in that of men; or that women in Greece, together with women in Portugal, are those who have experienced, at least during the first months of the pandemic, the largest losses in working hours at the European level. These findings should be viewed in conjunction with the increased pressure faced by Greek women during the pandemic, in their effort to cope with the expectations associated with both their professional and family lives. The concluding section summarizes the arguments made and discusses pathways for further research.

Keywords Covid-19 pandemic · Greece · Government responses · Women's employment and unemployment · Women's professional and family life

---

V. Lalioti (✉)
Department of Political Science and Public Administration, National and Kapodistrian University of Athens, Athens, Greece
e-mail: blal@pspa.uoa.gr

C. Aspalter (ed.), *Covid-19 Pandemic*,
https://doi.org/10.1007/978-981-99-2497-4_12

Introduction

Based on an extensive literature review and the use of data with an emphasis on aspects of women's employment in Greece, the present chapter seeks to attain a two-fold aim. Firstly, to provide the reader with an overview of the way in which the Covid-19 pandemic evolved in Greece and the government response. Secondly, to outline the main implications of the Covid-19 related crisis for women's employment in the country.

To this end, the chapter sheds light, inter alia, upon the highly centralized way the Greek government handled the crisis, the rhetoric adopted, as well as the policy measures undertaken, as a means to protect the jobs and the well-being of those employed, to encourage the creation of new jobs and to alleviate the impact of the slowdown in product demand that businesses were faced with. As discussed in detail in the main body of the chapter, examples of these measures include job retention schemes, measures to address work-life balance, repayable advance payments to enterprises and mandatory rent reductions for business properties in the sectors of the economy more harshly hit by the pandemic.

After outlining the government response to the pandemic, and also how this response has been evaluated by both researchers and public opinion, the discussion focuses on the effects of the pandemic on female employment in Greece. Within a context largely defined by the idiosyncratic features of the domestic labour market and the broader characteristics of women's employment in the country, a series of crisis-related effects are presented. These are exemplified by the fact that Greece is amongst the EU countries where women have experienced the highest, compared to men, losses in income from employment. Such findings should be viewed in conjunction with the increased pressure faced by women during the pandemic—in a country which is still broadly typified by a familistic social model—in their effort to cope with the expectations associated with both their professional and family lives (Markantonatou 2021).

The concluding section summarizes the main chapter findings and suggests pathways for further research, such as highlighting the 'real' value of work in society. This includes discussing the need to re-evaluate payments for positions in 'essential economy sectors'/'essential services,' in which women are 'traditionally' over-represented (Lalioti 2020a), as well as rethinking the value of domestic (and, more often than not, unpaid) work.

The Evolution of the Pandemic in Greece

The evolution of the pandemic in Greece included several waves, following the pattern of a small, initial wave between March and May 2020 and larger waves at least up to the end of 2021 and the first months of 2022. Over time, variants of Covid-19 made their appearance and would be linked to the emergence of new waves. The unprecedented increase in Covid-19 cases at the end of 2021, for instance, due to a variant of the virus (broadly known as Omicron, to be 'followed' by Omicron-2), was reversed to a large extent in January 2022, with the decline in the number of cases recorded continuing at a slower pace in February 2022.

The reported epidemiological data improved during spring 2022, allowing the gradual lifting of the majority of the restrictive measures that had been imposed until the beginning of the summer (FEIR 2022: 18–19). Yet, at the time of writing (June-July 2022) and more than three weeks after the lifting of the requirement to wear masks indoors (on June 1—and with exceptions), the rate of transmission of the Covid-19 variants has triggered, once again, fears for the outbreak of a new wave.

That being said, whilst in many other European countries, neighbouring Italy included, the pandemic progressed quickly, with cases and fatalities exploding within a short period of time, things in Greece evolved differently, that is, at a relatively slower pace. The period from December 2019/January 2020, when the outbreak of Covid-19 was reported in China, until the end of February 2020, when the first Covid-19 case was announced in Greece, may be defined as a 'preparatory' phase. During this phase, the foundations of the centralized approach that would characterize the Greek government's response to the pandemic, discussed in detail in the next section, were laid. This included, aside from following the WHO and EU health guidelines, establishing an expert committee of epidemiologists to monitor the evolution of the virus at the national level and to advise the government accordingly, as well as issuing an information package advising regular temperature testing for those who had travelled recently, amongst other things (Aspriadis 2021).

The return of a tourist group from Israel and the announcement of the first Covid-19 case (on 26 February 2020) signalled the end of the 'preparatory' phase and the beginning of the main crisis phase and what was to become the first small Covid-19 wave.[1] By 27 February 2020 there were three confirmed, i.e. registered, Covid-19 cases and carnival events throughout the country were cancelled. An effort began to identify potential spread networks, while also requiring a 14-day quarantine for individuals with Covid-19 cases and all those who had been in contact with them.

During the second week of March, with the number of confirmed/registered Covid-19 cases having risen to around 100 and the first virus-related death being recorded, educational institutions (primary and secondary schools, and universities) and cafés, restaurants and tourist spots nationwide were all ordered to close. By the end of March 2020, and as the number of Covid-19 cases in the country was increasing, all public religious services were suspended, and gatherings of more than ten people and all non-essential travel were banned. Citizens were required to have a special permit sent by SMS or signed by themselves in order to leave their house, for which there were only six possible reasons.

As will be discussed in more detail in the next section, although the management of the initial phase of the pandemic may be deemed to have been relatively 'successful,' as reflected in the number of Covid-19 cases being kept quite low compared to other EU countries of similar size/population, following the summer of 2020, and especially in October 2020, the number of cases suddenly began to increase rapidly.

The number of daily confirmed (registered) cases surged from 300–400 a day in mid-October, when the use of masks everywhere was made obligatory, to almost 3,000 a day at the end of October. The pressure on the National Health System (NHS), in a country that had already gone through at least ten years of economic austerity and with the NHS budget having been cut by three-quarters, was enormous, and the situation started to get out of control, particularly in northern Greece. In December 2020, the start of a vaccination programme marked a milestone in the evolution of the pandemic that would gradually result, up until the resurgence of Covid-19 cases in Greece during June-July 2022, in a decrease in the number of deaths and hospitalizations that were linked to Covid-19.

The evolution of the pandemic in Greece is largely reflected in the data collected and processed by the so-called Covid-19 Observatory,[2] headed by the Chairman of the Council of Economic Experts. The data were 'evaluated' by a small and flexible government committee, whose major task was to act immediately for the timely management of any emergency or regular need that would arise, so as to safeguard the health of the population, while also attempting to minimize the consequences for the Greek economy.

The Observatory produced weekly reports which citizens could access online. Based on information included in the 105th report issued by the Observatory,[3] at the beginning of June 2022 (between June 2–8), the average number of daily Covid-19 cases amounted to 3,713 cases; that is an increase of 3.8% compared to the previous week, when the relevant number was 3,578 (or 358 people per one million of citizens). During the reference period, 64.9% of the cases recorded were in Attica (which includes the Greek capital, Athens) and 5.8% in Thessaloniki (the country's second largest city), while the remaining cases were scattered throughout the country.

Furthermore, drawing on data from Google Mobility, the mobility of the population in the period following the second lockdown imposed on the country, that is data concerning the period between May 14 2021–29 April 2022, was characterized by an average increase of + 27.8 percentage points compared to the one-month period before the lifting of the lockdown (i.e. April 13-May 13, 2021). The biggest increase in mobility was recorded mainly in parks and outdoor spaces (+38.3%), public transport (+37.2%), and shops, restaurants and coffee bars (+29.6%). At the same time, the incidence of staying home decreased by 5.6%.

Overall, the average age of all the Covid-19 cases recorded in Greece since the beginning of the pandemic was 37 years old. Additionally, Greece, with 2,888 deaths per one million inhabitants, was ranked in the 11th place among the EU-27; the respective European average was 2,451. As far as the rate of vaccination is concerned, Greece, on the other hand, occupied the 12th position among the EU-27. Since December 27, 2020, when the vaccination programme started in Greece, and up to June 8, 2022 the total number of vaccinations equalled 21,038,379. These included a total of 7,916,816 vaccinations of at least one shot, 7,626,246 full primary vaccinations (depending on whether the complete course of vaccination required two shots or only one shot), and 6,071,425 booster shots (given to citizens who had 'completed' their primary course of vaccination with either two or one shots, depending on the vaccine).

Table 12.1 Daily average number of Covid-19 cases (per one million inhabitants)

Country	Daily average of Covid-19 cases per 1,000,000 inhabitants
Portugal	2,293.1
Germany	378.1
Greece	358.0
Spain	337.0
USA	332.9
France	297.1
Austria	290.0
Cyprus	289.2
Italy	288.1
EU	276.3
Belgium	149.1
Slovenia	124.0
United Kingdom	102.3
Denmark	92.6
Netherlands	79.2
Croatia	62.2
Serbia	35.7
North Macedonia	28.1
Russia	26.0
Bulgaria	23.8
Sweden	21.9
Albania	18.2
Romania	14.8
Turkey	1.6

Last, the following table (Table 12.1) presents information on how Greece compared to other countries, including most EU countries, in terms of the average number of Covid-19 cases per day and per one million inhabitants (on June 7, 2022 and after taking into account a 7-day rolling average).

Government Response and Its Evaluation

Similar to what happened at the international level, the outbreak of the Covid-19 pandemic at the start of 2020 prompted the Greek government to adopt restrictive measures. The basic tool utilized for the management of the Covid-19 related crisis, especially during the first waves of the pandemic, was a severe lockdown, as exemplified by school closures and the closure of all shops and markets, bars, cafés, and the international borders, as well as the adoption of distance working. Broadly speaking, social distancing played a key role, affecting, inter alia, the way the world of employment operated in the country (Aspriadis 2021).

Furthermore, as already mentioned in the previous section, the Greek government's response to the crisis was highly centralized, as reflected in the central roles assigned to two ministries (Civil Protection and Health), which took very stringent measures in order to slow down the spread of the virus. Largely because of the state of the public health system and the wider mistrust in institutions, and therefore the realization that it could not afford an epidemic of a magnitude similar to that of neighbouring Italy, Greece responded to the Covid-19 crisis by adopting a centralized top-down approach (Zahariadis et al. 2021).

This approach should be viewed in conjunction with the establishment of a major communications campaign to inform the public about Covid-19, with the government constructing, early on, a narrative to explain the measures and why they were initiated. This included televised addresses to the public by the Greek Prime Minister, Kyriakos Mitsotakis, but mostly daily television broadcasts about the situation, with briefings being left to experts.

Experts, such as Dr. Sotirios Tsiodras, spokesperson for the Ministry of Health and a professor of infectious diseases at the National and Kapodistrian University of Athens, were used to 'legitimate' the responses adopted to the evolution of the pandemic in Greece. In spite of changes in the communications strategy of stakeholders over the course of time, the relevant authorities would continue to advise those with increased social activity to avoid contact with people in vulnerable groups and the elderly, as well as to conduct self-tests and wear masks, whilst reiterating that vaccinated people were at less of a risk.

The above should be viewed in conjunction with the policy measures taken to help citizens and enterprises to cope with the significant economic effects of the pandemic. These measures were based on the same logic that characterized the relevant policy interventions in most countries, and largely drew on EU funds.[4] Furthermore, in terms of GDP, Greece is reported to be amongst the countries which had received the highest financial assistance from the EU for this purpose (Wieland 2022: 24).

A broad first distinction that can be made among the aforementioned measures is between 'direct measures,' targeted at protecting the jobs and the well-being of those employed and encouraging the creation of new jobs, on the one hand, and 'indirect measures' that aimed to alleviate the impact of the slowdown on the demand for goods that businesses were faced with, on the other hand.[5] Direct measures included, inter alia, job retention and job creation schemes, measures to protect employees' well-being in the workplace, as well as to address the work-life balance. Examples of job retention schemes were the temporary suspension of employment contracts and the so-called 'SYN-ERGASIA' employment support mechanism, i.e. a short-time work scheme under which employers in all sectors could reduce their full-time employees' working hours up to 50%, paying them the corresponding salary. One such job creation scheme was the employment subsidy programme, under which the state covered the employer and employee social security contributions of newly hired employees (either full-time or part-time) for a specific period of time, among other things.

Examples of measures targeted at protecting employees' well-being in the workplace are using teleworking, as well as providing employees who were members of vulnerable groups with special purpose leave (in case, for instance, that the exercise of their duties required contact with the public). Illustrative of a measure to address the work-life balance was a special purpose leave for employees with Covid-19 infected children.

The policy measures termed 'indirect' included measures which indirectly contributed to employment protection and/or required commitments by employers to keep the number of their employees stable. Examples are repayable advance payments to enterprises, mandatory rent reductions in business properties in the sectors hit by the pandemic, and the suspension of tax and social security obligations for enterprises active in these sectors.

Another distinction among the measures adopted during the Covid-19 related crisis could be made based on the specific objective pursued or the target group.[6] Hence, the measures were largely focused on providing financial support to enterprises and employees, safeguarding health and safety at the workplace, clarifying the timeframe and the type of work provided by enterprises and employees, etc.

The main target groups included employees (the self-employed are a very large category of employees in Greece) and the unemployed. Indicative of policy measures that aimed, for instance, to protect the income of employees were reductions in the rent paid for the employee's main residence and suspending (for a specific period of time) the collection of certified debts from employees working in enterprises whose operations had been affected by the pandemic (including those whose operations had been suspended by the government). Policy measures specifically targeting the self-employed and the unemployed included discounts in paying insurance contributions and time extensions in the allocation of regular and long-term unemployment benefits respectively.

The significant impact of the Covid-19 related crisis on the world of employment in Greece was also reflected in the new working arrangements set out and the shift in existing working conditions towards a more flexible basis. Examples of 'flexibility' are expanding special leave, part-time and shift/rotation work, staggered arrival times and online meetings, with special provisions covering vulnerable groups. Moreover, novel tools and facilities were made available, so as to enable distance working (e.g. user authentication tools and VPN/MFA connections, alongside organizing training programmes to strengthen the digital skills of employees) (Lampropoulou 2021: 7). Before the outbreak of the pandemic, Greece was notably amongst the countries with the lowest rates of teleworking in the EU (Tomei 2021: 261).

Given also the special reference made in this chapter to women's employment in the country, it should be noted that, broadly speaking, the policy measures adopted did not place any particular emphasis on gender. Exceptions concerned mostly the issue of violence against women during the pandemic (see e.g. UNWomen, undated).

Overall, the Greek government's response to the pandemic is deemed to have been, at least at the very first stages of the crisis, relatively timely. The government had been credited with reacting quickly to the pandemic, introducing various restrictions even when cases and fatalities were quite low and eventually managing to prevent a large and uncontrolled influx of cases (Betcherman et al. 2020).

When analyzing the handling of the pandemic's initial phase in Greece, a series of reasons have been put forward by policy analysts to explain the relative governmental 'success' in dealing with the crisis. These include the following: the predominance of evidence-informed policymaking; a timely and firm crisis response, driven by the prior experience of other European countries with the pandemic; the public sector's digital turn and quite effective intra-government coordination; and a communication strategy signaling that public health was a priority, which subsequently led to high citizen compliance with the restrictive measures (see e.g. Ladi 2021).

At the same time, the Greek response to the pandemic had also been presented, broadly speaking, by the international media as an 'unlikely' success story and was often compared to the relative Swedish 'failure' to cope with the crisis.[7] Being regarded as comparable, in terms of their population size and share of urban population, and considering the superiority of the Swedish health system vis-à-vis the Greek NHS, both Greece and Sweden had defied expectations in the first Covid-19 wave in contrasting ways. The key to the relative Greek 'success' seems to have been that government action was framed as a deliberate choice, aiming at prioritizing human lives over the economy and protecting 'at risk groups,' with a strong emphasis on intergenerational responsibility and a high level of personalization. By contrast, the rhetoric of the Swedish government was based on promoting the need to introduce proportional and sustainable voluntary measures and isolate 'at risk groups' (Zahariadis et al. 2021).

Things evolved in a quite different way during the second wave of the pandemic (starting in October 2020), when the delayed response (or the total absence of precautionary measures before the cases got out of control) led to a more severe crisis, whereas the government also failed to inform citizens in good time about the state of emergency. This was accompanied by a further shift towards the personalization of responsibility and individual social responsibility, which was largely criticized by the opposition parties and many citizens (Aspriadis 2021).

The views expressed by citizens with regard to the overall management of the Covid-19 related crisis by the Greek government are reflected in a series of surveys conducted on behalf of the think tank 'DiaNEOsis.'[8] More specifically, based on the findings of the 'seventh wave' of the relevant research (in October 2021), which investigated the attitudes of the population towards the pandemic and pandemic-associated issues, 42% of survey participants argued that the country was heading in the right direction, as opposed to 43.4% of survey participants who agreed with the exact opposite statement: that the country was heading in the wrong direction. Another 11.6% believed that the direction taken was neither right nor wrong, whilst 3.1% of survey participants said that they did not know the answer to the question asked by the researchers.

There was a 'transition' from the initial positive evaluation of the government response to the pandemic to a more negative evaluation. Illustrative of this change in public opinion as regards the way(s) the Greek government handled the Covid-19 related crisis is the significant decrease in the percentage of those claiming that the direction taken was the best: from 85.7% in April 2020, to 56.6% in September 2020, 54.4% in December 2020, 51.4% in January 2021, 45.8% in March 2021, 57.2% in May 2021 and, finally, 42% in October 2021.

In other words, the decrease was continuous, the only exception being the increase in the percentage of those claiming that the direction being taken was the right one in May 2021. Furthermore, when the question asked by the researchers conducting the relevant survey regarded the management of the crisis per se, then most survey respondents (48.4%) agreed with the statement that, generally speaking, the management was as it should be. By contrast, 45.8% of survey respondents believed that the management of the crisis was, overall, wrong. Another 5.8% of survey respondents claimed, on the other hand, that they did not know the answer to this question, whilst the percentage of women who responded that the management of the crisis was overall correct (50.9%) was higher than that of men (46%).

The evaluation of the policy measures adopted by the Greek government during the pandemic also sheds light upon findings which indicate the position of Greece compared to other EU countries. Hence, Greece is argued to have been one of the EU countries that focused more on directly budget-relevant measures (around 17% of GDP) (Wieland 2022: 18). Moreover, alongside Croatia and Malta, the country is reported to have provided less generous support to employees, in comparison to the majority of European countries, which introduced wage compensation at a relatively high percentage of earnings. The Greek government also appears to have prioritized, at least at the beginning of the Covid-19 related crisis, the provision of flat-rate benefits without support for reduced hours of work, as opposed to state support of 60 to 80% of wages (often up to a cap) normally provided by almost all European countries (with requirements for the employer to top up wages further in some countries) (Rubery and Tavora 2020: 77–78).

Additionally, based on the EUROMOD[9] simulation of the impact of the discretionary policy measures, exceptionally introduced or activated by national governments to address the Covid-19 economic challenges and, in particular as far as policies to preserve jobs (wage compensation schemes) and income support to the self-employed are concerned, Greece is one of the EU countries wherein an effort was made to protect the income of low earners. This is an income group that, broadly speaking, in most EU countries received the highest share of wage loss compensation.[10]

Greece is moreover reported to be one of the few European countries where no childcare arrangements were put in place, in order to support those working in health care and other 'essential' sectors and services. These sectors and services played a key role in preventing the collapse of the economy and society during the Covid-19 related crisis; and they are areas where women 'traditionally' outnumber men. On the other hand, Greece is cited as one of the countries that appears to recognize the importance of both parents' earnings for family income, as well as the right of both women and men to an independent income. This statement draws upon the idea that paying for parental leave at the same or higher level than job retention schemes, as was the case in Greece during the pandemic, might be an indication that the importance of care work is recognized; whilst also acknowledging, at the same time, the salience of specific dimensions of gender equality, such as those mentioned above (Rubery and Tavora 2020: 87, 90).

Lastly, the expansion of part-time employment and job rotation, along with the right given to enterprises to transfer their staff from one subsidiary to another (and the discussion on 'lending' employees to other enterprises during the pandemic), were arguably those policy interventions which triggered in Greece the strongest reactions from the opposition and associations representing employees. This stance was largely linked to the concerns about a potential worsening in the working conditions and the overall position of those 'covered' by such provisions (Lalioti 2020a).

Women's Employment During the Pandemic in Greece

Countries such as Greece, that is countries which were harshly hit by the 2008 global economic crisis and were still in the process of recovering at the outbreak of the 2020 pandemic, experienced, broadly speaking, worse economic outcomes during the pandemic compared to countries that were found to be in a better economic position at the beginning of the Covid-19 related crisis. Employment-related outcomes were not an exception.

Illustrative of these statements is the fact that, based on Eurostat data, Greece is one of the EU countries which experienced the greatest median employment income losses between the years 2019 and 2020.[11] Furthermore, the recession in the Greek economy peaked in the second quarter of 2020. While in other countries it was significantly reduced during the third and fourth quarters of that year, in Greece the decline in economic activity remained at high levels (see e.g. Nicolitsas and Filinis 2021: 169; IME-GSEVEE 2021: 12).

Against this backdrop, and before delving into the issue of women's employment during the pandemic in Greece, the first part of this section provides the reader with an overview of structural features of the Greek labour market, as well as key characteristics of female participation in that market. That being said, it is broadly acknowledged that the labour market in Greece suffers from long-term structural weaknesses, such as low participation and employment rates, low productivity and a relatively high degree of segmentation (see e.g. Gatopoulos et al. 2021).

Even before the 2008 crisis, labour participation and employment rates in Greece were among the lowest in the EU and, compared to other advanced European economies, they are still quite low.[12] More specifically, since 2009 the share of the active population in the country has remained relatively stable, fluctuating between 67–68%. In 2019, the (total) employment rate in Greece stood at 56.5%, back at its 2001 level, making it the worst performance in the EU (and 12 percentage points below the EU average). The low employment rate is partly due to the high unemployment rates characterizing the Greek labour market, especially after 2008.

Compared to most advanced economies, labour productivity in Greece is likewise low. Indicative of this outcome is that, in 2019, the value added produced per hour in the country corresponded to 56% of that produced in the EU (on average), and to less than 50% of that produced in northern European economies. The Greek labour market is also highly segmented, as reflected in two major lines of segmentation: first, the substantially higher—compared to most other European economies—share of self-employment; and, second, the division between declared and undeclared employment, with Greece estimated to have one of the highest shares of undeclared workers in the EU.

At the same time, the relatively low participation of women in the Greek labour market, vis-à-vis the respective performances of other European countries, largely explains the overall low labour market participation rate mentioned above. More specifically, based on Eurostat data, in 2021, women's employment rate in Greece, for those aged 20–64, was 52.7%, a percentage well below the EU-27 average of 67.7% for that year. During the fourth trimester of 2021, the activity rate for the same population group was 66% in the case of Greece, once again well below the 73.6% recorded for the EU-27.[13] Figs. 12.1, 12.2 below depict the aforementioned data.

Interestingly, the differences in the female participation rates between Greece and the advanced European economies of the EU-15[14] are concentrated among specific age groups (the younger age groups, i.e. 15–19 years and 20–24 years, and one of the oldest age groups, i.e. 55–59 years) (Lalioti and Nicolitsas 2021: 125). Greece is also one of the EU countries where the inactivity rate for women aged 15–64 exceeded 40% at the start of the Covid-19 crisis; which was much higher than the respective rate for men (EIGE, 2021: 13–14).

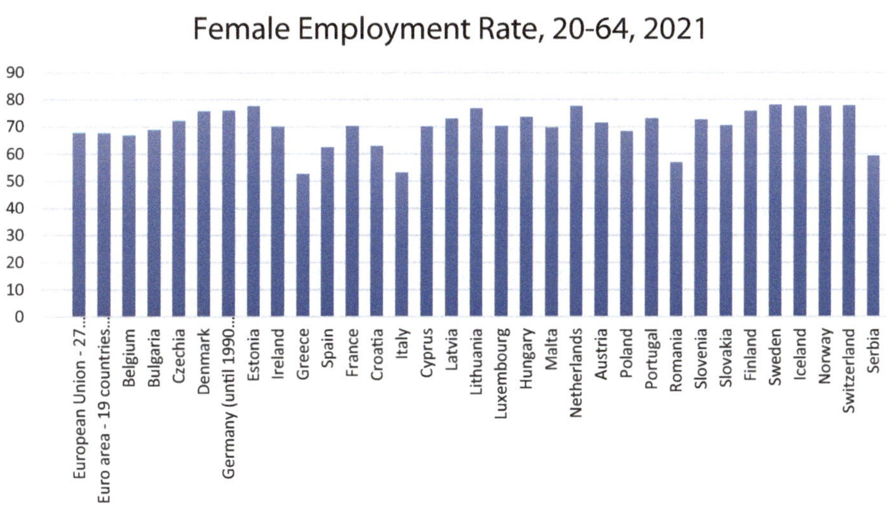

Fig. 12.1 Female employment rate, 20–64, Year 2021

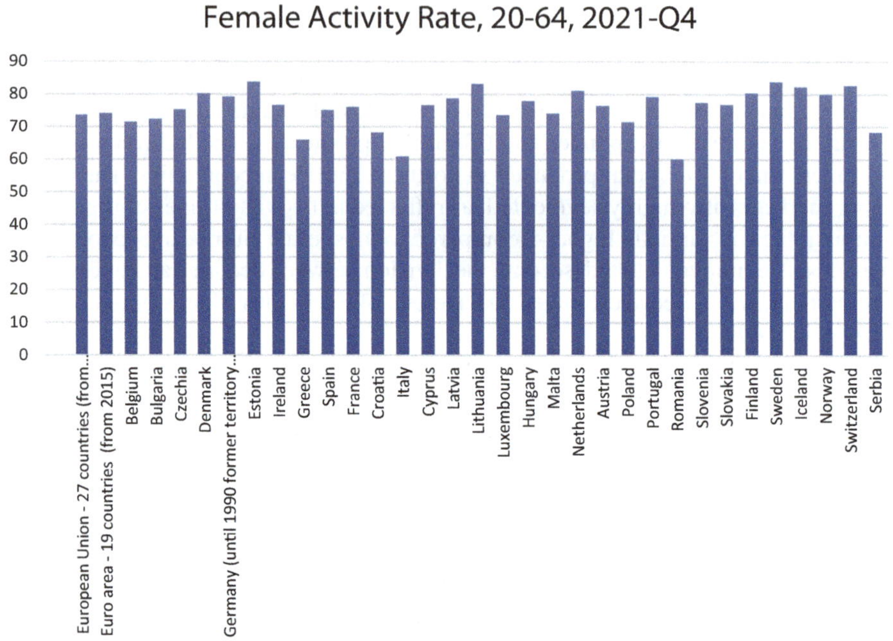

Fig. 12.2 Female activity rate, 20–64, fourth trimester 2021

The female participation rate in the Greek labour market is lower than the EU average and this is also reflected in the fact that Greece is one of the countries typified by the highest gender employment gaps in the EU, i.e. the difference between the employment rates of men and women of working age. For those aged 20–64, in 2020, the relevant percentage was 19.4%.[15] Unfortunately, in the coming decades, the employment gap between men and women in the country is arguably not expected to close (Fasianos and Karakitsios 2020). Greece is, moreover, amongst the EU countries with the highest overall gender earnings gap (40.4%).[16]

Despite the significant progress made, especially since the 1970s and 1980s, with regard to women's employment in Greece, the participation of women in the domestic labour market therefore remains quite low. Women in the country continue for example, to face unemployment rates that are higher than those of men, while also being over-represented in low-paid sectors of the Greek economy (e.g. education). Amongst the factors hindering female employment in Greece are arguably 'overlaps' between employment and family relationships, which are largely linked to the very high number of family businesses in the country and, within this context, women's direct dependence on the financial activity of the (male) spouse (Lalioti 2020b).

Hence, unfortunately, women are still incompletely integrated into the Greek labour market. The turning point for women seems to occur at the age of 25. Until then, men and women are both in education for the most part and differences in their labour market participation and employment rates are relatively small. After the age of 25, however, the situation changes, as exemplified by the greater increase in the male labour market participation rate. This outcome is linked to the substantial number of women who end up not joining the labour force due to family commitments, as well as to the lower demand for female workers, as opposed to male workers, in the post-25 age groups. In turn, these factors are linked to patriarchal attitudes, which are still widespread in Greek society (Katsikas 2021).

Illustrative of the dominance of such attitudes is the fact that the relatively limited presence of women in the Greek labour market does not seem to be heavily stigmatized. Among other things, this attitude is reflected in the findings of Round 4 of the European Social Survey (ESS),[17] according to which, in 2008, 49% of individuals in Greece agreed (strongly or otherwise) that women should be prepared to leave paid work to raise their family; a percentage significantly higher than the 37% of individuals in the EU-15, who agreed with the same statement.

In a similar vein, as the data collected during the 2013 Eurobarometer survey indicate, hiring criteria in the case of women are perceived as different from those for men, and are largely unrelated to their productivity.[18] After taking into account a sample of around 1,000 individuals, 47% of survey participants in Greece answered that they believe that, in the case of a woman, the most important criterion[19] considered by an employer in hiring her was her appearance. This was followed by whether she had children (45% of the survey participants) and her flexibility in terms of working hours (24% of the survey participants).

By contrast, in the case of men, the most important criteria reported by the survey participants were professional experience (55% of the survey participants), the level of qualifications (38% participants), flexibility in terms of working hours (26% participants) and ability for 'professional mobility' (e.g. travelling abroad) (25% participants). The respective European averages were 33, 49 and 35% in terms of the criteria mentioned for women; and 40, 38, 31 and 31% in terms of the criteria mentioned for men.

Since 2020, the pandemic has been a source of new stress in the labour market, in Greece and elsewhere, with women being, over the course of the Covid-19 related crisis, amongst the most harshly hit population groups. The impact of the pandemic on female employment has revealed increased vulnerabilities for women; and therefore arguably makes clear the need to adopt policy measures more directed towards them (see e.g. Katris 2021).

Leaving aside for the moment the (rather minimal) 'positive' effects of the pandemic on women's employment in Greece, such as the offer of permanent contracts to social care workers (in their vast majority women) (Rubery and Tavora 2020: 76), the above assertion on the increased vulnerabilities for women during the pandemic should be largely viewed alongside the fact that the so-called 'informal' economy and low-paid sectors (e.g. education, food services), where women often outnumber men, were amongst the most negatively affected during the Covid-19 related crisis (see e.g. Lalioti 2020a). Unlike in previous recessions, in which male-dominated manufacturing, construction, and other occupations were the most affected, the recession triggered by the pandemic (and the policy measures targeted at decreasing the health impact of the virus) affected female-dominated sectors more, such as hospitality, travel, education, and retail (Herod et al., 2021).

An example of the impact of the Covid-19 related crisis on women's employment in Greece is that, based on data included in a report of the National Institute of Labour and Human Resources (2021) on the effects of the initial stages of the pandemic on the domestic labour market, between 2019 and 2020, the reduction in the work positions occupied by women aged 25–34 equalled 185%.[20] The greatest loss was recorded in positions associated with the provision of personal services (mainly the food/catering sector).

When taking into account, moreover, data concerning salaried employment between January 2018 and October 2020, and without considering parameters such as employment trends at the local level, age or the employment regime (e.g. full- or part-time), the most extended losses in working positions for women were recorded in March and October 2020 and amounted to 17,672 and 15,316 positions respectively. If the focus is exclusively on full-time working positions however, then the negative effects of the pandemic on working positions for women, in October 2020, becomes even more pronounced.

In a similar vein, based on data from the Hellenic Statistical Authority (ELSTAT), during the first trimester of 2020, female unemployment in Greece equalled 19.3% and women were 43% of the workforce.[21] The respective percentages for men were 13.7 and 58.8%. During the second trimester of that year, female unemployment further increased to 19.9% and women comprised 43.3% of the workforce, whilst the respective percentages for men were 14.1 and 58.9%. During the fourth trimester of 2021, female unemployment fell to 17.5% and women were 44.4% of the workforce, with the respective percentages for men being 9.8 and 59.3%.

A higher level of education appears moreover to have worked as a shield against unemployment, more in the case of women than in that of men. Illustrative of this is the fact that, at the beginning of the pandemic, only for educational levels 0–2 the increase recorded in women's unemployment rates was higher than the one recorded for male employees with the same level of education[22] (Lalioti 2020b).

At the same time, the way female unemployment evolved in Greece during the Covid-19 related crisis arguably appears to confirm that, in spite of the clear, negative impact of the pandemic, the crisis may have also pushed women out of unemployment by affecting their availability or their job search. This outcome is, for example, reflected in the Eurostat data concerning unemployment for women aged 20–64. Although, since the second trimester of 2020 (23.6%), the changes recorded from trimester to trimester had been relatively small, unemployment for this category of the population experienced a continuous drop; and, in the fourth trimester of 2021, it came to 17.5%. Yet, these percentages were much higher than the EU-27 averages (7% in the second trimester of 2020 and 6.5% in the fourth trimester of 2021).

Eurostat data also reveal a drop in the percentage of women in Greece aged 20 to 64 who, between the second trimester of 2020 and the first trimester of 2021, had been in part-time employment and temporary contracts (14.5% in 2020-Q2, 12.9% in 2020-Q3, 11.8% in 2020-Q4, 11.2% in 2021-Q1).[23] A reversal to this trend started in the second trimester of 2021, when the respective percentage came to 12.5% (and then 12.5% in 2021-Q3 and 13.5% in 2021-Q4).

When compared to the first trimester of 2020, the data show, moreover, an increase in the percentage of women aged 15–29 belonging to the so-called NEET group (young people not in employment, education or training) in the second trimester of 2020 (from 16 to 18.9% of the total population). Following a fluctuation in the respective percentages, up to the third trimester of 2021 there was a drop, back to the rate reported at the beginning of 2020, only at the end of 2021 (at 15.9%). Still, the Greek performance was worse than the EU-27 averages, which were 16.6 and 14% in 2020-Q2 and 2021-Q4 respectively. Greece is, additionally, amongst the EU countries, where women have experienced the highest, compared to men, income losses from employment.[24]

Employment-related themes are also discussed in research efforts which put at their centre women and their views on a series of employment-related subjects (e.g. the pay gap between men and women, teleworking, etc.) over the course of the pandemic. An example is the survey undertaken by the European Parliament, the findings of which allow, inter alia, a comparison of the relevant situation in Greece to that in other European countries (EP 2022).

Greece is found to be one of the EU countries characterized by the lowest share of women (33%) who believe that the European Parliament should prioritize tackling the pay gap between women and men. Additionally, Greece, alongside other southern European, as well as Eastern European countries, is amongst the countries with the highest rates of women who agree with the statement that the pandemic has had a negative impact on their working lives. The share of women in Greece arguing that the pandemic has had a negative impact on their work-life balance (59%) is likewise one of the largest reported in the EU.

More than a quarter of women in Greece (31%) claimed, moreover, that the pandemic has made them either much more or somewhat more financially dependent on their partner, other relatives or friends. Furthermore, Greece is amongst the EU countries, where more than half of women (60%) agreed with the statement that the pandemic has had a negative impact on their income. Similarly, it is one of the EU countries with the largest shares of women (45%) saying that the pandemic's effects on the job market have reduced their opportunities for paid work, meaning less work for a salary or wage (more than they wanted to).

Greece is also one of the EU countries with the highest share of women (38%) arguing that they did less paid work than desired, because of the increase in work at home. Within this context, the country is, rather unsurprisingly, amongst those with the largest share of women (30%) who responded that, because of the pandemic, they are considering permanently reducing the amount of time allocated to paid work, or that they have already decided to permanently reduce it. The percentage of those arguing that, due to the pandemic, their professional decisions have changed is likewise quite high (47%) (EP 2022).

Additionally, taking into account that Greece has essentially maintained its so-called 'familistic' social model, the impact of the pandemic on women's employment should unavoidably be seen in conjunction with the effects of the Covid-19 related crisis on domestic work. Research conducted by the European Foundation for the Improvement of Living and Working Conditions (broadly known as Eurofound), part of which concerns documenting work experiences during the pandemic, reveals, among other things, a big difference (14 h) in the hours devoted by men and women in Greece to domestic work per week. Greece is placed at the very opposite end of the spectrum in relation to Scandinavian countries, but also countries sometimes included in the southern European social model, such as France. Furthermore, Greece is reported to be one of the EU countries where women, at least during the early Covid-19 crisis, were most affected in terms of the hours lost. More specifically, the respective decrease in Greece equalled 8.3% (EF 2020).

Considering, moreover, that the insufficient care infrastructure in Greece at least partly accounts for pushing women in particular to fill gaps in care (European Institute for Gender Equality, 2021: 38), the pandemic is deemed to have exposed the increased pressure faced by women, compared to men, in their effort to cope with the demands of both a professional and family life. This outcome appears to have become more pronounced, especially in the case of families with young children at home and when parents were in a teleworking regime.[25] The share of women who worked from home (on an exclusive or partial basis) was higher (75%) than the respective percentage of men (63%). This finding may be associated with the type of work and the employment sector (women, for example, outnumber men in office positions and in the education sector). Women were also more satisfied than men with teleworking (the respective percentages were 60.6 and 54.3%).

At the same time, the share of women who stated that, under the emergency measures adopted during the first wave of the pandemic in Greece, they would stop working if they could, was higher than that of men who made the same statement (14.2 and 9.3% respectively). This finding may be understood in light of the increased difficulties faced by women in combining their work with other activities, as reflected in the much higher percentage of women (33.9%), compared to that of men (23.6%), who reported that, due to work, they neglected their personal needs; or that, they have to use ‘some kind of magic’ in order to be able to combine work with other activities (36.8% of women compared to 23.2% of men who agreed with this statement).

The pandemic is also argued to have delayed women’s entry into the labour market (for those who had either planned to enter the labour market for the first time or after their children had reached school age). Furthermore, the policy measures taken during the pandemic, such as school closures, are expected to contribute, at least in the medium term, to (further) severe losses at the professional level for women (Markantonatou 2021).

Such arguments are closely linked to the idea that women, especially in familistic social models, continue to be regarded as responsible for the provision of care towards children and elderly family members, as well as for ‘home’-related issues in general. They are also related, however, to undeniable facts, such as the significant reduction observed during the pandemic in the provision of childcare services by older family members, such as grandparents, who often offered this type of assistance to working mothers (see e.g. Zamarro Perez-Arce and Prados, 2020).

Another aspect of women's employment over the course of the Covid-19 related crisis in Greece concerns the increased difficulties with regard to the labour market integration of 'specific' categories of women. These women tend to face significant problems in entering the labour market even under 'normal' circumstances, that is, not in emergency and/or crisis situations such as the outbreak of the virus in late 2019/ early 2020. The labour market situation of women who are victims of trafficking, for example, seems to have been aggravated during the pandemic. Job opportunities were fewer and many victims who had managed to secure a job before the Covid-19 related crisis were fired.[26]

Additionally, the rather limited, at this stage, research findings regarding the impact of the pandemic on gender-based discrimination in the labour market point to the sharp increase in this type of discrimination, and, therefore, in job insecurity for women in the workplace. In Greece (and elsewhere), the Covid-19 related crisis appears however to have been used as an excuse for further undermining women's rights in the labour market.[27]

The discriminatory treatment of women can take many forms: from not hiring a woman for a job (in spite of her having qualifications and experience that are higher or at least equal to the male employee who is eventually hired), to being offered unequal access, compared to men, to job-related benefits.[28] The expansion of flexible forms of employment, such as teleworking, has, moreover, often been criticized for being associated with low-quality work, as well as for paving the road for the further deterioration of women's labour market rights (Lalioti and Nicolitsas 2021).

Lastly, the pandemic has shed light upon how employment-related themes are closely linked and should therefore be viewed alongside issues such as mental health, which has been broadly acknowledged to have deteriorated during the crisis. Greece is amongst the EU countries with the largest share of women (41%) who believe that workplace and office closures and their effects (temporary/forced unemployment, homeworking, etc.) have had a major negative impact on their mental health (EP, 2022).

Overall, the Covid-19 related crisis has led to different outcomes in comparison to the 2008 financial crisis.[29] During the latter, and despite the intense pressure exerted on women to return to 'traditional' roles as mothers and caregivers, as well as the extension of labour market precariousness, when it comes to female participation in employment, there was 'resilience.' The financial crisis arguably failed to overturn equality gains for women, embedded in both work and everyday practices.

The Covid-19 pandemic, on the other hand, along with the policies adopted to restrain the health impact of the virus, has had negative effects on gender equality, as reflected in the fact that, for most women, the 'return' to care during the pandemic was not a decision emanating from their refusal to participate in the insecurity prevailing in the domestic labour market. By contrast, the prevalence of conservative stereotypes about the role of women as selfless caregivers, which emphasizes, inter alia, reconciliation between work and family life as an issue concerning exclusively women, is found at the centre of the long-term problem of the relatively low female participation in the Greek labour market.

Conclusions

Based on extensive desk research and data concerning different aspects of female employment in Greece, this chapter provided the reader with an overview of the pandemic and the relevant government response in the country, with special reference to women's employment. Hence, the chapter has highlighted the relative 'success' in dealing with the initial phase of the Covid-19 related crisis, compared with the later stages of the pandemic, but also the effects on female employment, as exemplified by the fall in women's income from employment and the increased pressure exerted on them to combine work and family life.

Elaborating on the discussion in this chapter, in Greece, as also in the case of other countries, it is therefore likely that the crisis triggered by the pandemic will aggravate the existing polarization in the domestic labour market, by means of further widening the gap in participation in it, among other things. Gender will be at the centre of this gap, and women with children in particular are expected to be the ones who, in addition to being more likely than other categories of workers to accept a reduction in their working hours (short-time working), will then have to deal with the possibility of being trapped in low-paid work. Furthermore, as women drop out of the labour market, there is a good chance that many will never return, meaning that the effects of the recession on female employability are likely to be felt for years.

At the same time however, taking into account that women make up, broadly speaking, the majority of employees in sectors harshly hit by the Covid-19 related crisis (e.g. health, care, education, etc.), the crisis may also arguably function as a 'window of opportunity' for women to become more involved in decision-making on ways out of the crisis, as well as on the relevant recovery processes. Similarly, the pandemic may open the road towards policy interventions, which will enhance women's employability, whilst also dealing with issues hindering female labour market participation, in a way that will reassure the equal treatment of all citizens regardless of their gender. This means strengthening, for example, childcare policies.

The state and all stakeholders should also become, however, more engaged in the effort to remove negative stereotypes; against women in general and women's degree of commitment to professional life in particular. These stereotypes are directly linked to the severe shortcomings of the Greek welfare state, such as the limited scope of social care services. They are mostly rooted, nevertheless, in patriarchal perceptions and norms, which often appear to be almost unshakable and certainly lead to the perpetuation of discrimination against women.

The above should, moreover, all be viewed in conjunction with the need to rethink the types and the content of work in contemporary society, and especially how these types and content are assessed. This includes acknowledging the necessity of 'positively' re-evaluating the work performed by women. The Covid-19 related crisis arguably made the unequal division of work in private spaces between men and women more visible, with unpaid-domestic work, often carried out by women, to have grown to the point that it triggered an international debate on a transition to an 'economy of care.'

The work done by the so-called 'essential occupations,' which played a key role during the pandemic and where women are over-represented, likewise needs to be re-evaluated. Examples are occupations in the fields of education and social care, which are not regarded as being on the front-line of the economy and are low-paid. Broadly speaking, the pandemic arguably opened up opportunities for re-negotiating gender roles at home, but also in the world of employment in general (Kambouri, 2022).

Women's 'vulnerabilities' with regard to the labour market, in Greece and elsewhere, should therefore be discussed alongside various themes highlighted under the impact of the Covid-19 pandemic; some are put at the centre of other chapters in this collective volume. As Marcel Gauchet, the prominent French historian and philosopher, put it we should now pay more attention to understanding issues that before the Covid-19 related crisis we essentially chose to ignore. In his own words: 'We were moving like sleepwalkers: the pandemic woke us up' (Gauchet, 2020).

Notes

1. This and the next paragraph are based on Petridou and Zahariadis (2021).
2. See https://covid19.gov.gr.
3. The information in this and the next two paragraphs is based on https://covid19.gov.gr.
4. The website of the European Commission includes detailed information on the support measures adopted by the Commission under the state aid and EU state aid rules. Also see European Commission, Greece.
5. This and the next two paragraphs are based on Nicolitsas and Filinis (2021).
6. This and the next paragraph draw mainly on Lalioti (2020a). Otherwise the source is given.
7. This paragraph is based on Narlikar and Sottilotta (2021). Otherwise the source is given.
8. This and the next two paragraphs are based on DiaNEOsis (2021).
9. EUROMOD is a tax-benefit microsimulation model for the EU that enables researchers and policy analysts to calculate, in a comparable manner, the effects of taxes and benefits on household incomes and work incentives for the population of each country and for the EU as a whole.
10. See https://ec.europa.eu/eurostat/statistics-explained.
11. See https://ec.europa.eu/eurostat/statistics-explained.
12. This and the next paragraph draw on Katsikas (2021).
13. See https://ec.europa.eu/eurostat/databrowser/view.
14. The member states of the European Union prior to the accession of ten candidate countries on 1 May 2004.
15. See https://ec.europa.eu/eurostat/statistics-explained/index.php.

16 This synthetic indicator measures the impact of the three combined factors on the average earnings of all women of working age—whether employed or not employed—compared to men: (1) the average hourly earnings; (2) the monthly average of the number of hours paid (before any adjustment for part-time work); and (3) the employment rate. See https://ec.europa.eu/eurostat/statistics-explained/index.php.
17 See European Social Survey.
18 This and the next paragraph are based on European Parliament, (2013).
19 The survey participants were offered the opportunity to provide multiple answers.
20 This and the next paragraph draw on National Institute of Labour and Human Resources (2021) and Lalioti (2020b).
21 This paragraph is based on the Labour Force Survey (LFS) data published by ELSTAT (in Greek) in the period between June 2020 (for labour force information on the first trimester of 2020) and March 2022 (for labour force information on the fourth trimester of 2021).
22 Based on the classification of the 'International Standard Classification of Education' (ISCED, 2011). More specifically, ISCED 0 accounts for 'Early childhood education' ('less than primary,' for educational attainment), ISCED 1 for 'Primary education' and ISCED 2 for 'Lower secondary education.'
23 See https://ec.europa.eu/eurostat/databrowser/view.
24 See also https://ec.europa.eu/eurostat/statistics-explained.
25 This and the next paragraph are based on Symeonaki et al. (2021).
26 See https://www.kmop.gr.
27 See https://www.amnesty.gr/news.
28 See e.g. https://www.synigoros.gr.
29 This and the next paragraph are based on Kambouri (2022).

References

Aspriadis, N. 2021. Managing Covid-19 pandemic crisis: The case of Greece, *Journal of International Crisis and Risk Communication Research* 4 (2): 387–412.

Betcherman, G. et al. 2020. Reacting quickly and protecting jobs: The short-term impacts of the Covid-19 lockdown on the Greek labour market, *IZA Discussion Papers*, No. 13516, Bonn: Institute of Labour Economics (IZA).

DiaNEOsis. 2021. *Panhellenic public opinion survey on the Covid-19 pandemic 7th wave.* Athens: DiaNEOsis (in Greek).

Eurofound. 2020. *Living, working and Covid-19,* Covid-19 series. Luxembourg: Publications Office of the European Union.

European Institute for Gender Equality. 2021. *Gender equality and the socio-economic impact of the Covid-19 pandemic*, Research note, Vilnius: EIGE.

European Parliament 2013. *Women and gender inequalities in the context of the crisis*, European Parliament, Eurobarometer Flash Survey, Brussels: European Parliament.

European Parliament. 2022. *Eurobarometer flash survey: Women in times of Covid-19.* Brussels: European Parliament.

Fasianos, A., and A. Karakitsios. 2020. *Female force participation in Greece,* Presentation. Athens: Council of Economic Advisors.

Foundation for Economic and Industrial Research. 2022. The Greek economy, *Quarterly Report*, No. 1/22, (in Greek).

Gatopoulos G. et al. 2021. Evaluating the impact of labour market reforms in Greece during 2010–2018, *GreeSE Paper*, No. 156, Hellenic Observatory Papers on Greece and Southeast Europe.

Gauchet M. 2020. We were moving like sleepwalkers: The pandemic woke us up, *To Vima tis Kyriakis*, May 10, (in Greek).

Herod A. et al. 2021. The impact of the Covid-19 pandemic upon employment and inequality in the Mediterranean EU: An early look from a labour geography perspective, *European Urban and Regional Studies*, 1–18.

IME-GSEVEE 2021. *The impact of the pandemic upon enterprises*, Report produced by the Institute of Small Enterprises of the General Confederation of Professional Craftsmen of Greece, (in Greek).

Kambouri, N. 2022. Gender, care and policies reconciling work and family during the pandemic. *Social Policy* 16: 76–93 (in Greek).

Katris, C. 2021. Unemployment and Covid-19 impact in Greece: A Vector Autoregression (VAR) data analysis. *Engineering Proceedings* 5: 41.

Katsikas, D. (2021). The Greek labour market: Key features and trends before the pandemic, In: *Youth Inclusion and Gender Equality in the Greek Labour Market: Trends, Challenges, and Lessons from the Nordic Countries*, eds. D. Katsikas, D. Nicolitsas, and T. Fløtten, Athens: Papazissis.

Katsikas, D.; Nicolitsas, D., and Fløtten, T. (2021). Summary and conclusions, In: *Youth Inclusion and Gender Equality in the Greek Labour Market: Trends, Challenges, and Lessons from the Nordic Countries*, eds. D. Katsikas, D. Nicolitsas, and T. Fløtten, Athens: Papazissis.

Ladi, S., A. Angelou, and D. Panagiotatou. 2021. Regaining trust: Evidence-informed policymaking during the first phase of the Covid-19 crisis in Greece. *South European Society and Politics*. https://doi.org/10.1080/13608746.2021.1983932.

Lalioti, V. 2020a. *Employment at the time of Covid-19: An attempt to outline policy interventions relevant to the world of employment and the discussion on the next day of the pandemic*. Athens: National Institute of Labour and Human Resources (in Greek).

Lalioti, V. 2020b. *Aspects of discrimination against women in the Greek labour market*. Athens: National Institute of Labour and Human Resources (in Greek).

Lalioti, V. and Nicolitsas, D. (2021). Young women in the Greek labour market, In: *Youth Inclusion and Gender Equality in the Greek Labour Market: Trends, Challenges, and Lessons from the Nordic Countries*, eds. D. Katsikas, D. Nicolitsas, and T. Fløtten, Athens: Papazissis.

Lampropoulou, M. (2021). Public administration in the Era of Covid-19: Policy responses and reforms underway, Greek and European Economy Observatory, *ELIAMEP Policy Paper*, No. 74/2021.

Markantonatou, M. 2021. From austerity to the pandemic and back again? Lockdown politics in Greece, *Historical Social Research* 46 (4): 143–162.

Narlikar, A., and C.E. Sottilotta. 2021. Pandemic narratives and policy responses: West European governments and Covid-19. *Journal of European Public Policy* 28 (8): 1238–1257.

National Institute of Labour and Human Resources 2021. The impact of the Covid-19 pandemic on the labour market, *Thematic Bulletin*, No. 5, March, (in Greek).

Nicolitsas, D., and Filinis, K. 2021. The impact of the pandemic on the Greek labour market, In: *Youth Inclusion and Gender Equality in the Greek Labour Market: Trends, Challenges, and Lessons from the Nordic Countries*, eds. D. Katsikas, D. Nicolitsas, and T. Fløtten, Athens: Papazissis.

Petridou, E., and N. Zahariadis. 2021. Staying at home or going out? Leadership response to the Covid-19 crisis in Greece and Sweden. *Journal of Contingencies and Crisis Management* 29: 293–302.

Rubery, J., and Tavora, I. 2020. The Covid-19 crisis and gender equality: Risks and opportunities, in: Vanhercke B., Spasova, S., and Fronteddu, B. (eds.), *Social policy in the European Union: State of play 2020 facing the pandemic*, Brussels: European Trade Union Institute (ETUI) and European Social Observatory (OSE).

Symeonaki, M., et al. 2020. Work, family, companionship and parenting during the first wave of the Covid-19 pandemic. *Social Policy* 13: 5–43 (in Greek).

Tomei, M. 2021. Teleworking: A curse or a blessing for gender equality and work-life balance? *Intereconomics* 5: 260–264.

UNWomen (undated), Implementation of the agreed conclusions of the 60th session of the Commission on the Status of Women on Women's Empowerment and the link to sustainable development: Contribution by Greece, https://www.unwomen.org.

Wieland, V. 2022. *Overview of how major economies have responded to the Covid-19 pandemic: Growth trajectories, debt sustainability, best practices*, Brussels: European Parliament.

Zahariadis, N., et al. 2021. Policy styles and political trust in Europe's national responses to the Covid-19 Crisis. *Policy Studies*. https://doi.org/10.1080/01442872.2021.2019211.

Zamarro, G., Perez-Arce, F., and Prados, M.J. 2020. *Gender differences in the Impact of Covid-19*, https://ktla.com/wp-content/uploads/sites/4/2020/06.

Chapter 13
The Covid-19 Pandemic in Austria: With Special Reference to Migrant Care Workers

Kai Leichsenring, Selma Kadi, Andrea E. Schmidt, and Heidemarie Staflinger

Abstract This chapter presents the experiences of a country with a well-established welfare state during the Covid crisis. Unprecedented policy measures stabilized the labour market, key infrastructures and the health system. However, the Pandemic also highlighted a number of major shortcomings of the regulatory framework of social and health policy responses. A special focus is being put on long-term care as this sector has been hit particularly in terms of mortality, related structural shortcomings and political debates. On average, 25% of deaths during the pandemic have occurred in residential care settings, long-term care settings were badly equipped with protective gear, and the isolation of residents in care homes triggered ample discussions about human rights. One of the idiosyncrasies of the Austrian long-term care system is its reliance on migrant care workers both in the formal delivery of services and in the sector of so-called private live-in care. Although Austria is one of few countries where some kind of regulation of personal carers was implemented, this "dualisation of the workforce" keeps low-skilled migrant personal carers in the secondary labour market and continues to divide the care workforce. While working conditions and wages are already critical in formal care delivery, the situation of migrant live-in carers, in their majority female, is often precarious. The chapter exposes this specificity in quantitative terms as well as in its partly dramatic consequences during the Pandemic when lockdowns and travel restrictions showed the limits of this type of care delivery. In the long run, it is argued, shortages of the workforce in long-term have to be addressed by systemic reforms that strengthen integrated care delivery with decent working conditions, and ethical recruitment strategies that ensure equal rights for all care workers.

K. Leichsenring (✉) · S. Kadi
European Centre for Social Welfare Policy and Research, Vienna, Austria
e-mail: leichsenring@euro.centre.org

A. E. Schmidt
National Public Health Institute, Vienna, Austria

H. Staflinger
Chamber of Labour for Upper Austria, Linz, Austria

C. Aspalter (ed.), *Covid-19 Pandemic*,
https://doi.org/10.1007/978-981-99-2497-4_13

Keywords Covid-19 Pandemic · Austria · Long-term care system · Migrant workers · Working conditions · Wages · Equal rights

Introduction

Assessing the performance of countries and governmental strategies during the pandemic has become a widespread exercise which is, however, hampered by poor and scarcely comparable data-bases. Tables on excess mortality may offer a more comprehensive picture (see Fig. 13.1 for Austria and selected European countries) as the pure glance at SARS-CoV-2 incidence, prevalence and death rates remains laden with a wide range of confounding variables such as testing rates, vaccination rates and diverse data gathering methods. Moreover, the fixation on epidemiological data has often overshadowed issues of everyday life that had been in 'crisis mode' already before the onset of the pandemic.

Notwithstanding the country's well-equipped hospital sector, also Austrian health care staff had to face serious bottlenecks and years of unconceivable stress. While the acute health sector thus was immediately in the spotlight of the pandemic, it took some time until the long-term care sector gained attention. On the one hand, this caused a high incidence and deaths in residential care homes because of, among other things, lack of hygiene procedures and protective gear (altogether, more than 40% of deaths during the pandemic had occurred in care homes by February 2021; Leichsenring et al. 2021); day-care facilities and home care services, too, were suspended to a large degree.

On the other hand, with the onset of the first lockdown and related travel restrictions, an area that has become a distinguishing specificity of long-term care in

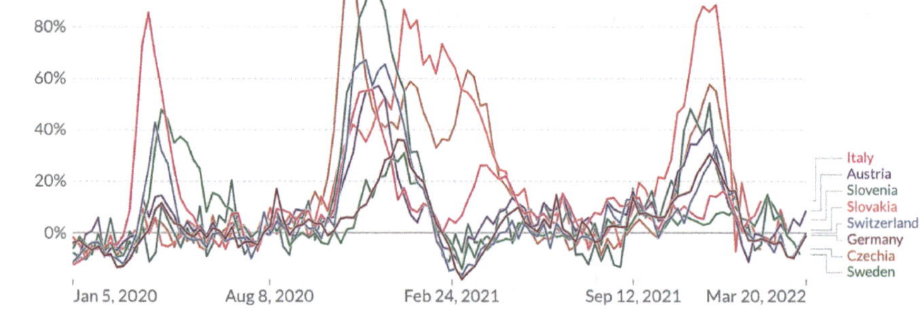

Fig. 13.1 Excess Mortality in Selected European Countries, 2020–2022. *Note* Comparisons across countries are affected by differences in the completeness of death reporting. *Sources*: Mathieu et al. (2020), Human Mortality Database (2022), World Mortality Dataset (2022); see also Karlinsky and Kobak (2021)

Austria hit the headlines—live-in care provided by mainly female migrant workers from Romania, the Slovak Republic and other East European countries. Although Austria is one of few countries where some kind of regulation of personal carers was implemented, the low-skilled migrant personal carers' working conditions and wages had been criticized as precarious already before the pandemic (Bachinger 2016; Leiblfinger and Prieler 2018; Winkelmann et al. 2015). Moreover, Austria also relies heavily on migrant and/or foreign-born workers in the formal long-term care workforce, where staff shortages have generally increased during the pandemic.

This chapter will therefore focus on the challenges and consequences of the pandemic on migrant care workers. We will discuss the significance of migration for the LTC sector in Austria (for an overview of the Austrian LTC system see Bachner et al. 2018; Leichsenring 2017) and particularly the situation of the about 59,000 live-in migrant carers. Before doing so we shall provide, first, an overview of the pandemic in Austria, and secondly, a brief outline of the unprecedented public support measures of a developed welfare state to stabilize the economy, the labor market, key infrastructures and the health system. The chapter will conclude with some considerations regarding the future of migrant carers under conditions of ongoing crises.

The Pandemic Development in Austria

On 27 January 2020, SARS-CoV-2 (labelled '2019 new type of coronavirus') was classed as a notifiable disease in Austria (BMSGPK 2022a). The first case was detected in January 2020 in Tyrol (Kreidl et al. 2020). The Austrian government issued travel warnings for China, Iran, Israel and South Korea in March. This was followed by further travel restrictions and efforts to support citizens in returning to Austria (Schmidt et al. 2020). The first lockdown was imposed on 16 March after cases had climbed to 1,192 (Łaszewska et al. 2021).

The development of the pandemic between 1 January 2020 and 31 January 2022 can be described in seven different phases (BMSGPK 2022a): The first phase lasted until 15 March 2020 and included the detection of the first cases. The second phase starts with the first lockdown on 16 March 2020 and lasted until the relaxation of rules after 11 April 2020. The third phase, from 12 April to 31 August was characterized by increased relaxation of rules. During the fourth phase from 1 September 2020 to 14 February 2021 case numbers were rising again. On 14 November 2020, Austria had the highest rate of new infections worldwide (APA 2020). The fifth phase from 15 February to 6 June 2021 included mass vaccinations, increased testing and the reopening of schools (BMSGPK 2022a). Phase six from 7 June until 31 of December 2021 included again increased relaxation of rules, more vaccinations, more tests and screenings in schools. Phase seven, which started at the beginning of 2022 was characterized by the dominance of the Omicron variant of SARS-CoV-2 and again rising case numbers. On 1 February 2022, daily new infections were at an all-time high of 44,183 cases (Kleine Zeitung 2022).

The pandemic highlighted fractures in the Austrian long-term care sector. In particular, in care homes (nursing and residential care) residents were considered as risk groups for being affected by severe cases of Covid-19. Striking a balance between residents' right to self-determination versus protection of their health was challenging also in care home settings. Overall, by February 2022 the cumulative number of deaths linked to Covid-19 among care home residents amounted to 6.35% in Austria, as a share of the number of residents living in care homes (Comas-Herrera et al. 2022). This places Austria in the middle range by international comparison for the countries where data are available, with approximately 13% in Scotland, and less than 1% in South Korea.[1]

Overall, international analyses show that overall incidence correlates with incidence in care homes: In countries where deaths of people living in the community were low, deaths of care home residents were also low. In Austria, while the number of cases in Austrian care homes during the first wave was estimated to be low in comparison with other countries, by February 2021 about 43% of deaths due to Covid-19 had occurred in care homes (Comas-Herrera et al. 2021, 2022; Leichsenring et al. 2021; Schmidt et al. 2021).

As the pandemic spread and with vaccination rates rising, the share of all deaths among care home residents due to Covid-19 amounted to 28.4%[2] by July 2022 (as a share of all deaths) in Austria.[3] Among long-term care staff in nursing homes, two people had died by 20 July 2022 in Austria according to data from the states (Bundesländer).

Government Response and Its Evaluation

The government response included mandatory reporting of Covid-19 cases, isolation of those who were infected, lockdowns, social distancing and a fund to support measures in various areas (e.g. healthcare, economy, public order, education) (Antony et al. 2021).

The measures can also be distinguished based on their main aims. Some measures aimed at limiting the spread of the virus, others at monitoring and information on the SARS-CoV-2 situation, some at strengthening healthcare, others at mitigating the effects of measures to confront SARS-CoV-2, and some at the evaluation of measures. We cannot discuss all of them in detail, but provide an overview with examples in Table 13.1.

The Austrian government introduced measures based on the *Epidemiegesetz* (law concerning epidemics) and subsequently the Covid-19 Maßnahmengesetz (Covid-19 measures law) (Antony et al. 2021). While the former regulates which diseases have to be registered and enables the government to close e.g. schools, the latter includes various mitigating measures. The Covid-19 Maßnahmengesetz includes the introduction of a fund to finance mitigating measures addressing various areas of the welfare state: the stabilization of the health system, revitalization of the labor market, support of public order and safety, measures to support the education system, measures to

Table 13.1 Types of measures to confront SARS-Cov2

Aim of measure	Examples
Limit the spread of SARS-CoV-2	Travel warnings, mandatory reporting of cases, isolation in case of infection, lockdowns, social distancing, home office, distance learning, testing, vaccination campaign
Monitor and inform about the SARS-CoV-2 situation	Dashboard by the Austrian Agency for Health for humans, animals & plants (AGES); 'Gecko crisis committee' to evaluate, provide advice, and support the government; map with traffic lights to communicate about the SARS-CoV-2 risk in different regions in Austria
Strengthen healthcare	Tests, vaccinations; long covid centers
Mitigate the effects of measures to limit the spread of Covid-19	Financial support; changes in regulations of isolation to keep critical infrastructure going; corridors for 24 h-carers
Evaluation of the government response	Analysis of 'saved lives', effects on other health issues in terms of access to healthcare, effects on mental health

mitigate the loss of income and to support the economy. The law also enabled the government to restrict access to specific areas except for specified activities (e.g. helping someone in need).

Policies included the Austrian short-time work scheme, in which the working hours of employees can be reduced to zero hours for three months and 80–90% of the loss of income is compensated by public subsidies (Schnetzer et al. 2020; EF 2020a). The scheme consists of 5 different phases with varying regulations (phase 1 lasted until end of May 2020, phase 5 started in July 2021) (AK 2022). A version of this measure was already negotiated by social partners to avoid unemployment following the Great Recession in 2008. To deal with the effects of SARS-CoV-2, this was renegotiated. By 1 April 2020, applications for short-time work had been submitted for about 250,000 workers.

This meant that a significant number of workers in Austria could keep their job and did not have to drastically reduce consumption. The government also introduced a top-up of the emergency assistance allowance (EF 2020c), a family hardship fund (EF 2020f) and a measure to avoid energy shutdowns in case of payment difficulties (EF 2020g). It implemented a 15 billion Covid-19 fund from which companies that had experienced at least 40% sales loss due to Covid-19 measures would receive subsidies (EF 2020d) and a 3 billion fund to pay subsidies for companies starting new investments (EF 2020e). To keep critical infrastructure running, some employees at the Viennese energy provider Wien Energie self-isolated (EF 2020h). Several professions received bonus payments (e.g. EF 2020i).

At the beginning of the pandemic, LTC workers faced shortages of PPEs, and were at times even explicitly exempted from protection regulations. As the pandemic progressed, legislation and regulations were adapted to better account for safety of both residents and staff. High requirements resulted in increased burden for LTC staff. For instance, due to changing work schedules, additional efforts required to support otherwise lonely residents, to communicate with informal carers and family members of residents, and to deal with increased hygiene regulations (BMGSPK 2020; Staflinger and Schmidt 2020).

The Ministry of Social Affairs, Health, Care and Consumer Protection (BMSGPK) issued recommendations for the LTC sector focusing on protective equipment (May 2020), dealing with essential staff who had contact with someone who tested positive (March 2020), relief of visiting restrictions in care homes (April 2020) and return to everyday life in these institutions (June 2020) (BMSGPK 2020). Workers in the social and health care sectors received bonus payments (EF 2020j), medical prescriptions could be issued electronically (EF 2020k), and working parents and carers could access subsidized care time (EF 2020l),

In terms of LTC, the government immediately introduced the *Covid-100 Millionen €Sonderfonds für Pflege* (Covid-19 100 million €special fund for care) (EF 2020b) that consisted of financial transfers from the federal state to the provinces, which are responsible for procuring LTC services and facilities. The funds should be used, for example, to employ extra staff, and to provide information. At a later stage, these funds were also used to facilitate travel from and to Austria of personal carers (see below).

Measures in the LTC sector in Austria included those supporting preparedness (e.g. creation of taskforce, keeping spas empty in case of need for more space, recommendations from the ministry), prevention (restriction of visits, isolation of inhabitants returning from hospital), control and management of infections (supervision for staff, support from external staff), support to mitigate the deteriorating quality of life of residents in care homes, e.g. by enabling virtual communication with relatives (BMSGPK, 2020). To expand workforce capacities in the health and long-term care sector in Austria, the following measures were taken (Schmidt and Bachner 2020):

Childcare facilities/schools remained open for children of health and care staff (critical professions).

The requirements in licensing and registration of health and care professionals were abridged.

Medical students were recruited and could work in return for ECTS points.

Conscientious objectors in civilian service as well as people in military service were hired to support staff in hospitals and care homes.

Staffing plans in hospitals and long-term care facilities were adapted, e.g. by establishing separate teams.

Medical staff was recruited to analyze which specific tasks could be carried out by non-medical staff, e.g. students and/or retired people.

Additional safety measures were promoted for health care workers in private practice, including the use of telemedicine.

By April 2020, some ad-hoc initiatives were started to facilitate travel of 24-hour carers from Eastern European countries to ensure that people with live-in carers continue to receive care, but with marginal impact only (Bachmann 2020a, b).

Many measures were not organized federally, but locally. As an example, the Viennese *Kuratorium Wiener Pensionisten-Wohnhäuser* (Holicek 2020) which is the largest, (quasi-)public provider of care homes in Vienna, had to organize training for staff on topics such as dealing with people living with dementia in case of the need of isolation, preparation of isolations, dealing with deceased inhabitants who were tested positive before passing away, care for those who tested positive and those who had contact with someone who tested positive as well dealing with laundry and waste from those who tested positive.

The pandemic board prepared various communication formats for care homes, residents received a biweekly magazine and could often also listen to, for instance, radio programs produced locally in care homes. Leisure activities (concerts, phone calls) were increased to combat loneliness while lockdown measures prohibited usual activities. Child care, discussion rounds and psychological support were offered to staff. The Kuratorium prepared videos on hygiene management in eleven languages for staff. However, care homes in general felt widely neglected and/or disadvantaged as against acute health care facilities when it came to support measures, coordination or the delivery of protective gear. This was underlined drastically by the umbrella organization of Austrian care homes (Lebensweltheim 2020).

Socioeconomic factors influenced who was affected in which way by the pandemic more directly but also who was particularly affected by the measures to manage the pandemic (Haas et al. 2021). The evaluation of the management of the pandemic (Antony et al. 2021) found that particularly older people living with dementia receiving care were additionally disoriented due to the pandemic. People receiving care had reduced access to therapies. Individuals living in senior and care homes were in the early stages faced with severe restrictions, in particular by the limitation or even complete prohibition of receiving visits. Those who worked in LTC were burdened through the need to wear protective gear, and the additional lack of staff due to infections. Research on the experiences of care staff in Tyrol (Flatscher-Thöni et al. 2022) found that the measures (temporarily) weakened the paradigm change towards person-centered care in residential homes. Isolation of those who were in contact with someone who tested positive, loss of routines through the prohibition of personal visits and visits from therapists, mandatory testing as well as the wearing of masks meant that the provision of person-centered care was challenging and created situations of moral distress for staff.

The Ministry of Social Affairs, Health, Care and Consumer Protection described the prevalence and reviewed the response to Covid-19 in care homes, showing the substantial lack of protective gear in care homes: only one third of them were able to provide FFP2 masks, in 30% of care homes there was even a lack of disinfectant (BMSGPK 2020). The report suggested five areas to improve preparedness for similar situations in the future:

> General framework conditions for care in times of crisis need to ensure the involvement of representatives of the sector in local, regional and national crisis task forces to discuss different perspectives in the tension between safety and personal freedom.
>
> Staffing in residential care facilities needs to be addressed by regional workforce management across facilities and organizations, by additional and more specialized workforce

(e.g. Covid-19 experts, hygiene specialists), and by ensuring the involvement of families, volunteers and other potentially supportive resources.

Cooperation of LTC facilities and services with primary and secondary health care, including therapists, needs to be improved, starting from more and enhanced mutual information, and the improvement of telemedicine and e-health, including related training of staff.

Participation and self-determination of residents as well as the de-medicalisation of LTC have been promoted and improved over the past decades in Austria. The pandemic has contributed to a sudden backlash that undermined quality of life and the involvement of residents and their families in decision-making, the access to information and the possibility to meet with friends and family.

Further research on the impact of Covid-19 is needed, including a better link of data bases (registry data) and studies about the impact of the pandemic on different stakeholders.

Migrant Care Workers During the Covid Crisis

To understand migrant care work in Austria, it is necessary to distinguish between employees in the formal care sector with a migrant background (that might include commuters from neighboring countries), and those who provide care in private households, usually living-in with the person being cared for. The former group constitutes about one third of nurses and other health professionals in the acute health care sector, and about 25% of all LTC workers in residential and mobile care services, with significant variation between Vienna (up to 50% of foreign-born LTC staff) and the remaining regions (Bauer et al. 2018; Mairhuber and Allinger 2021). The latter group comprises of about 59,000 personal carers from Romania, Slovakia and other East European countries (WKO 2022). We will first discuss those who are registered as healthcare workers and then those who work as live-in carers.

Overall, the number of health and long-term care professionals with a third country nationality increased from 4,410 to 4,553 between 2019 and 2020 (Holzweber et al. 2021; Rappold et al. 2020), corresponding to a 3.2% increase. A slightly larger percentage increase was observed among EU citizens, amounting to 4.7% (from 10,517 to 11,019 workers). At the same time, the share of nostrifications (first-time registrations that were based on recognition of foreign diplomas) almost stagnated between 2019 and 2020 (increasing from 12.7 to 13% as a share of all first-time registrations). Overall, first-time registrations among health and long-term care professionals increased by 3.7% from 2019 to 2020 (from 99,006 to 102,629 workers) (cf Tables 13.2 and 13.3).

In Austria, live-in care workers have to register as 'personal carers' with the Austrian Economic Chamber. Live-in personal carers are usually called '24-h carers' in Austria, legally the terminology of 'personal carers' (Personenbetreuer) is applied. This type of care provision had developed at the aftermath of the fall of the 'iron curtain' and following the introduction of the LTC allowance during the 1990s. People in need of care and their families took advantage of the wage differential

Table 13.2 Nationalities of registered care professionals in Austria 2019 and 2020

	DGKP (nurse with diploma) 2019	DGKP (nurse with diploma) 2020	PFA (nursing assistant level 2) 2019	PFA (nursing assistant level 2) 2020	PA (nursing assistant level 1) 2019	PA (nursing assistant level 1) 2020
Austria	86,838	89,986	840	1,902	48,646	50,699
EU/EEA/ CH	8,599	8,990	95	132	1,823	1,897
Third country	3,578	3,672	59	106	773	775
Total	99,015	102,648	994	2,140	51,242	53,371

Sources GBR, GÖG; Rappold et al. (2020); Holzweber et al. (2021)

Table 13.3 Professional first qualifications of registered nurses in 2019 and 2020

Professional qualification	Number 2019	Percentage 2019 (%)	Number 2020	Percentage 2020 (%)
Bachelor degree	1,506	1.5	2,039	2
Certificate of recognition/ nostrification	12,615	12.7	13,100	13
Diploma	84,885	85.7	87,490	85
Total	99,006	100	102,629	100

Sources GBR, GÖG; Rappold et al. (2020); Holzweber et al. (2021)

and the lack of employment opportunities in neighboring countries to hire (usually untrained) personal carers, initially in the form of moonlighting. At that time the majority of personal carers originated from Slovakia. Therefore, it became a general standard that personal carers took turns of two weeks resulting in each person in need of care being catered for by two personal carers each month.

Following some scandals and political debates, a range of legal measures were developed in 2007 to turn these private arrangements into a more regulated area of care. Namely, the 'Personal Care Act' (BGBl. I Nr. 33/2007) stipulated some basic standards regarding a minimum of training, access to social security, working times and forms of employment. As a result, hiring a personal carer became more costly for families, even if the additional costs for social insurance contributions were partly compensated by dedicated subsidies (see below).

As a corollary, hitherto 'illegal' care arrangements widely vanished and personal care became an important 'pillar' of the Austrian LTC system. If a care recipient or a family wants to employ a live-in carer rather than the live-in carer being self-employed, this is still possible based on the 'home helpers and home employees law' (Hausgehilfen- und Hausangestelltengesetz) (Markovic 2021). In this case, the employers have to pay social security contributions and this is hardly ever an option that is chosen.

As of to date, this type of care is covering about 7% of persons in need of care, i.e. about 30,000 out of ca. 460,000 beneficiaries of the Austrian long-term care allowance. Since 2007, the number of personal carers continued to rise steadily until 2018 and remained relatively stable in the ensuing years, even during the pandemic. Based on the membership statistics of the Austrian economic chamber, in which live-in carers share a 'specialist group' with coaches, the numbers of those active in the sector have changed slightly since the start of the pandemic. In 2019, the group included 98,961 members rising to 99,462 in 2020 and then falling again to 98,227 in 2021 (WKO 2022). Of these, 68,926 were active members in 2019, 67,396 in 2020 and 67,301 in 2021. By the end of December 2021 there were 59,488 individuals active as live-in carers.

Table 13.4 shows the age structure of personal carers in Austria. The development over time reveals a tendency towards an ageing workforce, with increasing shares of personal carers in higher age groups, and even rising shares beyond pension age.

Table 13.5 provides an overview of the number of personal carers that are actively registered with the Austrian Economic Chamber and the persons in need of care eligible for a subsidy that amounts to €275 per carer per month, i.e. max. €550 if two self-employed carers are hired, which is the general rule. For fully employed carers, a subsidy of up to €1,100 would be granted. Eligibility criteria include an income threshold of €2,500 per month, and care needs of at least level 3 of the LTC allowance as well as a confirmation that the live-in carer has a theoretical training as at least a home helper or respective practical experience or is working under supervision of a registered nurse.

Given these criteria, there is about one third of families engaging personal carers without a subsidy as they do not comply. Moreover, as the subsidy has not been valorised since 2007 it has lost in purchasing power by more than 20% up till today. Some regional governments have therefore increased subsidies based on their competences, respectively.

Table 13.4 Personal carers in Austria by age groups

Age groups	2015	2016	2017	2018	2019
70+	0.2	0.2	0.2	0.3	0.4
61–70	7.5	8.8	10.1	12.0	14.0
51–60	33.7	35.5	35.9	38.3	40.3
41–50	34.2	34.3	34.5	32.9	31.0
31–40	17.6	15.7	14.3	12.6	11.0
20–30	6.8	5.5	5	3.9	3.3

Source Schober (2020)

Table 13.5 Number of registered personal carers (active), number of subsidised beneficiaries and public expenditures, 2015 and 2020

	Beneficiaries of subsidies for personal care	Expenditures for public subsidies (in mio. €)	Registered and active personal carers
2015	21,940	138.6	50,159
2020	24,031	161.4	59,488

Note Some additional families engaging personal carers are receiving subsidies at the regional level in Lower Austria where a specific scheme has been established
Source WKO (2022)

As almost all personal carers are registered as self-employed with the Austrian Economic Chamber (only very few are directly employed by families), many regulations regarding working time and protection against unfair dismissal do not apply (Schmidt et al. 2016; AI 2021).

Personal care is organised by agencies that connect supply and demand in Austria and across borders. These brokering agencies also organise travels to and from the workplace, and they administer individual contracts and invoices. The number of these brokering agencies increased both in source countries and in Austria. To date, there are more than 900 of these agencies (WKO 2022).

Following recommendations of the Austrian Audit Commission regarding quality assurance (RH 2018), some additional mechanisms were introduced, namely the "Austrian Quality Certificate 24" (ÖQZ-24) for brokering agencies (https://oeqz.at). To obtain this certificate the agency has to submit a number of documents and the description of key processes from recruitment and contracting to support and emergency services. Auditors of the 'Association for the promotion of quality in care for older persons' will then visit the organisation and assess their compliance with defined standards. For instance, certified agencies need to ensure one visit per year by a registered nurse to assess the quality of care provided. The ÖQZ-24 is however a voluntary audit with related costs so that currently no more than about 5% of agencies have been certified.

Another quality assurance mechanism in the Austrian LTC system consists in yearly visits by registered nurses of a small sample of beneficiaries of the long-term care allowance and of all recipients of the means-tested public subsidy for personal carers. In 2020, there were 10,067 of such visits in households receiving the subsidy. The quality of care was assessed as 'thorough and reliable' in more than 90% of all cases, in particular regarding hygiene, personal care and nutrition, only 0.05% (personal care) to 0.33% (nursing care) of assessed cases were regarded as problematic or improvable (BMSGPK 2021). As these decidedly positive results of announced visits were often criticised, an ongoing project is based on unannounced visits to get better insights.

Another way of improving the quality of personal care is being promoted by self-organised mutual support in organisations such as 'Institut für Personenbetreuung' or 'DREPT pentru îngrijire' (Leiblfinger and Pieler 2018). The association DREPT was founded in 2020 by live-in carers from Romania. Together with 'iniciativa24,' an association by live-in carers from Slovakia, it founded the IG 24 Syndicate for 24-h Carers (IG 24 2022). IG 24 is currently campaigning to contest the self-employment status of live-in carers in court (Respekt.net 2022).

Also, the Union 'vidaflex' is getting involved increasingly in this area, for instance by accepting personal carers as members and by developing a platform to better match the needs of (potential) users and personal carers (see below). Several other projects are ongoing that aim at supporting the quality of personal care by means of digitalisation. For instance, the goal of the project "24 h QuAALity," coordinated by the University of Applied Studies Vienna, is to develop an application to enhance the quality of 24-h care. The software is offering an information and training portal on recurrent care and nursing situations in relevant languages, an electronic care documentation to support quality assurance and a function to respond professionally to emergency situations (https://projekte.ffg.at).

Notwithstanding these endeavours and small improvements, working conditions of personal carers remain highly precarious and fail to meet general labor standards, in particular concerning working time, wages and the status as 'self-employed.' Personal carers are decidedly dependent on both brokering agencies and the families for whom they are working.

A study by Amnesty International published a study that criticizes the lack of rights and the low wages paid to self-employed personal carers between €10,000 and €12,000 per year, which is about a third of the average wage in Austria. Personal carers can hardly decide autonomously on their working time, breaks or absences, and sickness leave is only paid in case of long-term sickness of more than 42 days; contracts are often concluded between the brokering agency and the family, rather than with the personal carer her-/himself (AI 2021). Most personal carers must travel an entire (unpaid) day to get to and from their place of work in Austria, so that many have changed from fortnightly to monthly turns (in particular Romanians, see Hopfgartner et al. 2022).

Another issue is that live-in carers frequently sign off collecting powers to the agencies when signing their contracts (Markovic 2021). In case of disputes, the agencies then often don't pay out the full payment to carers. The prevailing legality narrative regarding 24-h care has also been contended by Steiner et al. (2020) since it tends to undermine the focus on working conditions, the structural precarity and power inequalities in live-in care.

According to a study on the quality of care and related working conditions from care workers' perspectives that included also interviews with personal carers (Leichsenring et al. 2015), the (unpaid) travel times and the separation from their own family are perceived as major burden as well as the fact that autonomous working comes with isolation and the lack of support in case of emergencies. Generally, personal carers' informed that their working conditions are substantially dependent on and restricted to the household in which they are working, and the fact that 24-h care basically means to be available around the clock on seven days per week. Even if the Personal Care Act stipulates a right to three hours break per day, in practice this cannot be realised in many cases as nobody else is available to take over.

This is particularly burdensome in case of clients' care needs during night-time and/or if the living environment is not sufficiently appropriate or adapted to personal care, e.g. due to small bathrooms that cannot be accessed with a wheelchair. Personal carers nevertheless generally appreciate the regulations specified in the Personal Care Act. Still, they feel pressure as they can be dismissed and sent away from the household at any moment. A crucial aspect is of course the communication with the family of the person in need of care that is usually seen as the employer, and this relationship depends a lot on mutual understanding and 'luck' whether agreements and successful communication mechanisms can be established with the key contact person and other family members.

Most personal carers do not consider themselves as part of the LTC system, their contact with the formal care system is reduced to monthly quality assurance visits by registered nurses of the brokering agency (and even these are not always ensured) or the family doctor. It is also perceived as problematic that there is often no proper handover between personal carers as the departing carer is usually leaving with the same minibus with which the other carer is arriving, leaving no time for mutual exchange. A key challenge consists in finding the correct balance between proximity and distance with the person in need of care—having too close a relationship could result in being accused of inheritance fraud, while too much distance might be perceived as carelessness.

Although some personal carers are even registered nurses or social workers, most of them have various other professional backgrounds, ranging from teachers to waiters or other service-related professions. Personal carers mainly rely on learning from experience regarding their caring skills. Even if some agencies also offer further training, it mainly depends on personal initiative to acquire specific skills. Finally, and in spite of often asserted statements that 24-h care exemplifies a win–win-situation for all involved parties, personal carers often get the impression that their situation in the home countries (unemployment, low wages) is being capitalised on, and that wages paid for their challenging work are rather low (Leichsenring et al. 2015).

Similar findings were reported by a more recent study based on focus groups with selected groups of personal carers from Croatia, Hungary and the Slovak Republic—wages are independent from clients' care needs, it is often difficult to get along with the household budget allocated by families, which are in many cases also requesting additional services such as gardening or cleaning also those parts of the house, in which the rest of the family is living. Contacts with the GP are also often managed by the family alone, while they are required to take care of medication, which is not always specified as a remit (Reichmann 2021a).

Reichmann carried out an online survey commissioned and supported by vidaflex, a Union-initiative for single-person companies, showing that personal carers do not feel themselves and their work sufficiently appreciated—only 10% feel appreciation by political decision-makers, only 44% by families, and 51% by clients. More than 70% report major burden by working conditions (lack of sleep, lack of household budget or aids), the severity of clients' care needs, lack of or wrong information, or clients that press for price cutting. Almost 60% are not or even not at all satisfied with their brokering agency, and only about one third feel well informed by the agencies (Reichmann, 2021b) (cf Table 13.6).

With the onset of the Covid-19 Pandemic, the ensuing lockdown and related travel restrictions all these challenges got an additional bend. Above all, the mechanism of fortnightly or monthly shifts had suddenly been disrupted. Personal carers who worked their turn in Austria had to stay and continued to care under the given conditions, i.e. the already significant social isolation that characterizes live-in care became even more pronounced. At the same time, those who were in their home countries remained without work and income. This situation exacerbated with the first lockdown continuing into April and May 2020.

Regional governments and Economic Chambers therefore started to intervene by organizing charter flights and trains for personal carers to and from Romania, Bulgaria and Croatia (Leiblfinger et al. 2020). However, according to the Covid-19 rules at that time, the newly arrived carers had to spend two weeks in quarantine—and rather than earning, they had to contribute to accommodation costs (Bachmann 2020b). Altogether, this intervention had no significant impact. Most agencies did not participate as they were not able to guarantee for a replacement. Additional costs occurred for protective gear and tests both in Austria and in the home country. These costs could eventually be reclaimed, but this became obsolete when testing became a free service across Austria.

Eventually, the regional governments and the Federal Ministry offered a premium of €500 to those who continued to stay in Austria, but it turned out that not all personal carers were able to claim it because many of them do not dispose of an Austrian bank account that was a necessary requirement. Additional challenges consisted in

Table 13.6 Appreciation of performance and key aspects of burden as perceived by personal carers

	Very much (%)	Rather (%)	Partly (%)	Not at all (%)	Don't know or N/A (%)
Appreciation of care work					
… by persons being cared for	12	39	41	5	3
… by family members	8	36	47	5	3
… by political decision-makers	1	9	53	24	13
Types and extent of burden					
Wrong information by agency about client	48	24	11	9	8
Lack of sleep	43	29	16	9	4
Mental stress	42	35	16	4	2
Bad working conditions in the household	42	22	16	16	5
Clients pressing for price-cutting	41	24	11	15	9

Note Based on an online survey (N = 2,275 personal carers), April–May 2021
Source Reichmann (2021b)

the risk of infection during travel or within the families as well as in costs of testing and regionally different hygiene and lockdown regulations (Dallinger et al. 2021).

The Economic Chamber as the legal interest representation of self-employed personal carers has started to campaign for higher public subsidies for personal carers up to a threshold that amounts to the alleged average subsidy paid by public authorities for a place in a care home (around €1,650 per month) so that personal carers can claim higher wages. Other requests by the Austrian Economic Chamber concern a better involvement of personal carers and their interest organisation in debates of the Austrian LTC reform and a rather strict repudiation of the 'employment model' of personal care—this would only increase costs and make personal care unaffordable for many families (Janisch 2021), and it would certainly menace the role of the Economic Chamber as representative body of self-employed personal carers.

However, also the Chamber of Labour and vidaflex, the already mentioned Union-initiative for 'single-person companies' such as personal carers, have become active in this field. They promote the creation of an online-platform to match supply and demand on a non-profit basis to reduce the dependency of personal carers on brokering agencies. Personal carers welcome this new opportunity that should also be combined with the establishment of standardised contracts to specify tasks, rights and responsibilities of all involved parties (Reichmann 2021a).

Outlook and Conclusion

The pandemic has certainly contributed to widening existing societal fractures and to raising awareness of social phenomena that have been invisible for many citizens that are not directly affected by, for instance, caring for a relative with long-term care needs, by unemployment or by needing special treatment in a hospital. It led to unprecedented support measures in various welfare policy areas (short-term work, increase in emergency assistance allowance, family hardship fund, halt to energy shutdowns) and various subsidies for companies which faced a loss of sales. Particular measures were introduced for LTC (bonus for social and healthcare workers, fund to support LTC). SARS-CoV-2 also demonstrated the extent to which the Austrian LTC system relies on informal carers and the need for their support. The measures announced by the Austrian government include an annual payment of €1,500 for informal carers who are not able to work because of caring obligations and a legal entitlement to a care leave of three months (increased from one month previously) in case this is part of collective agreements or works agreement (BMSGPK 2022b).

Researchers have repeatedly highlighted the need to improve working conditions for professional carers (Brückner et al. 2022). Calculations by the National Public Health Institute (Rappold and Juraszovich 2019) suggest that 76,000 individuals need to be recruited as professional carers by 2030 which means that enormous efforts have to be made in terms of attracting staff to the LTC sector. To recruit such a large number of individuals to work in LTC, various policy measures are necessary. One example is targeted training as it is done in the 'migrants care' project for individuals who are interested in working in the LTC sector but do not have the necessary language skills through a tailored language course which includes learning strategies to confront discrimination and basic knowledge of the care sector; participants are thus better prepared when starting their professional training (Greindl 2022).

The measures included a bonus payment for some professional carers for two years, an additional week of annual leave for those who are 43 years and older, and the permission for care assistants to carry out additional tasks (BMSGPK 2022b). In order to recruit care workers from abroad to the LTC sector, the measures stipulate easier access to a work permit (Rot-Weiss-Rot-Card) and an accelerated recognition procedure (nostrification) of foreign qualifications. While those with other than Austrian nationalities make up about 10% of professional carers (Holzweber et al. 2021), they comprise around 98% (Kirchner 2018) of live-in carers. Thus, those with other than Austrian nationalities provide almost all care in the lowest paid care jobs with particularly difficult working conditions. The pandemic has brought working conditions of professional carers and live-in carers into the public debate and demonstrated the need for improvements, even more considering the need to recruit additional workers to the sector.

In a mid-term perspective, it will be necessary to discuss and address the issue of the LTC care workforce, including professionals, migrant (live-in) carers and informal carers in a wider European context. Rather than finding national solutions that do not consider consequences in source countries, and rather than entering into a European-wide competition for foreign care workers, it would be recommended to elaborate on a European strategy to professionalize care work, to improve working conditions and to work towards a convergence of regulatory frameworks, including quality assurance. Respective funding mechanisms would need to be developed to incentivize Member States that remain responsible for their health and long-term care systems according to the subsidiarity principle.

The EU Care Strategy published in September 2022 calls however for the exploration of legal migration pathways for long-term care workers and refers to the skills and talents package in the Pact on Migration and Asylum (EC 2022). It remains to be seen whether Member States will follow these recommendations and contribute to the implementation of fairer and better shared rules, together with major investments in the development of integrated LTC systems.

Notes

1. Please note that data were collected between October 2021 and April 2022 depending on the country. Data were collected and compared by the LTCCovid.org network.
2. Own calculations by the Austrian National Public Health Institute based on data provided by the states.
3. The share of 28.4% corresponds to 5,392 deaths recorded among care home residents out of a total of 18,971 deaths due to Covid-19 in Austria on July 20, 2022.

References

AI, Amnesty International. 2021. *"Wir wollen nur ein paar Rechte"—24-Stunden-Betreuer*innen werden ihre Rechte in Österreich verwehrt*. London: AI.

AK, Arbeiterkammer. 2022. *Corona Kurzarbeit*. https://www.arbeiterkammer.at.

Antony, G., J. Antosik, M. Weigl, C. Marbler, and A. Laschkolnig. 2021. *Gesundheitsfolgenabschätzung zu Auswirkungen des Lockdowns und Social Distancings zur Eindämmung von Covid-19 auf die Bevölkerung in Österreich*. Vienna: Gesundheit Österreich.

APA. 2020. Österreich aktuell mit höchster Neuinfektionsrate weltweit. *Der Standard*. November 14. https://www.derstandard.at.

Bachinger, A. 2016. 24-Stunden-Betreuung In Österreich—Die Nutzung migrantischer Arbeitskraft: Vorzeigemodell oder Arbeitsausbeutung? *Femina Politica* 1: 39–51.

Bachmann, A. 2020a. 24-Stunden-Betreuung: Viel Ärger um die Flüge aus Rumänien. *Moment*, April 7. https://www.moment.at.

Bachmann, A. 2020b. 24-Stunden-Betreuung: Ein Flug, kein Zug, viele Irrtümer. *Moment*, May 4. https://www.moment.at.

Bachner, F., et al. 2018. Austria health system review. *Health Systems in Transition* 20 (3): 1–256.

Bauer, G., R. Rodrigues, and K. Leichsenring. 2018. *Arbeitsbedingungen in der mobilen und stationären Langzeitpflege in Oberösterreich*. Vienna: European Centre for Social Wefare Policy and Research, Linz: AK Oberösterreich. https://doi.org/10.13140/RG.2.2.29338.18886.

BMSGPK, BM für Soziales, Gesundheit, Pflege und Konsumentenschutz. 2022b. *Betroffene und Angehörige in der Pflege*. https://www.sozialministerium.at.

BMSGPK, BM für Soziales, Gesundheit, Pflege und Konsumentenschutz. 2020. *Covid-19 in Alten- und Pflegeheimen*. https://goeg.at.

BMSGPK, BM für Soziales, Gesundheit, Pflege und Konsumentenschutz. 2021. *Pflegevorsorgebericht 2020*. Vienna: BMSGPL.

BMSGPK, BM für Soziales, Gesundheit, Pflege und Konsumentenschutz (ed.). 2022a. *Die Covid-19-Pandemie: Bestandsaufnahme und Handlungsrahmen*. https://www.sozialministerium.at.

Brückner, M., et al. 2022. Clean up time! Redesigning care after Covid-19: A position paper on the care crisis from Austria, Germany and Switzerland, *International Journal of Care and Caring* 6 (1–2): 247–251.

Comas-Herrera, A. et al. 2021. *LTC-Covid International Living Report on Covid-19 and long-term care*. https://doi.org/10.21953/lse.mlre15e0u6s6.

Comas-Herrera, A. et al. 2022. *International data on deaths attributed to Covid-19 among people living in care homes*. February 22. https://ltccovid.org.

Dallinger, L., L. Brentjens, N. Schulze, and M. Weichselbraun. 2021. 24-Stunden-Betreuung in Österreich: Ausländische Kräfte kämpfen während der Coronakrise mit alten Problemen und neue Belastungen. *Moment*, February 15. https://www.moment.at.

EC, European Commission. 2022. *Proposal for a council recommendation on access to affordable high-quality long-term care*. https://op.europa.eu.

EF, Eurofound. 2020a. *Covid-19 short-time work scheme, measure AT-2020a-10/229*. Dublin: EU PolicyWatch. https://static.eurofound.europa.eu.

EF, Eurofound. 2020b. *Covid-19 €100 million special fund for 24-hour nursing care, measure AT-2020b-13/585*. Dublin: EU PolicyWatch. https://static.eurofound.europa.eu.

EF, Eurofound. 2020c. *Online application for unemployment benefit and top-up of emergency assistance, measure AT-2020c-12/576*. Dublin: EU PolicyWatch. https://static.eurofound.europa.eu.

EF, Eurofound. 2020d. *Entrepreneur's wage, measure AT-2020d-16/789*. Dublin: EU PolicyWatch. https://static.eurofound.europa.eu.

EF, Eurofound. 2020e. *Investment premium, measure AT-2020e-36/1238*. Dublin: EU PolicyWatch. https://static.eurofound.europa.eu.

EF, Eurofound. 2020f. *Covid-19 family hardship fund and family crisis fund, measure AT-2020f-16/577*. Dublin: EU PolicyWatch. https://static.eurofound.europa.eu.

EF, Eurofound. 2020g. *No energy shutdown when payment difficulties occur, measure AT-2020g-12/580*. Dublin: EU PolicyWatch. https://static.eurofound.europa.eu.

EF, Eurofound. 2020h. *Self-isolation Vienna Energy, measure AT-2020h-12/552*. Dublin: EU PolicyWatch. https://static.eurofound.europa.eu.

EF, Eurofound. 2020i. *Recommendation for Corona bonus in retail collective agreement, measure AT-2020i-43/1310*. Dublin: EU PolicyWatch. https://static.eurofound.europa.eu.

EF, Eurofound. 2020j. *Corona hazard bonus in collective agreements in the social and health-care sectors, measure AT-2020j-27/1307*. Dublin: EU PolicyWatch. https://static.eurofound.europa.eu.

EF, Eurofound. 2020k. *Electronic prescriptions, measure AT-2020k-12/583*. Dublin: EU Policy-Watch. https://static.eurofound.europa.eu.

EF, Eurofound. 2020l. *Special subsidized care time for working parents and carers, measure AT-2020l-12/545*. Dublin: EU PolicyWatch. https://static.eurofound.europa.eu.

Flatscher-Thöni, M., E. Holzer, M. Pallauf, and C. Kreyer. 2022. Covid-19 Schutzmaßnahmen in Alten- und Pflegeheimen: Zwischen Autonomie und Fürsorge—Ergebnisse einer Interview-studie. *Ethik in Der Medizin* 34 (2): 221–238.

Greindl, C. 2022. Nachschub an Pflegekräften durch "migrants care." *Tips Freistadt*. https://www.tips.at/nachrichten/freistadt.

Haas, S., D. Antony, G. Antony, S. Gaiswinkler, R. Griebler, C. Marbler, M. Weigl, and P. Winkler. 2021. *Soziale Faktoren der Pandemie*. Vienna: Gesundheit Österreich.

HMD, Human Mortality Database. 2022. *Website*. https://www.mortality.org.

Holicek, M. 2020. Stationäre Pflege und Corona-Krise. In: *Frauengesundheit und Corona: Schriftenreihe Frauen Gesundheit Wien*, ed. Stadt Wien, No. 1. https://www.wien.gv.at.

Holzweber, L., M. Zach, A. Gruböck, B. Juraszovich, S. Mathis Edenhofer, E. Rappold, and A. Wallner. 2021. *Jahresbericht Gesundheitsberuferegister 2020*. Vienna: Gesundheit Österreich. https://www.sozialministerium.at.

Hopfgartner, L., C. Seubert, F. Sprenger, and J. Glaser. 2022. Experiences of precariousness and exploitation of Romanian transnational live-in care workers in Austria. *Journal of Industrial Relations* 64 (2): 298–320.

IG 24. 2022. *IG24—Interessengemeinschaft der 24-Stunden-Betreuer_innen*. https://ig24.at.

Janisch, H.G. 2021. Politik will 24-Stunden-Betreuung einschränken! *ORF Nachlese* 5: 4.

Karlinsky, A., and Kobak, D. 2021. Tracking excess mortality across countries during the Covid-19 pandemic with the world mortality dataset. *eLife* 10: e69336. https://doi.org/10.7554/eLife.69336.

Kirchner, M. 2018. *Die 24-Stunden-Betreuung in Österreich—Registrierung und Qualitätssicherung Presentation*. https://www.euro.centre.org.

Kleine Zeitung. 2022. Corona: 39.493 Neuinfektionen und 47 Todesopfer in 24 Stunden. *Kleine Zeitung*, March 2. https://www.kleinezeitung.at.

Kreidl, P., et al. 2020. Emergence of Coronavirus disease 2019 (Covid-19) in Austria. *Wiener Klinische Wochenschrift* 132: 645–652.

Łaszewska, A., T. Helter, and J. Simon. 2021. Perceptions of Covid-19 lockdowns and related public health measures in Austria: A longitudinal online survey. *BMC Public Health* 21: 1502. https://doi.org/10.1186/s12889-021-11476-3.

Lebensweltheim. 2020. Covid-19 in Alten- und Pflegeheime—Lehren aus der Krise müssen in Pflegereform einfließen. *Presseunterlage*, June 29.

Leiblfinger, M., and V. Pieler. 2018. *Elf Jahre 24-Stunden-Betreuung in Österreich: Eine Policy- und Regime-Analyse*. Linz: Katholische Privat-Universität Linz.

Leiblfinger, M., et al. 2020. Impact of Covid-19 policy responses on live-in care workers in Austria. *Germany, and Switzerland, Journal of Long-Term Care* 2020: 144–150.

Leichsenring, K., A.E. Schmidt, and H. Staflinger. 2021. Fractures in the Austrian model of long-term care: What are the lessons from the first wave of the Covid-19 pandemic? *Journal of Long-Term Care* 2021: 33–42.

Leichsenring, K., K. Schulmann, K. Gasior, and M. Fuchs, 2015. *Gute Pflege aus Sicht der Beschäftigten: Bedingungen, Ziele und Perspektiven der Qualitätsverbesserung in der Langzeitpflege.* Vienna: AK Wien & Europäisches Zentrum für Wohlfahrtspolitik und Sozialforschung.

Leichsenring, K. 2017. The Austrian welfare state system: With special reference to the long-term care system. In: *The Routledge international handbook to welfare state systems*, ed. C. Aspalter. Oxon: Routledge.

Mairhuber, I., and B. Allinger. 2021. *Transnationale Betreuungs- und Pflegekräfte in europäischen Privathaushalten.* Vienna: AK Wien & FORBA.

Markovic, F. 2021. *24-Stunden-Betreuung—Die Ausbeutung muss beendet werden*, June 21. https://awblog.at.

Mathieu, E., H. Ritchie, L. Rodés-Guirao, C. Appel, C. Giattino, J. Hasell, B. Macdonald, S. Dattani, D. Beltekian, E. Ortiz-Ospina, and M. Roser. 2020. *Coronavirus pandemic (Covid-19).* https://ourworldindata.org.

RF, Rechnungshof Österreich. 2018. Förderung der 24-Stunden-Betreuung in Oberösterreich und Wien. Bericht des Rechnungshofes. Wien: Rechnungshof Österreich.

Rappold, E., and B. Juraszovich. 2019. *Pflegepersonal-Bedarfsprognose für Österreich.* BMSGPK. https://jasmin.goeg.at.

Rappold, E., B. Juraszovich, M. Zach, A. Gruböck, and A. Wallner. 2020. *Jahresbericht Gesundheitsberuferegister 2019.* Gesundheit Österreich. https://www.sozialministerium.at.

Reichmann, A. 2021a. *Erhebung der Situation in der 24-Stunden Betreuung in Hinblick auf die Entwicklung einer gemeinwohlorientierten Vermittlungsplattform.* Vienna: Reichmann Research Consulting (unpublished).

Reichmann, A. 2021b. *Berufliche Situation von 24-Stunden-BetreuerInnen in Österreich.* Vienna: Reichmann Research Consulting (unpublished).

Respekt.net. 2022. *24h-Betreuer*innen ziehen vor Gericht.* https://respekt.net.

Schmidt, A. E., J. Winkelmann, R. Rodrigues, and K. Leichsenring. 2016. Lessons for regulating informal markets and implications for quality assurance—The case of migrant care workers in Austria. *Ageing & Society*, 36(4), 741–763. https://doi.org/10.1017/S0144686X1500001X.

Schmidt, A. E., and F. Bachner. 2020. *Workforce—health system response monitor: Austria.* https://eurohealthobservatory.who.int.

Schmidt, A. E., K. Leichsenring, H. Staflinger, C. Litwin, and A. Bauer. 2020. *The impact of Covid-19 on users and providers of long-term care services in Austria.* International Long-Term Care Policy Network. https://LTCcovid.org.

Schmidt, A. E., L. Rainer, M. Zuba, G. Gredinger, and F. Bachner. 2021. Aktuelle Zahlen zu Infektionen und Todesfällen in Alten und Pflegeheimen. *Press conference*, February 4. https://goeg.at.

Schnetzer, M., D. Tamesberger, and S. Theurl. 2020. Mitigating mass layoffs in the Covid-19 crisis: Austrian short-time work as international role model. *VOX Eu*, April 7. https://voxeu.org.

Schober, M. 2020. Die 24-Stunden-Betreuung in Österreich: Eine Analyse der Arbeitsbedingungen von selbstständigen Personenbetreuerinnen, *Master thesis.* Linz: Johannes Kepler Universität.

Staflinger, H., and A. E. Schmidt. 2020. Frauen in der stationären Langzeitpflege—Lehren und Lektionen aus der Covid-19-Krise. In: *Frauengesundheit und Corona*, ed. Stadt Wien. Vienna: Büro für Frauengesundheit und Gesundheitsziele.

Steiner, J., V. Prieler, M. Leiblfinger, and A. Benazha. 2020. Truly legal!? Legal framing and legality narratives in live-in care in Austria, Germany and Switzerland. In: *Towards a scarcity of care?*, eds. N. Katona and A. Melegh. Budapest: Friedrich-Ebert-Stiftung.

Winkelmann, J., A. E. Schmidt, and K. Leichsenring. 2015. Regulating migrants as a low-cost solution: The formalisation of a dual care labour market in Austria. In: *At your service? The political economy of household services in Europe*, eds. N. Morel and C. Carbonnier. Basingstoke: Palgrave Macmillan.
WKO. 2022. *Personenbetreuung und Personenberatung: Branchendaten.* http://wko.at/statistik.
WMD, *World mortality dataset*. 2022. https://github.com/akarlinsky/world_mortality.

Part IV
Concluding Part

Chapter 14
Analyzing Problem-Cum-Policy Cycles and Evaluating Policy Strategies in the Covid-19 Pandemic: A Meta Conclusion

Christian Aspalter

Abstract This concluding chapter, rather than summarizing all conclusions to be drawn from the above chapters, chooses to look for a meta conclusion, a conclusion that hovers above other (or all other) conclusions. What has struck the author are the partitionings of the Covid-19 Pandemic into either waves or distinct policy response periods. While these are straightforward and simplistic terms that do enable the discussion of the Pandemic in a descriptive (and here and there explanatory) manner, these are missing the point when it comes to social problems and health problems per se. That is, policies and policy strategies have addressed the virus, and its direct consequences, i.e. associated deaths and hospital occupancy, but not the wider range of social and health problems that have arisen and are still arising from this Pandemic. This conscise chapter, hence, throws up the ball for further discussion and elaboration down the road, and theory making perhaps, on this subject matter. The chapter also shortly refers to the best country responses in global comparison, by pointing out the positive policy experiences of Nordic European countries, which not only looked at the virus, but more so also on maintaining human dignity and human freedom.

Keywords Covid-19 pandemic · Policy responses · Problem-cum-policy cycles · Social problems · Health problems · Human dignity · Human freedom

Wow what a week! Just finished the a-bit-more-than-a-week emotional and psychological roller coaster ride of getting out of a very long, dark, uncomfortable and winding *rabbit hole*, in warp speed. I am talking about being in China, and at the beginning of the third week in December, 2022. In other words, with the cancelling of the travel code (as we know it here in China), just a few hours ago, the Covid-19 Pandemic has been de facto declared 'officially' over! Covid-19 so the government

C. Aspalter (✉)
Department of Social Sciences, Beijing Normal University-Hong Kong Baptist University United International College, Zhuhai, Mainland China, China
e-mail: christian@uic.edu.hk

C. Aspalter (ed.), *Covid-19 Pandemic*,
https://doi.org/10.1007/978-981-99-2497-4_14

maintains, now, is just another form of a common cold (*ganmao*). For sure, for the world, for the people of China, and the ones that are living in China, roughly about one fifth of the earth's population, the Covid-19 Pandemic is over. Fears have gone, new ones have come, and many, for many, have stayed.

The end of a problem is not the end of problems.

The (one) medical Covid-19 problem has gone, for most. However, other medical problems have stayed: (i) Long-Covid, (ii) the mental health knock-on pandemic (of the Covid-19 Pandemic) and (ii) the yet very long persisting PTSD pandemic that was brought on by single or multiple traumas, including health disasters of oneself or one's loved ones, plus policy-measures-initiated/caused disasters, such as personal (employment and other economic) disasters.

On top, inequality has and is worsening all over the planet, and so is, therefore, poverty, in all its forms and dehumanizing aspects, including health deprivation, health care deprivation (mental and physical health included) (Therborn 2013; Piketty 2014; Aspalter 2023a, b).

Only for people who have lived in China through the Pandemic, it becomes feelable; these people have just witnessed a *paradigm shift* of Kuhnian proportions (Kuhn 1970a, b), shifting from Newtonian to Einsteinian physics in a matter of good a week!

And deep and wide, on the inside, people keep wondering and wondering a lot of things. Medicines, and all sorts of herbal teas in the form of medicine bottles, have been sold out, and working-class families have spent a fortune for things like simple assorted Chinese flower tea (similar to chamomile tea). But, China is back to live! People are living their lives again. Lives have changed, but lives are lived again. They are still feeling uncomfortable. I have not seen so many students wearing a mask in class, as I did yesterday, ever; and now the Pandemic is over. Barricades, border barriers, border tents, public testing stations, and different kinds of all-overpowering (local, provincial and national) QR codes at walls and entrances have disappeared over the course of the last week.

This is a *new normal* for China, for most people in China, for now. A super scary, yet more and more joyful, transition to a new live, a new-found normal. The *lifeworlds* of people (cf Habermas 1981) have completely altered in a matter of days. And it is with a great sense of insecurity that people look for and walk their ways throughout their new lives, day for day, trying to make sense and find new ways for each step and situation ahead. This is what they are, new lives, and not just life chapters. *New lifeworlds, new lives.*

As a policy expert, I kept wondering how perfect, i.e. resolute, China's path out of the *rabbit hole* was, over the last days. But, it was not wisdom per se (not when looks behind the curtain of politics), but sheer utter necessity, one could say self-preservation, a last-hour-move so to speak, each step of the way. More important than the why, was the how. Literally about every two days a major (before unthinkable) change, or compound of changes was announced, and implemented within hours, across a country that is home to 1.4 billion people. What a feat!

What have we learned during and throughout the Pandemic? What is the take-away? One can think of an endless number of things. So, rather than summarizing an endless number of things, or randomly picking conclusions, out of the many that have been reached throughout this book, by the most accomplished and most wonderful contributors of this book(!), I here purposefully choose to try to find and/or instigate a meta conclusion of sort:

In public administration science, policy cycles have been the feature of a great many textbooks. But, besides the fact that these policy cycles are utterly boring (and useless in policy practice in general), they are also completely missing the point, and they are utterly useless when trying to cope to understand and learn from the Covid-19 Pandemic—what happened to people, to countries, to entire world populations, and why politicians did what they did (and how they come to decide to do the things they did and not do the things they did not do, at this or that time, in this or that country or place).

As the title of this book highlights, there are many problems that are arising from the Pandemic, many were there before, but got spurred and flared up in a progressively cumulative manner. Social problems spur one another, they are cumulative and catalytic (being a catalyst to one another). Health problems are social problems, and social problems lead to health problems. Social policy is covering, and has to cover, health problems; and as such health policy is always social policy, all of health policy is (also of course mental health policy).

> The problems are not over, the train of social (including health) problems is yet on course!

Policy, and policy strategies, and each policy measure on the way, played a big part not only in addressing social (incl. health) problems, but also, in a greater than ever visible manner, *created* social (and health) *problems* along the way. People died. Not only because of the virus, or the additional effect of the virus on their already more or less dire health conditions. People died and people suffered. People encountered before-unseen, before-unfelt, before-unthinkable losses and hardships throughout the Pandemic, due to both the virus itself, but also—*and this is key*—policies and measures, and the systems put in place, themselves, and that all over the world.

The policies and measures, and systems in place, also led to step-by-step surveillance of people and public data mining of epic proportions. The process of collecting speech data and most personal, including contextual data (e.g. location and time, and people nearby), started, to be sure, earlier. But now, smart phones, smart TVs, smart all sort of things are jointly collecting and robbing data from people, to make them in the future not only more helpless, but also more unequal, and more dependent (cf Zuboff 2019; Eubanks 2018, 2014; Marcuse 1964).

The super-super rich get yet so much richer, and the poor and the near-poor get yet so much poorer. The game of super inequality (Aspalter 2022), the rigged game, the rigged matrix, we all find ourselves and find ourselves competing and working in, is ever spun further by the super-super-rich elites and technology elites, and has ever spun further out of control of normal politics *and* the people at large alike. Inequalities, powerlessness and poverty have widened and reinforced themselves through the Pandemic, in the places where people live (cities, counties, regions, and countries), but also globally (Aspalter 2023a). The intellectual cultural elites, the political elites and technical elites, all being controlled and steered by the super-super rich, joined forces to cut out political capital from the Pandemic and its knock-on crises (cf e.g. Aspalter 2022, 2023b; Holcombe 2018, 2021, 2022).

Intellectually organized political hate, name-calling and us-versus-them-like thinking and political agitation have flared up an existing cultural/intellectual/political civil war in the Foucauldian sense (cf Foucault 1975, 1976, 2009, 2010, 2014; Nietzsche 1887; as well as Piketty 2020; Rabinow 2010; Lukes 2005; Galbraith 1992; Marcuse 1964). This has become a commonplace all over the world, more in the Western developed countries than anywhere else. The public and social media was full in, and gone deeper into fear-triggering and fear-maintaining mode (cf the basic conclusions made by Herman and Chomsky 2002; cf also Chomsky, Foucault 2022a, b).

All in all, therefore, to conclude, we are to study policy cycles not for the fun of it, or for the intellectually insatiable thirst a scientist may have.

> We have to study policy cycles in tandem with social problem cycles.

Thus, we have to study—and this is perhaps the greatest takeaway on top of all the other takeaways that of course there are—*problem-cum-policy cycles*; and, there, problems are the most important (leading and guiding) aspects of these.

A full evaluation of the Covid-19 Pandemic policies across the globe will have to endure years of analyses, with a full set of global data on everything (as much as possible of course), including the full year of 2022, and thereafter, covering all countries and regions in the world. But first major and more important results are in, and throughout this book one can plunge into many sub-aspects of the Pandemic, problems faced by older people, women, families; different problems like employment, mental and physical health, poverty, lack of care, and so forth.

The very recently published *Health at a Glance: Europe 2022* by the OECD, when one looks through the first and second round of data included from the Pandemic and its outcomes, clearly points to the winner in terms of Covid-19 policies that had—*in total*—least negative effects and—*in total*—most (possible) positive effects, i.e. Northern European countries. In Chapter 2 (see Fig. 2, and Appendix of Chapter 2), the author has uped the game and applied his SRP Index to judge aggregate performances of countries. And here, Iceland is the overall best performer—or winner, if it were contest; and actually it is a contest, a race for defending people's lives from all sorts of problems and dangers, incl. loss of quality of life, loss of human decency, and of course our long-fought-for freedoms. And as a group, by and large, Northern European countries, Iceland, Norway, Finland, Denmark and Sweden can now with strong empirical evidence be declared as having applied the best overall policy strategy-mix and policy-mix, as least when looking at the earlier parts of the Pandemic.

> Just looking *alone* at '*so-called case*' numbers, and '*so-called Covid deaths*' is highly misleading due to the fact of very different cut-off lines (at which virus count exactly a test has a 'positive' test result), very different definitions (of Covid deaths), and very different report systems, and report incentives and disincentives, plus all the political censorship and

intervention (how to report and or not report, or how to publish or not publish the collected data).

Just looking at *the* Covid Problem is also misleading, as (as this book here shows) suicide and other forms of deaths of despair, mental health issues, long-term care issues, loneliness and isolation, poverty, unemployment, social deprivation, etc., are at least as devastating (and some may dare say it, *even more*) *when* combined altogether, and *when* looked at a long-term perspective that spans the Pandemic period per se, and the post-Pandemic period (incl. e.g. exit waves or after waves, such as waves that are caused by relative absence of normal seasonal flu and other viruses). All in all, we see, and will see, also ripple effects and long-poverty and long-inequality waves long after Covid has gone, plus additional mental health waves that come with the exit wave and last long thereafter, as e.g. highly visible now in China.

And with all this happening, one also ought *not to forget freedom, human dignity and human decency*, which are to be the mainstay of social policy and, with it, health policymaking all along, all the times, also in extremely difficult and testing times, in all places.

It can be learned from the Pandemic that many developed liberal democracies (other than the ones in the very North of Europe) plunged, in a sheer automated fashion, into authoritarian behavior, undemocratic behavior, unfreedom-causing behavior, just like that, as if a switch had fallen, and turned from good to I-don't-care-I-tell-you-what-to-do (authoritarian, i.e. 'super bad') kind of behavior, plus systems of oppression and legal mandates on top of endless (including a long list of Constitutionally illegal *and* unethical) measures and policies. Other countries elsewhere of course suffered much worse, that is needless to say.

But the lack of freedom and the heartless and ignorant drive to domination of all (including all formerly sacred) people's life aspects, in a most disgraceful and dehumanizing manner, by (a) bureaucrats, (b) randomly appointed (and self-proclaimed) experts, and (c) the politicians themselves in the heart of the Western Half of Europe and elsewhere was *extremely remarkable*, which ought to spark strong feelings of shame (or decency a posteriori) and a strong need of philosophical, political and institutional reflection.

When it comes to the first wave of the Pandemic, Sweden made a most-striking impression of having applied by far the most-overperforming policy response strategy and methods. The final words will lay with the data that is yet to come in from all over the world, that in the end will include all countries, and all aspects of all phases of all waves of the Pandemic.

Self-responsibility was the *trump card* early on during and throughout the Pandemic, and it is also at the late phase of the last Omicron Wave, as e.g. witnessed on formerly unimaginable scale, at formerly (and up-to-date) unseen speed, here in China.

Freedom also needs assistance from the government, especially e.g. for older citizens' homes and care facilities; the shocking numbers of e.g. the United Kingdom, New York, and partially also Sweden (later on), and many places elsewhere, have shown this. But, in any case, anywhere, and at all times:

freedom is irreplaceable, and must be irrevocable, under no circumstance, with no excuse or whatsoever well-meant pretext and rationale.

And, yes, with freedom comes responsibility, a lot of it, *and* a great deal of sufficient, big enough public investments in the health care delivery systems is absolutely needed, so that they are effectively sufficiently equipped to handle the (any possible) job in health care, at any whatsoever challenging times. We are talking about large-scale universal—and preemptive—*supply-side investments by governments* into the health infrastructure of every country, province, city and county, and that around and in all corners of the globe.

References

Aspalter, Christian. 2022. Super inequality: A general theory of mass poverty. *Social Development Issues* 44 (2): 1–19.

Aspalter, Christian. 2023a. *Ten worlds of welfare capitalism: A global data analysis.* Singapore: Springer.

Aspalter, Christian. 2023b. *Super inequality: Theoretical essays in economics and social policy*, Singapore: Springer.

Chomsky, Noam. 2002a. *Media control: The spectacular achievements of propaganda.* New York: Seven Stories Press.

Chomsky, Noam. 2002b. *Understanding power: The indispensable Chomsky*, ed. Peter R. Mitchell and John Schoeffel. New York: New Press.

Eubanks, Virginia. 2018. *Automating inequality: How high-tech tools profile, police, and punish the poor.* New York: St. Martins Press.

Eubanks, Virginia. 2014. How big data could undo our civil-rights laws. *The American Prospect*, April 22.

Foucault, Michel. 1975. *Surveiller et punir: Naissance de la prison.* Paris: Èditions Gallimard.

Foucault, Michel. 1976. *Histoire de la sexualité: La volonté de savoir*, vol. 1. Paris: Èditions Gallimard.

Foucault, Michel. 2010. *The government of self and others.* London: Palgrave Macmillan.

Foucault, Michel. 2009. *Security, territory, population*, ed. M. Senellart. London: Palgrave Macmillan.

Foucault, Michel. 2014. *Wrong-doing and truth-telling: The function of avowal in justice*, ed. F. Brion and B.E. Harcourt. Chicago: University of Chicago Press.

Galbraith, John K. 1992. *The culture of contentment.* Boston: Houghton Mifflin.

Habermas, Jürgen. 1981. *Theorie des kommunikativen Handelns: Zur Kritik der funktionalistischen Vernunft*, Volume 2. Frankfurt a.M: Suhrkamp.

Herman, Edward S., and Noam Chomsky. 2002. *Manufacturing consent: The political economy of the mass media.* New York: Pantheon.

Holcombe, Randall G. 2018. *Political capitalism: How political influence is made and maintained.* Cambridge: Cambridge University Press.

Holcombe, Randall G. 2021. Elite influence on general political preferences. *Journal of Government and Economics.* https://doi.org/10.1016/j.jge.2021.100021.

Holcombe, Randall G. 2022. Capitalism, cronyism, and inequality. In *Capitalism and inequality: The role of state and market*, ed. G.P. Manish and S.C. Miller. Oxon: Routledge.

Kuhn, Thomas S. 1970a [1962]. *The Structure of Scientific Revolutions.* Chicago: University of Chicago Press.

Kuhn, Thomas S. 1970b. Logic of discovery or psychology of research? In *Criticism and the growth of knowledge*, ed. I. Lakatos and A. Musgrave. Cambridge: Cambridge University Press.
Lukes, Steven. 2005. *Power: A radical view*. London: Palgrave Macmillan.
Marcuse, Herbert. 1964. *One-dimensional man: Studies in the ideology of advanced industrial society*. Boston: Beacon Press.
Nietzsche, Friedrich W. (1887). *Zur Genealogie der Moral: Eine Streitschrift*, C.G. Leipzig: Naumann.
OECD. 2021. *Health at a Glance 2021*. Paris: OECD.
OECD. 2022. *Health at a Glance: Europe 2022*. Paris: OECD.
Piketty, Thomas. 2020. *Capital and ideology*. Cambridge: Harvard University Press.
Piketty, Thomas. 2014 [2013]. *Capital in the Twenty-First Century*. Cambridge: The Belknap Press of Harvard University Press.
Rabinow, Paul, ed. 2010. *Michel Foucault: The Foucault reader*. New York: Vintage.
Therborn, Göran. 2013. *The killing fields of inequality*. Cambridge: Polity.
Zuboff, Shoshana. 2019. *The age of surveillance capitalism: The fight for a human future at the new frontier of power*. New York: Public Affairs.